T0255017

Introduction to Augmentative and Alternative Communication

Second Edition

Introduction to Augmentative and Alternative Communication

Sign teaching and the use of communication
aids for children, adolescents and adults
with developmental disorders

Second Edition

STEPHEN VON TETZCHNER AND HARALD MARTINSEN

UNIVERSITY OF OSLO

W
WHURR PUBLISHERS
LONDON AND PHILADELPHIA

© 2000 Whurr Publishers
First published 1992 as Sign Teaching and the use of
Communication Aids by Whurr Publishers Ltd
19b Compton Terrace, London N1 2UN, England and
325 Chestnut Street, Philadelphia PA 19106, USA

Reprinted 2001

All rights reserved. No part of this publication may be
reproduced, stored in a retrieval system, or transmitted in
any form or by any means, electronic, mechanical,
photocopying, recording or otherwise, without the prior
permission of Whurr Publishers Limited.

This publication is sold subject to the conditions that it
shall not, by way of trade or otherwise, be lent, resold,
hired out, or otherwise circulated without the publisher's
prior consent in any form of binding or cover other than
that in which it is published and without a similar
condition including this condition being imposed upon
any subsequent purchaser.

British Library Cataloguing in Publication Data
A catalogue record for this book is available from the
British Library.

ISBN: 1 86156 187 3

Preface

An increasing number of families and professionals are involved with severely communication-impaired children, adolescents and adults who use alternative communication systems to compensate and supplement delayed or limited development of spoken language. These families and professionals need to have sufficient knowledge about the various alternative communication systems and their practical use in intervention and everyday conversations. The present book may serve as an introductory text for speech and language therapists, teachers in school and preschool, psychologists, care nurses, etc., as well as for families with members who have severe developmental speech and language disorders, and to facilitate collaboration between different groups of professionals, and between professionals and families.

The purpose of the book is to provide information about the diverse groups of users with developmental disorders, as well as a variety of non-speech communication systems and intervention strategies, that can be used to increase the communicative possibilities of people with limited spoken language. It is a guiding principle that communication intervention should include all parts of the usual environment of a communication-impaired individual and aim to enhance the initiative and self-reliance of the individual.

The first edition of this book was written in 1991. At that time, the field of 'augmentative and alternative communication' was quite new and the terms so little known that we chose not to use them in the book's title, as we do now. In the 10 years that have passed since the first edition, a large body of research has been published, and many new ideas and insights have been developed. The present volume is a total revision of the original manuscript, in line with the theoretical and clinical developments within the field, including a new chapter on multi-sign utterances. A textbook on visual communication needs an abundance of illustrations in order to relay the essence of these communication forms, and the rich illustrations of the first edition have been kept. The first version was translated by Kevin M.J. Quirk whereas the revision has been made by the authors. The revision was completed in January 2000.

We want to express our thanks to Nicola Grove and Kaisa Launonen for their many insightful comments on draft versions of this revision.

STEPHEN VON TETZCHNER

HARALD MARTINSEN

Contents

Preface   v

Chapter 1

Introduction   1

Terminology   4
Notation   5

Chapter 2

Augmentative and alternative communication   7

Manual signs   9
Graphic signs   10
    Blissymbols   10
    Pictogram Ideogram Communication   17
    Picture Communication Symbols   18
    Rebus   18
    Lexigrams   20
    Sigsymbols   21
Pictures   22
Orthographic script   24
Tangible signs   24
    Premack's word bricks   24
    Tactile signs   26
Choosing a sign system   27
    Manual, graphic or tangible signs   27
    Use of the systems   29
    Manual signs   30
    Graphic signs   31
    Tangible signs   33

Chapter 3

Communication aids   34

Traditional aids   35
High-technology aids   37
  Artificial speech   43
  Telecommunication aids   45
Pointing   46
Keyboards   48
Switches   50
Choosing a communication aid   51
  Mobility   53
  Direct selection and scanning   53
  Manual and electronic aids   55
Some characteristics of aided communication   57
  Articulation   57
  Time   57
  The role of the conversational partner   60

Chapter 4

Children, adolescents and adults in need of augmentative and alternative communication   62

Three functional groups   62
  The expressive language group   63
  The supportive language group   63
  The alternative language group   65
  Distinguishing between the groups   66
The most common groups in need of augmentative and alternative communication   66
  Motor impairment   67
  Developmental language disorders   70
  Learning disability   73
  Autism   77
  Rett's syndrome   82
Some common problems   87
  Learning takes time   87
  Generalisation   88
  Learned passivity and dependency on others   88
  Behavioural disorders   89

Chapter 5

Assessment   90

The need for total intervention   90
Assessment methods   91
   Tests   91
   Checklists   94
   Information from those in contact with the individual   95
   Systematic observation   95
   Experimental teaching   95
Basic information   96
   Overview of the day   97
General skills   99
   Interest in objects, activities and events   99
   Attention and initiation of communicative contact with others   99
   Self-help skills   100
   Self-occupancy   101
Motor skills   101
Vision and hearing   104
Diagnosis   104
The family's need for support, relief and help   105
Language and communication   106
   Use   106
   Comprehension   109
Evaluating the language intervention   113
   Specific goals   114
   Generalized effects   115
Information transfer when changing school, work and home   116
Defining areas of responsibility   119

Chapter 6

The teaching situation   122

Joint attention   123
Designing the teaching situation   124
Planning for generalization   127
Duration and location of teaching sessions   129
Structuring   130
   Frame structure   130
   Situational structure   131
   Cues   132

Initiating the intervention   133
The effect of sign teaching on speech acquisition   133

Chapter 7

Teaching strategies   135

Structured overinterpretation and total communication   136
Implicit and explicit teaching   136
Comprehension and use of signs   138
Teaching comprehension   140
  Natural situations   140
  Special training   145
Teaching sign use   146
  Watch, wait and react   146
  Reacting to habitual behaviour   149
  Build-and-break chains   149
  Reacting to signal-triggered anticipatory behaviour   150
  Fulfilling wants   151
Focusing on expression and comprehension   155
Incidental teaching   158
Structured waiting   160
Naming   162
Structured and unstructured situations   163
Preparatory training   165
  Eye contact   167
  Gaze direction and attentiveness   168
  Sitting still   169
  Behaviour chains   170
  Imitation   171
  Motor skills   173
Facilitating techniques   173

Chapter 8

Choosing the first signs   178

Existing communication   181
General and specific signs   182
Repetitions   185
Motor skills   186
Perception   189
Iconicity   191
  Manual signs   192
  Graphic signs   194

Tangible signs   198
Simple and complex concepts   198
What to expect   204

Chapter 9

Further vocabulary development   207

Alternative and supportive language groups   207
   Contrasts between signs   211
   Signs for proper names   213
   Expanding use   214
   Individual sign dictionaries   216
The expressive language group   217
   User involvement   217
   Expanding the situations in which signs may be used   218
   Increased access to signs   223
   Expanding the vocabulary by using sign combinations   261
Ready-made vocabularies   228
From graphic signs to orthographic script   236

Chapter 10

Multi-sign utterances   240

Vocabulary   244
   Pivots   245
   Verb island constructs   247
   New sign categories   249
   Inflections   249
Sentences   250
   Horizontal and vertical structures   250
   Topic-comment   252
   Semantic roles   253
   Negation   256
   Fill-in   256
   Chaining   257
   Ready-made sentences   259
Cognitive effort   260
Comprehension   262
   Bootstrapping   263
   Perspective   263
   Comprehension of spoken language   264
Variation   264

Chapter 11

Conversational skills   266

Alternative language group   267
  Routines, plans and scripts   268
Supportive language group   273
Expressive language group   276
  Environmental strategies   278
  Partner strategies   282
  Conversational strategies   287
Narratives   294

Chapter 12

The language environment   297

Adapting the environment   298
  The simultaneous use of speech and signs   299
  Simplified language   300
  Models   301
Teaching families   302
Teaching peers and friends   306
Teaching staff   308
Cost and benefit   311

Chapter 13

Overview of case studies   312

List of sign illustrations   319
References and citation index   323
Index   352

Chapter 1
Introduction

A significant minority of the population is unable to communicate fully through speech. They may be totally unable to speak or speech may not be enough to fulfil all communicative functions; they may also need a non-speech mode of communication as a supplement to, or a substitute for, spoken language. This minority includes children, adolescents and adults with motor impairment, learning disability, autism, delayed speech, and other developmental or acquired language disorders. The size of this group is not fully known. People with acquired impairments constitute an extensive group, including many elderly people.

This book is mainly concerned with *developmental* language and communication disorders. There may be large differences between, on the one hand, the consequences of congenital and early acquired impairments and, on the other, the consequences of impairments acquired at a later age. Inclusion of acquired impairments would need a separate volume. A congenital or early acquired impairment may make it difficult to develop skills that are only indirectly related to the impairment. For example, people who lose sight and hearing as adults can usually still speak and write, whereas those who are born deaf and blind rarely learn these skills. Many children with motor and speech impairments develop reading and writing difficulties, whereas adults who have comparable motor and speech impairments rarely acquire such difficulties. Moreover, as a result of the diverse developmental experiences of the two groups, their cultures and life styles will also differ. It can be estimated that the developmental group includes at least 0.5 per cent of the population, although this estimate is probably low. As more attention is paid to language and communication disorders, the number of cases has increased. The growing interest in language and communication disorders has also led to an increased awareness of the need for alternative communication systems. Today, there are a large number of such systems available.

This book is concerned with the use of manual, graphic and tangible signs in language intervention. The largest group of people who use

1

manual signs are those who are deaf. Deaf children, however, acquire sign language in the same informal manner as most hearing children learn to speak. Growing up in a signing environment, they do not need any special teaching to learn to sign. Consequently, the present book is *not* concerned with deaf people. The exception to this is deaf people who need a communication aid as a result of motor impairment, making expressive signing impossible.

There are large differences among people in need of alternative communication systems. Many children will develop speech and the need for such systems will disappear. To varying degrees, they also adapt to society and become ordinary members of a social community.

For people with a life-long need for an alternative communication system, language comprehension and motor skills may determine their course of life and the degree to which they will acquire ordinary life qualities. One particular subgroup understands what other people say and the events that take place around them, and shares the values and norms of the prevailing culture. Their need for alternative communication systems is the result of motor impairments that hinder speech. Usually, they have motor disorders that hinder other activities as well, making them dependent on technical aids and assistance from others.

Another subgroup is made up of people who fail to acquire speech and do not profit from traditional speech and language therapy. For most of the people in this group, the language disorder is part of a more general impairment that also influences other intellectual and social skills.

Difficulty in communicating with other people produces widespread consequences and affects people in all aspects of life and at all ages. In the prelingual period, communication difficulties influence the interaction between the children and their caregivers, and disturb or destroy natural processes of culturalization. Parents of children with extensive communication disorders often experience impoverished contact with their children. They have problems understanding their children's interests and are often confused about what to do. The children risk losing opportunities for natural learning, which normally form part of any social environment. Most of what children learn as they grow up is co-constructed with more competent members of society; what they learn is conveyed through: shared focus, reactions from adults and other children, what others explain and tell them about things, and seeing and hearing what others say and do. In this manner, children learn language and acquire the knowledge, values and norms of their culture. Children with language and communication disorders will have less exposure than others to such learning opportunities.

From childhood and throughout life, feelings of self-sufficiency, self-respect and worth are closely related to the ability to express oneself. The perception of oneself as independent and equal to others is related to the ability to express one's needs, ideas, concerns and feelings. When this ability is compromised, people may have difficulties making themselves 'heard' and lose control over their own fate. They risk alienation and exclusion from the social norms. They may experience that other people underestimate them – talk down to them and make decisions for them – thus reinforcing their feeling of being second-class citizens. Alternatively, they find that people overestimate them, assuming that they have an understanding and control of the situation, which in fact they do not have, and hence attribute meanness and badwill to them, rather than a reduced ability to respond appropriately in social interactions. For people with the most severe disability, such negative experiences may – together with inconsistent and infrequent reactions to their initiations and wants – lead to learned passivity and extensive dependency on others, as well as frustration and behavioural problems. For them, the ability to communicate means an increased understanding of the world and what is going on around them, the possibility of expressing their needs and a higher level of activity.

Providing an alternative mode of communication to children and adults with no or limited speech may increase their quality of life, provide them with better control over their own lives and greater self-respect, and give them the opportunity to feel equal in society. Moreover, for people with extensive motor impairments, language and communication may be easier to develop than other skills. For them, the non-vocal expressive language skills that they acquire may have a dual function – enabling them also to participate more in all kinds of social and societal activities.

The choice of an alternative communication system must be viewed in a broad perspective. The system should improve everyday life and make the user feel less disabled and more able to control life. The choice of communication system must therefore be based on the total situation of the individual. Most people who need an alternative communication system also need other forms of intervention. The teaching of a new communication system must be co-ordinated with the whole range of habilitation services on offer, such as education, training, help, etc. Language and communication intervention must not be isolated from other forms of intervention. In the same way as for other forms of language and communication, alternative communication systems should function as a tool to be used in all life situations.

Many new communication systems and aids have come into use, and it may be difficult to get descriptions and evaluations of them. The various groups of people in need of alternative or supplementary communication often require different communication systems and, although the newest model is not always the best, knowledge about what systems are available is crucial in order to be able to make the right decisions. It is also necessary to know how to adapt the different systems and aids to the needs of individual users. Thus, the main aims of this book are to:

- give an overview of manual, graphic and tangible communication systems and communication aids that can be used with children, adolescents and adults in need of alternatives and supplements to speech
- give an overview of the principal groups of people in need of an alternative communication form, and the major differences between the individuals within the various groups
- describe the assessment and important factors for the choice of communication system and individual signs, and discuss how the choice can be based as much as possible on the user's particular characteristics, interests and needs
- describe the most important principles for teaching and giving environmental support to different alternative communication systems, including discussion of how language and communication intervention may best be adapted to enhance the initiative and self-reliance of the individual.

Terminology

The use of graphic and manual signs by non-deaf people with language and communication disorders is fairly new and hence there is a need for new terms. The terminology used in this book is in accordance with the modern professional literature. However, at one point the terminology differs from most of the literature within the field. The term 'sign' is used as a generic term for linguistic forms that are not speech, and includes both manual and graphic forms. The reason for this is that, although in the literature on augmentative and alternative communication, graphic signs have often been described as 'symbols', in the field of linguistics, both speech and manual and graphic signs are referred to as language symbols (Lyons, 1977). Peirce (1931), among others, distinguishes between 'symbolic' and 'iconic' signs. Most graphic signs described as 'symbol systems' (Picture Communication System [PCS], Pictogram Ideogram Communication [PIC], etc.) would not have been regarded as 'symbolic' by Peirce. Using the term 'symbol' to describe only one type of communication system seems imprudent. 'Sign', referring to the form of the expression, appears to be a more neutral concept.

In keeping with international terminology, words and phrases such as *to speak*, *to say something*, *speaker*, *listener*, etc., are used fairly loosely. An *aided speaker* uses a communication aid, whereas a *natural speaker* speaks in the normal manner. A *listener* is the same as a conversational partner. A *listener* does not necessarily hear somebody speak, but may 'read' a graphic or manual sign, or interpret another form of communication. The term 'non-speaking' is used to indicate that the individual lacks speech, whereas the term 'non-verbal' indicates that the person in question lacks any kind of language: spoken, manual, tangible or graphic.

Although most of the individuals who receive this form of intervention are children, many adolescents and adults with developmental disabilities are also taught to use alternative communication systems. One reason for this is that many people with severe disabilities need intervention into adulthood – and some throughout their lives. Another reason is that there is still a substantial group of adults who never had the opportunity to learn an alternative communication system in childhood. We therefore use the term 'individual' to refer to the person who receives intervention, unless it is clear from the context that it is a child, an adolescent or an adult. We use the term 'teacher' for all professionals involved in teaching the individual. Thus, a 'teacher' may be a nursery school teacher, teacher, care nurse, speech therapist, psychologist, etc. The term 'significant people' is used to refer to family, friends, daily carers in sheltered housing, and others who are close to the person or responsible for his or her interests. It does not usually comprise teachers and other educators.

Notation

The notation used in this book follows von Tetzchner and Jensen (1996). In accordance with this, *naturally spoken utterances* are italicized, whereas *'words and sentences in machine-produced digitized or synthesized speech'* are italicized and in quotes. In written presentations of sign language, every sign has a *gloss*, i.e. a name or translation. Such glosses are written in capital letters, for example, SHOP (Figure 1). The gloss of *GRAPHIC SIGNS* and *PICTURES* are in capital letters and italicized. (Many of the examples in this book do not refer specifically to manual *or* graphic signs. In these examples, capital letters are used.) The same notation is used for *TANGIBLE SIGNS*. When the gloss of a single manual or graphic sign needs more than one word in translation, these will be hyphenated, for example, YOU-AND-ME or *YOU-AND-ME*. Indications of whole words and written ready-made sentences are underlined. Also s-p-e-l-l-e-d words are underlined. Quotation signs are used for 'interpretations or translations of meaning' of manual or graphic sign utterances. They are also used for the meaning of facial expressions, gestures, pointing, etc., e.g. 'yes' (nodding) and 'no' (shaking the head). Parentheses {. . .} indicate simultaneous expressive forms, e.g. speech and manual signs, or manual and graphic signs. {HAPPY. *I am happy*} means that the manual sign HAPPY is produced simultaneously with the naturally spoken sentence *I am happy*.

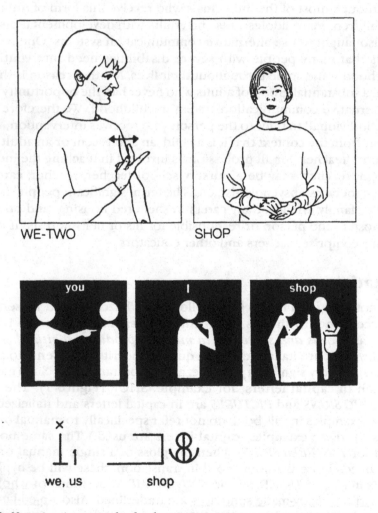

Figure 1. *Notation in use in this book. WE-TWO SHOP, or YOU I SHOP, may mean 'We are going shopping'.*

Chapter 2
Augmentative and alternative communication

Speech is the most common form of human communication and therefore the preferred mode for people with normal hearing. However, some people are not able to speak, no matter how much training they are given. For these individuals, alternative communication will be their main form of communication. Others have more limited speech disorders. They may need alternative communication while learning to speak or to augment their communication and make their speech easier to understand. Augmentative and alternative communication thus implies the use of non-speech modes as a supplement to, or a substitute for, spoken language:

- *Alternative communication* is used when the individual communicates in face-to-face communication in ways other than through speech. Manual and graphic signs, Morse code, writing, etc., are alternative forms of communication for individuals who do not have the ability to speak.
- *Augmentative communication* means supplementary or supportive communication. The word 'augmentative' emphasises the fact that intervention with alternative forms of communication has a dual purpose: to promote and supplement speech and to guarantee an alternative form of communication if the individual does not begin to speak.

The units of alternative communication systems are manual, graphic and tangible signs. The term 'sign system' may be used to describe collections of these signs:

- *Manual signs* include the sign languages of deaf people and other signs performed with the hands (e.g. systems such as Signed Norwegian and Signing Exact English). The verb 'to sign' refers to the use of manual signs. Sign language comprises only manual signs used by deaf people.

7

- *Graphic signs* include all graphically formed signs (Blissymbols, Picture Communication Symbols [PCS], Pictogram Ideogram Communication [PIC], Rebus, etc.).
- *Tangible signs* are usually made of wood or plastic (e.g. Premack's word bricks). Some tangible signs are designed for blind and severely visually impaired people, and may be termed 'tactile signs'. They are also usually made of plastic or wood, and have distinctive shapes and different surface textures.

The division between *aided* and *unaided* communication designates different forms of alternative communication:

- *Aided communication* includes all forms of communication in which the communicative expression exists in a physical form outside the user. The signs are selected. Pointing boards, synthetic speech machines, computers and other forms of communication aids all belong to this category. Pointing at a graphic sign or picture is a form of aided communication because the sign or picture is the communicative expression.
- *Unaided communication* is communication in which the disabled individuals make the communicative expressions by themselves. The signs are *produced*. This chiefly encompasses manual signs, but Morse code also belongs to this category because the users make every single letter in Morse. Blinking with one's eyes to indicate 'yes' and 'no' is also a form of unaided communication. The same applies to ordinary pointing and other gestures, because in these instances the pointing is the communicative expression.

The division between *dependent* and *independent* communication relates to how the alternative communication form is used and the contribution of the conversational partner:

- *Dependent communication* means that the disabled individual relies on another person to put together or interpret the meaning of what is being expressed. Dependent communication forms may be boards with single letters, words or graphic signs, but also people using manual signs may need a partner to interpret and put the meaning of the signs together.
- *Independent communication* means that the message is wholly formulated by the disabled individual. For people using graphic communication, this may be achieved with the help of synthetic speech machines that speak whole sentences or technical aids where the message is written on paper or a screen.

Manual signs

In most countries there are two types of manual signs. The first type is found in the sign languages used among deaf people. These sign languages are often named after the country, e.g. Norwegian Sign Language (NSL), American Sign Language and British Sign Language (BSL). The sign languages are *primary*, i.e. not derived from a spoken language. They have their own grammar, with inflections and word orders (syntax), which differ from that of spoken languages. The sign languages of the various countries differ in much the same way as spoken languages do. The topography (articulation) of the signs differs, they are inflected differently and the sentences have a different word order. There are also dialectal variations. Sign languages have developed naturally and have undergone change through contact with other sign languages, as well as with spoken and written languages (compare Klima and Bellugi, 1979; Woll, Kyle and Deuchar, 1981; Siple and Fischer, 1991).

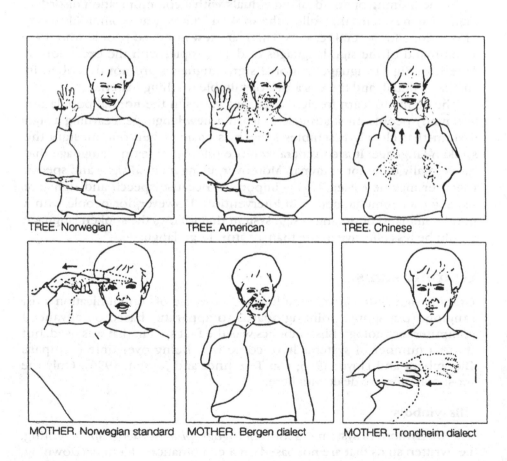

TREE. Norwegian   TREE. American   TREE. Chinese

MOTHER. Norwegian standard   MOTHER. Bergen dialect   MOTHER. Trondheim dialect

The other type of signs may also be called *manual sign systems*. They are constructed so that they follow speech word for word, and are inflected in the same way as the national spoken language. Accordingly, these also differ from one country to the other, and include, for example, Signed Norwegian (Norsk tegnordbok, 1988), Signing Exact English (Gustason, Pfetzing and Zawolkow, 1980) and the Paget–Gorman Sign System (Paget, 1951; Paget, Gorman and Paget, 1976). These manual sign systems are often devised by teachers of deaf children as a means of representing the spoken language through signs. Usually, many of the signs in the constructed systems are borrowed from the national sign languages, whereas inflections and syntax are modelled on the national spoken language. These systems have never been used widely among deaf people because the inflections and syntax of spoken languages are not well suited to a visual and manual language.

In the training of non-deaf individuals with a communication disorder, manual sign systems that follow the spoken language are commonly used. This is done for several reasons. There are few non-deaf people who have a command of the sign languages of deaf people; with the exception of American Sign Language, national sign languages are not described in sufficient detail, and there is a lack of suitable teaching material.

The ability to learn foreign languages varies in the normal population and many people must struggle to learn a new language. Learning a sign system that closely resembles speech is easier when one masters the spoken language. It is considerably more difficult to learn a language that has a totally different grammar. Moreover, using manual signs and speech together may be easier. This is important because speech and signs are usually used simultaneously in intervention. However, for people with a good command of signing, a sign system that follows the spoken language would be less effective in use than a natural sign language.

Graphic signs

Graphic sign systems are often linked to the use of communication aids, ranging from simple pointing boards to apparatus based on advanced computer technology. Blissymbolics was the first system that was used, but quite a number of systems have come into being over time (compare Bloomberg and Lloyd, 1986; von Tetzchner and Jensen, 1996). Only the most common are dealt with here.

Blissymbols

The Blissymbolics system is a form of *logographic* or *ideographic* writing, i.e. written signs that are not based on a combination of letters (Downing,

1973). Blissymbolics were originally constructed as an international written language with Chinese as a model. The aim was to promote peace by enabling statesmen from different countries to communicate more easily with one another (Bliss, 1965). The system was never put to such use. It was first used in Toronto as a system of writing for motor-impaired children who were unable to speak, and who also had difficulty in learning to read and write (McNaughton and Kates, 1974; McNaughton, 1998).

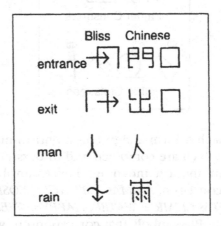

The Blissymbolics system consists of 100 basic signs, or *radicals*, which can be combined to form words for which there are no basic signs. A number of these sign combinations are conventional. The Blissymbolics Institute in Toronto and the International Blissymbolics Committee have adopted a number of fixed English glosses, or 'translations', which can be adapted to fit different English-speaking cultures, as well as other national languages. A specific Blissymbol or a given combination may be used slightly differently in different countries, in the same way as a word in the spoken language, when translated, is not exactly the same in another language. Where a conventional combination has not been decided on, it may be possible to construct several Blissymbols that correspond to the same spoken word, as can be seen in the example of *FATHER CHRISTMAS*.

Communication boards with Blissymbols usually consist of both basic signs and sign combinations that the user often needs. For most words in the spoken languages, however, there are no established Blissymbol conventions and, in many cases, the user either would not know the accepted form or not have the necessary elements. Thus, it is up to the users to find a suitable Blissymbol combination to express what they wish to say. It is quite common for the interventionists to give different background colours to Blissymbols with glosses referring to different word classes. However, some Blissymbol users complain that this limits their creative use of the system (Kollar, 1999).

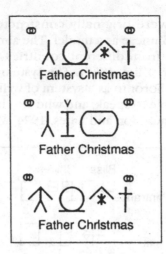

The Blissymbols that form a sign combination may be regarded as *semantic elements* which are combined and understood by analogy. This gives the sign combination meaning. For example, the Blissymbol *ELEPHANT* usually consists of *ANIMAL + LONG + NOSE. HOME* is *HOUSE + FEELINGS. TOILET* is *CHAIR + WATER. HAPPY* is *FEELING + UP* (Figure 2). In addition to the Blissymbols that correspond to whole words, there are also a number of markers that constitute grammatical inflections and denote parts of speech, such as *PAST, PLURAL, ACTION, OPPOSITE-MEANING*, etc. Thus the Blissymbolics system has a fairly complex construction, based on combinations of signs (compare Schlosser, 1997a, 1997b).

The basic signs and sign combinations may also be joined together to form sentences. Bliss (1965) gives information about syntax, but in principle any word order may be used. In most countries, the word order taught will resemble the word order of the spoken language as closely as possible.

The graphic formation of many Blissymbols can be fairly complex. In addition, many of them have one or more basic signs in common. For individuals with normal vision and good linguistic and intellectual skills, this may not matter, but for learning-disabled individuals, this complexity can be a great barrier. With the exception of cases in which only the simplest signs have been taught, experiments in teaching Blissymbols to this group have not been very successful. Intellectually well-functioning people with speech impairments and reading difficulties have gained most benefit from Blissymbols (McNaughton and Kates, 1980; Sandberg and Hjelmquist, 1992).

The Blissymbolics system is no doubt the most advanced graphic system available for non-speaking people. However, its relative

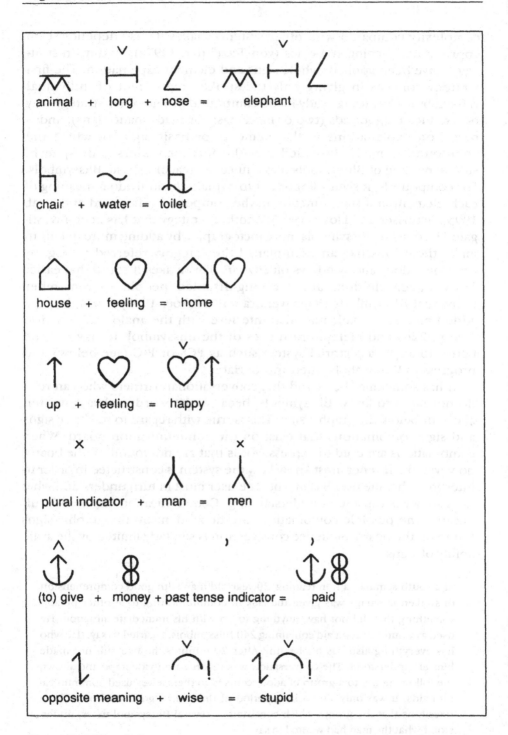

Figure 2. *Blissymbols.*

complexity compared with other systems makes its use dependent on appropriate teaching strategies (von Tetzchner, 1997a). Two main strategies have been applied: whole signs and element explanation. The first strategy consists in giving only the spoken equivalent of individual Blissymbols (including ready-made compounds). The other strategy may be used for compounds (two or more basic or ready-made signs), and is based on explanations of the elements or basic signs of which the compound is made. Provided that the learner understands speech, simple naming of Blissymbols may suffice for teaching basic Blissymbols. For compounds, it seems important to explain the individual meaning of each element and their function in the compound (Shepherd and Haaf, 1995; Schlosser and Lloyd, 1997). Another strategy that has been investigated is to make Blissymbols more pictographic by adding more details to make them look like an exemplar of the category referred to, e.g. by drawing a door and windows on *HOUSE*. This makes it somewhat easier for younger children and learning-disabled people to remember individual Blissymbols (Raghavendra and Fristoe, 1990, 1995), but the added pictorial details may also interfere with the analogical function (see p. 226) and metaphorical uses of the Blissymbol. It may thus be better to apply a pictorial system such as PCS or PIC (see below) and progress to Blissymbols when appropriate.

It has sometimes been said that conversational partners who can read do not need to know Blissymbols, because the word is always written above or below the graphic sign. This is true with regard to the basic signs and sign combinations that exist on the communication board. When combinations are used to express words that are not found on the board, however, the listener must know how the system is constructed in order to interpret what the user has meant. The user must in turn understand what the listener is capable of understanding. Communication can be difficult because the possible combinations are dependent on the graphic signs found on the board. Sentence construction is similarly limited by the availability of signs.

At a youth seminar, a non-reading, 20-year-old man with good comprehension of spoken language was given the task of communicating to another person something that did not have anything to do with his immediate situation. He used a communication aid containing 240 Blissymbols. He tried to say: 'He who has everything also has his health.' After 20 minutes, he had still not made himself understood. The conversation was recorded on videotape and shown the following day to a group of adolescents who themselves used communication aids. It was only after a long period of time and a good deal of probing questions that the group, which consisted of several Blissymbol users, understood what the man had wanted to say.

An adolescent who used Blissymbols told his teacher at school: *MOTHER ALMOST-SAME-AS COCA-COLA*. It was only when his mother came to school later that day and explained that she had been angry with him that morning that it was understood that the utterance was intended to mean 'Mum was angry'.

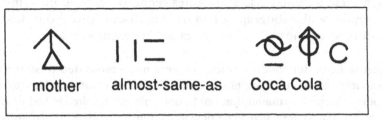

mother   almost-same-as   Coca Cola

In retrospect it is easy to understand that the youth expressed that 'mother almost bubbled over', but the example clearly shows how difficult it can be to make the graphic signs suffice, and how creative both the user and the listener must be when conversation has nuances.

Blissymbolics was the first graphic system to be used in many countries (von Tetzchner and Jensen, 1996), but there seems to be a steady decrease in the use of Blissymbols in Europe and North America. In a recent Norwegian epidemiological study comprising 25 per cent of the population, among children aged under 10 years who used graphic communication as their main form of intervention, there was a total absence of Blissymbols (von Tetzchner, 1997a). Studies in Sweden (Sandberg and Hjelmquist, 1992) and Scotland (Murphy et al., 1995) indicate a somewhat wider use of Blissymbols in these countries than in Norway, but the decline also seems to take place in these countries. One reason for the decline is that, for a number of the early users, Blissymbols proved too difficult. Instead of improving communication, they lead to frustration for both the users and those close to them. This tended to happen before other systems had come into use, and today individuals with learning disability or severe language disorders are given more appropriate systems. On the other hand, there have also been examples of children being given a board with Blissymbols despite the fact that they could read and write, and would have got greater benefit from a board with letters and words (compare Conway, 1986; Smith et al., 1989).

Perhaps the pendulum has moved too far in the opposite direction. The result may be less appropriate communication and developmental opportunities in general for some children. It is important that those who can benefit from an advanced system are given the opportunity to learn Blissymbols. As indicated above, this is not always the case. However, many parents and professionals have reacted negatively to Blissymbols. It is not uncommon for them to use the Blissymbols only when the child is in for assessment or control at the habilitation centre that prescribed its use. This may be the result of a lack of introduction to, and guidance in using, the system, and because no clear explanation has been given for the choice of Blissymbols (Frafjord and Brekke, 1997). Professionals (and through them parents) also sometimes seem to perceive Blissymbols as a rival to traditional orthography. Referring to discussions about Blissymbols at the time when the child was 4 years old, a parent said:

> Because he understood so much, we were more motivated to start with a computer, to start teaching him the alphabet and go that way, instead of via another alternative communication. In our opinion, he already had that. And we had begun to hope that some time in the future – maybe very far away – he would learn to read and write (von Tetzchner, 1997a, p. 229).

Teaching Blissymbols may also be considered so time consuming that it will interfere with other activities. The teacher of another boy, referring to a discussion in the boy's fifth year of life, said:

> There was still a need for expanding the vocabulary and the communicative competence. Then the issue of reading and writing was raised and his possibilities in relation to that. And how should we spend the time? If he were to learn Blissymbols, how much time would be left for play? This was the real issue. If he could jump from PIC to reading quite fast, before first grade, we will not spend the time on teaching Blissymbols. We will use it for play (von Tetzchner, 1997a, p. 229).

If a child has to rely on a less advanced system than he or she can possibly master, the consequence may be that he or she remains unnecessarily long at a plateau in expressive language development while waiting for the introduction of traditional orthography. Moreover, children with speech and motor impairments are at risk of developing reading disorders (Koppenhaver and Yoder, 1992), and lack of access to an advanced form of non-orthographic graphic communication may hinder their general language development. Neither of the boys referred to above was taught to read and write before attending school at the ordinary starting age of 7 years (in Norway). Acknowledging the importance of play, the teacher cited above seemed to overlook the fact that, for motor-impaired children, language is the key to participating in play as well as in conversations.

Pictogram Ideogram Communication

Pictogram Ideogram Communication (PIC) originates from Canada (Maharaj, 1980). This system has become very popular in the Nordic countries and has to a great extent replaced the use of Blissymbols among those with severe learning disability. PIC consists of stylized drawings which form white silhouettes on a black background (Figure 3). The gloss is always written in white lettering above the drawing. There are presently around 1300 PIC signs, including 300 designed in Japan.

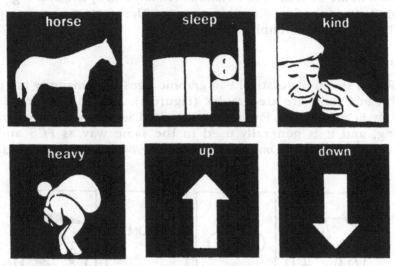

Figure 3. *Pictogram Ideogram Communication.*

PIC signs do not yield the same problems found with Blissymbols. Both parents and professionals feel that they are easier to understand, and have taken to them quickly. PIC signs are, however, less versatile and in some respects more limited than Blissymbols. Also PIC signs may be used to form sentences, as well as new words but, with the relatively small number of signs, this is not always easy. When the user needs more opportunities than those given by PIC signs, the signs may be supplemented with graphic signs from other systems, which have a more general use.

The use of PIC signs has been of great benefit to many people, but the popularity of these graphic signs may also have led to overuse. PIC signs have sometimes been recommended for people who could have used Blissymbols or normal writing.

Picture Communication Symbols

Picture Communication Symbols (PCS: Johnson, 1981, 1985, 1992) originate in the USA. The system consists of about 3000 signs. They are simple black-and-white line drawings with the gloss written above them (Figure 4). Some function words, such as articles and prepositions, e.g. *OF*, *FOR* and *WITH*, are represented in traditional orthography without any line drawing. The signs are easy to draw, and PCS can therefore even be copied by hand. PCS is probably the most widely used graphic system today. It is common in the USA, the UK, Ireland, Germany and Spain, and is growing in popularity in the Scandinavian countries. The greatest asset, compared with PIC, is the larger number of signs.

Rebus

The Rebus system consists of 950 graphic signs. The majority are pictographic and some are ideographic (Figure 5). As with Blissymbols, the Peabody Rebus Reading Program was devised as a system of logographic writing, and it is generally used in the same way as PCS and PIC (Woodcock, Clark and Davies, 1969; Clark, 1984). The system originated

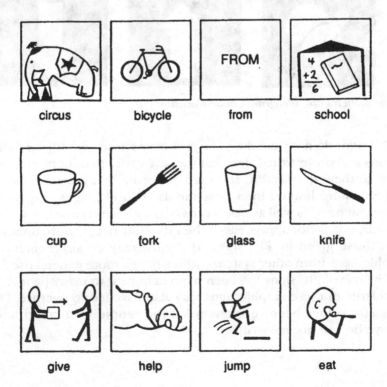

Figure 4. *Picture Communication System.*

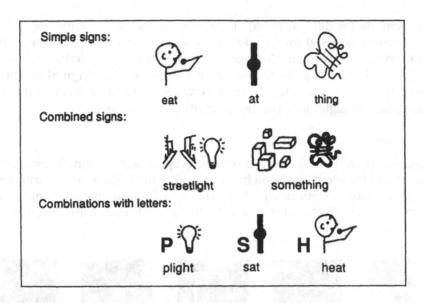

Figure 5. *Rebus signs.*

in the USA, and a British version has been developed, closely linked with the Makaton project (van Oosterom and Devereux, 1985; Walker et al., 1985).

Rebus signs may be combined in the usual way: *STREET* + *LIGHT* becomes *STREETLIGHT*. In addition, the pronunciation of the sign's gloss may also be used, e.g. *LIGHT* can mean both 'bright' and 'not heavy'.

The Rebus system was originally designed to help people with a mild-to-moderate degree of learning disability to learn to read. At a later stage, its use was extended to be used as a means of communication (Jones, 1979). Thus, in traditional teaching of Rebus, emphasis is placed on using letters as well as graphic signs. One or more letters are combined with the pronunciation of glosses, so that the combinations of graphic signs and letters form new words. When a sign is combined with a letter, it is the pronunciation of these two elements together that expresses the new word. The meaning of the graphic sign plays no part. *C* + *OLD* becomes *COLD*. *P* + *LIGHT* becomes *PLIGHT*, and *C* + *AT* becomes *CAT*.

This use of the Rebus system has proved to have a positive effect on an individual's reading skills (Kiernan, Reid and Jones, 1982), and this is related to the practice of using corresponding sounds as well the ordinary meanings of the graphic signs. At the same time, the Rebus system places few demands on reading skills, because it is not necessary to be able to read all the letters in a word. Investigations into the teaching of reading and sound recognition show that, initially, children are able to say what the first sound or syllable is in a word, without being able to identify the other sounds (Skjelfjord, 1976). Thus, it seems as though this use of the Rebus system is based on a mid-stage in the acquisition of reading skills, and thereby enhances the further development of these skills. Although this use of Rebus at present is quite uncommon, the original reading-oriented strategies is one of the system's important contributions. Of course, the strategies may be adopted with any other system.

Lexigrams

Lexigrams do not constitute a complete graphic sign system. They consist of a set of nine elements, which may be combined in different forms and assigned glosses (Figures 6 and 7). The stated aim is that the signs shall not be pictographic. As there are no fixed or allocated meanings, each

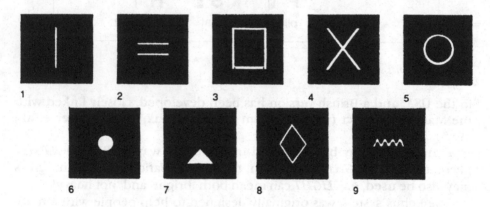

Figure 6. *The nine main elements in Lexigrams.*

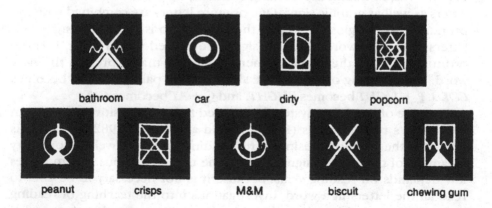

Figure 7. *Examples of Lexigrams.*

sign's gloss is assigned on the basis of an assessment of the individual and his or her environment. Lexigrams have mostly been used in the USA and their use seems to have been limited to research (Romski and Sevcik, 1996).

Sigsymbols

These graphic signs are based on both graphic iconicity (see p. 191) and sign language. There are three types of signs: pictographic, ideographic and manual sign-linked. It is the use of graphic representations of manual signs that is the most distinctive feature compared with other systems (Figure 8). The name 'sigsymbol' or 'Sigsym' is an abbreviation of sign-symbol (Cregan, 1993). As manual signs differ from country to country and between the various systems, it is essential that the sigsymbols are designed on the basis of the sign language or a manual sign system in use in the particular area. The design of the pictographic and ideographic sigsymbols is based on similar principles to most other graphic systems.

The British sigsymbol system consisted of 240 items when it was developed in 1982 (Cregan, 1982; Jones and Cregan, 1986). The American version consists of 390 items, and about half of them are based on Signed English (Cregan and Lloyd, 1984, 1990). Sigsymbols may be particularly useful for individuals who use both graphic and manual signs, and as a possible written language for people who learn manual signs. Sigsymbols based on manual signs may also be used with other graphic systems.

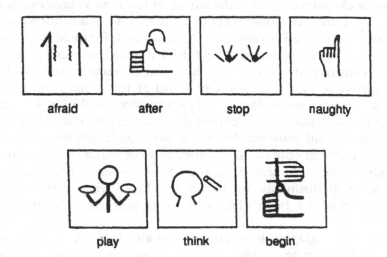

afraid   after   stop   naughty

play   think   begin

Figure 8. *Sigsym.*

Pictures

Pictures, i.e. drawings and photographs, are commonly the first graphic communication form provided for young children. However, the understanding of pictures is an important cognitive skill that normally emerges slowly and that may not be easily achieved by people with learning disability. Small children show a limited comprehension of pictures (Kose, Beilin and O'Connor, 1983). For example, in early language development the names of learned objects are not transferred to pictures of those same objects (Lucariello, 1987). Picture comprehension is also limited among many learning-disabled people, and photographs may be more difficult to comprehend than line drawings (Dixon, 1981; McNaughton and Light, 1989). If the individual does not understand what the pictures are supposed to represent, then there is little point in using pictures instead of a graphic sign system.

The desire to use something that the individual can recognize and react to is generally the argument used in favour of pictures. However, picture use is not a goal in itself. The question is whether the visual content of pictures helps the disabled individual to use them communicatively. Pictures have both advantages and disadvantages. A *general* interest in pictures may be an argument for using a sign system based on iconicity, providing that the person does not have fixed routines related to the act of 'looking at pictures'. If disabled individuals are interested in *particular* pictures, the use is dependent on what they associate with these images. Looking at and reacting to pictures is not a *linguistic use*, and the use of pictures as *words* may necessitate the individuals unlearning their original use of such images. Unlearning established reactions to known pictures is the same as removing part of the basis that forms an already existing social interaction, and this would seem to be neither necessary nor wise.

Most people are surrounded by pictures and, for those who are to use pictures as words, it can be difficult to distinguish between pictures used in the ordinary manner – to look at and remember, to talk about, as decoration and illustrations, etc. – and pictures that form part of the individual's own vocabulary. Using pictures that are distinctive and totally different from others, and defining these as the individual's vocabulary, is therefore helpful. Most graphic sign systems are largely based on iconicity, and the pictorial content may sometimes confound their use as a word (Smith, 1996). At the same time, they do have some special characteristics that may help distinguish them from usual pictures (e.g. PCS and PIC). It may therefore be beneficial to use a graphic sign system instead of pictures.

The use of graphic sign systems may also facilitate naming, which is often difficult when a child has to communicate with pictures. For example, parents and children often sit with picture books and tell each other the names of things that they see in them. If the pictures on the communication board are fairly similar to those in the books, there is little purpose in indicating both the one in the book and the one at the communication board. This would only be a form of matching, and would not imply a linguistic use. Indicating a picture on the communication board would be simple pointing, difficult to perceive as naming of the objects and activities in the picture in the book, which is a condition for calling it a linguistic use.

In addition, it seems that pictures are not generally regarded as an individual's language. The experience of users is that they are not taken seriously when they communicate with pictures, and that pointing at a picture is not taken as meaning that they have something to say (Conway, 1986). Parents often act as though the child pointed only at an ordinary picture, and may begin to talk about what is in the picture, what is happening in it, etc. (C. Basil, personal communication, 1989).

When making communication boards, many people use photographs of things in the child's environment. For example, the parents may take a photograph of their car and try to teach the child to use it as the generic term for 'car'. This may make it difficult for the child to use the picture to talk of cars other than the parents' car. The picture is treated as a proper name: 'Mummy and Daddy's car', instead of as a generic name for a class of objects, 'cars'. If one imagines that photographs of a child's mother and father were used as general expressions for 'man' and 'woman', i.e. to represent all men and women, the problem becomes even clearer.

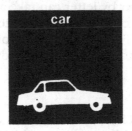

Sometimes pictures are cut out of magazines and placed on the communication board without taking into account how difficult it sometimes is to distinguish between such pictures. Some severely learning-disabled individuals are either colour-blind or unable to use colour information (J.F. Fagan, personal communication, 1987). There are also considerable general cultural differences with regard to perception of pictures. In some cultures, people understand black-and-white line drawings but are incapable of recognizing photographs in colour

(Stephenson and Linfoot, 1996). These are arguments in favour of using a sign system in black and white with good contrast, because the likelihood that the user will perceive and comprehend the differences between the signs is greatest in such a system.

The most important function of photographs may be as names of people. As a name refers only to a particular person, photographs fill this function well. However, when photographs are applied as communication aids, the child is often present in the photograph. This may make it difficult to interpret the meaning of the picture that is indicated, whether it refers to the actual location, the situation, the person or several of these aspects. It also becomes difficult to use the photograph to communicate about what other children and adults are doing or want. In order to avoid these problems one may introduce a separate photograph of the child together with one or more photographs or signs from a graphic system that denote objects, activities, etc. By combining a photograph of the child and a photograph or graphic sign, instead of integrating them in the same item, it will be possible to change the activity, object, etc., while keeping the photograph of the child; alternatively, insert the photograph of another child or adult with the item relating to an activity or object. In this way, a basis is made for multi-sign utterances even if the pictures denoting the activity and the child are presented together at first (von Tetzchner et al., 1998).

Orthographic script

Many communication aids are based on normal writing. As spelling out words and sentences letter by letter can take a long time, an aid that uses letters will often contain combinations of letters, words and sentences in addition to single letters. For users who have only a limited vocabulary, the communication aid may consist of single words.

Tangible signs

Some children may benefit from being able to touch as well as see the shape of the sign. In addition to tangible sign systems, objects that symbolize events, and more or less object-like models of objects, may serve as tangible signs, as well as shapes that do not resemble objects in the category that they refer to (Rowland and Schweigert, 1989; Bloom, 1990). They may also have different textures. The oldest and most extensive tangible communication system was made by Premack (1971).

Premack's word bricks

Premack's word bricks form a system that has been used fairly extensively in the UK and the USA for teaching both learning-disabled and autistic individuals. The word bricks were originally devised in order to investigate whether apes could learn a language that was not based on speech. It was therefore important for Premack (1971) that the word bricks did not resemble those objects that they were used to refer to. This was because he wished to show that apes could learn non-iconic signs. Deich and Hodges (1977) made additional word bricks, and a number of these resemble the objects that they are used to represent. The word bricks are made of plastic or wood and differ in form (Figure 9). What sets these signs apart from others is the fact that they can be physically investigated, manipulated and moved.

Premack's system was chiefly aimed at teaching single signs, even though they were also strung together to form sentences. Carrier developed the use of Premack's word bricks by producing a systematic, pedagogical programme for the teaching of sentence building (Carrier, 1974; Carrier and Peak, 1975). The word bricks were marked with coloured tape to denote the part of speech that the word brick belonged to. Articles were marked with red, verbs with blue, nouns with orange, etc. As well as learning how to use single bricks, users would also learn a

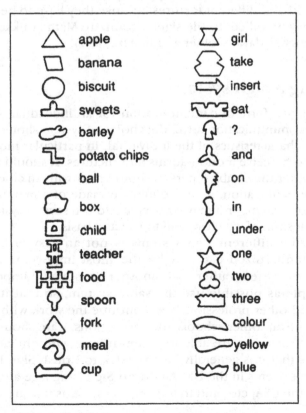

Figure 9. *Premack's word bricks.*

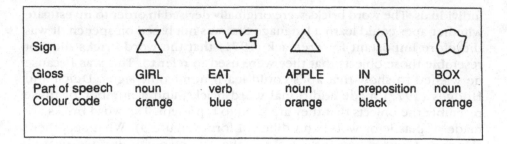

Figure 10. *Carrier's sentence building with Premack's word bricks.*

simplified syntax from the fact that different types of sentences consisted of different colour sequences (Figure 10).

Tactile signs

Some tangible signs have been designed to serve people with blindness or severe visual impairment. They typically have forms that can be easily discriminated and different textures because they have to be identified by feel, and may be called 'tactile signs' (compare Mathy-Laikko et al., 1989; Murray-Branch, Udavari-Solner and Bailey, 1991).

Choosing a sign system

To find the best form of communication for an individual who needs an alternative communication form, the choice of system should be based on the known characteristics of the individual, in particular motor skills and the ability to perceive motion, forms and pictures. It should first be determined whether the disabled person should start with an aided or unaided form of communication. A choice may be made of a manual, graphic or tangible sign system, or it may be decided to use several systems. There is then the question of which system to use as a basis.

Comparing different sign systems is not an easy task. Within one country, standardized use may be the most important argument for choosing one system rather than another. It is highly important that as many people as possible use the same system, so that it is easier for teachers and other professionals to continue the work with children and adolescents from other schools and institutions. Care should be taken to ensure that the users are able to communicate with one another direct. This means that it is generally best to stick to British Sign Language and British sign systems in the UK, American Sign Language and manual sign systems in the USA, etc., and to the graphic systems that are in general use within the country (Blissymbols, PCS, PIC and Rebus). Convincing proof of the need for a particular new sign system would be required in order for that sign system to be put into use. Standardized use also increases the possibilities of gaining broad experience with a system, and thereby revealing both its strong and weak points.

Manual, graphic or tangible signs

When choosing between manual and graphic signs, the individual's perceptual abilities should be taken into account. Visually impaired individuals can often comprehend the movements of manual signs more easily than they can perceive a drawing. The movements can also be understood kinaesthetically, as in communication among people with a combined visual and hearing impairment where the manual signs of the conversational partner are performed with the user's hands. For some users, technical aids with graphic sign systems and synthetic speech will be helpful. Many learning-disabled people get little benefit from pictures; for others graphic signs have great attention value. Some people seem to benefit from being able to feel and manipulate the tangible signs such as Premack's word bricks, but in general little is known of how this may influence learning and use.

The ability to use one's arms and hands is also an important factor in the choice of communication form. One significant difference between manual and graphic signs is the fact that graphic signs are selected whereas manual signs must be produced. Manual signs therefore appear to place greater demands on memory. Moreover, for comprehension of both types of signs, the individual has to pay visual attention to the sign produced by the communication partner and the communicative consequence related to these signs. However, for production, the demands on attention are somewhat different. Manual sign users may be attentive to the communication partner or the person, object or event that they refer to while signing. Graphic sign users have to pay attention to and indicate a graphic sign, which makes it difficult for them at the same time to attend to the communication partner and other aspects of the situation (Martinsen and von Tetzchner, 1996).

There are a number of factors that may be of importance for the choice between a manual and graphic system, but about which little is known. Assertions about the functional differences between the systems are often based on suppositions. Experiments have predominantly shown that, for people without communication disorders, Rebus and Blissymbols are easier to learn than Premack's word bricks (Clark, 1981). There are, however, no comparisons of the use of PIC signs and Premack's word bricks in the teaching of learning-disabled people.

Few studies have compared aided and unaided communication. The best investigation is that carried out by Hodges and Schwethelm (1984). They compared the learning of manual signs and Premack's word bricks among 52 children and adolescents (aged 5–17 years) with an average non-verbal IQ score of 13. There were four groups with 13 individuals in each group. In an initial 3-month period, one of the groups was taught to use Premack's word bricks, as prescribed by Hodges and Deich (1978). Another group was taught to use the bricks using the method prescribed by Carrier and Peak (1975). The last two groups were not given any training for the first 3 months. In the next 2 months the first two groups, plus one of the others, were taught manual signs (Table 1).

Table 1. *The teaching of Hodges and Schwethelm's groups (1984)*

Group	First period of training (3 months)	Second period of training (2 months)
1	Training in the use of Premack's word bricks according to the method prescribed by Deich and Hodges (1977)	Training in the use of manual signs
2	Training in the use of Premack's word bricks according to the method prescribed by Carrier and Peak (1975)	Training in the use of manual signs
3	No training	Training in the use of manual signs
4	No training	No training

To begin with, both of the groups that began with the word bricks were trained in matching, and they were taught to use the tangible signs only when they had managed the matching tasks. Only 7 of the 26 children in these two groups managed the matching tasks and were able to continue with the word bricks. Of the 19 children who were not sufficiently adept at matching, 12 learned from 1 to 11 manual signs in the second phase. Only one of the children who learned to use word bricks did not learn to use manual signs. Having been taught the use of the word bricks, signs did not appear to have any significance to the use of manual signs. The children in the first two groups learned an average of 4.3 manual signs, whereas the group that had not been taught during the first 3 months learned an average of 5 manual signs.

The experiment reflects not only the difference between manual and tangible signs, but also that the teaching methods differed. Carrier places great emphasis on the matching of colours and numbers as a criterion for teaching Premack's word bricks. Hodges and Deich also emphasize skills in matching. The extent to which the matching tasks were accomplished did not, however, prove to be crucial to whether or not the manual signs were learned. It is not unlikely that several of the children could have learned to use Premack's word bricks if another, more functional teaching method had been used. On the other hand, it may be easier to establish a functional teaching situation with manual signs.

It is difficult to draw reliable conclusions from this experiment. Nevertheless, it does suggest that it is best to begin with manual signs if the individual does not have any special difficulty in using his or her hands. There are, however, also examples of children who have learned to use aided communication after manual sign teaching had been unsuccessful. One of the children in Hodges and Schwethelm's experiment (1984) learned to use the word bricks, but did not learn to use manual signs during the course of the second teaching period. In another experiment (Deich and Hodges, 1977), a 9-year-old boy rapidly learned to use Premack's word bricks, despite the fact that manual sign teaching beforehand had proved unsuccessful. Afterwards, he also learned to use manual signs. It is conceivable that learning to use word bricks laid the foundations for learning manual signs. Von Tetzchner and associates (1998) describe two pre-school children with autism who acquired comparable, large, expressive vocabularies of photographs and PIC signs after having shown little progress in manual signing. One of these children also acquired both spoken words and some manual signs after the initial success with graphic communication. In an experimental setting, Rotholz, Berkowitz and Burberry (1989) found graphic communication intervention to be more effective than manual signs for two adolescents with autism.

Use of the systems

When factors related to learning do not indicate which sign system is best suited to an individual, other circumstances should be given more emphasis. One of the great advantages of manual signs is that they can be taken everywhere. The individual does not need to carry a board or another form of communication aid. On the other hand, many graphic signs are easier to understand for people who are unfamiliar with the system. The desires for mobility, a large vocabulary and to be easily understood by many people are often contradictory when choosing an alternative or supplementary form of communication. What should be given most priority depends on the individual user of the system. For a well-functioning adolescent who cannot write, who is in the company of many friends and relations, or who often meets new people, a graphic system may prove to be the most beneficial. For a severely disabled, autistic adolescent who is seldom in contact with people outside the home, school and institution, manual signs may be the best choice because their acquaintances can be expected to learn to comprehend and produce the manual signs, and because the individual does not have to remember to carry a communication board around at all times.

It is not always necessary to choose *between* graphic and manual signs. In some cases graphic signs can supplement the use of manual signs.

> A 13-year-old boy with moderate learning disability had learned to use a small communication aid that enabled him to write messages on paper (Memowriter). This he used when he met people who did not know manual signs. He also learned to ask people first in writing whether they knew manual signs. If the answer was positive, he began to use manual signs, which were quicker to use. If the answer was negative, he continued to write. He had approximately the same size vocabulary in manual signs as he did in writing, a little over 300 words (Reichle and Ward, 1985).

> An 8-year-old girl with mild learning disability had a good understanding of spoken language but great problems expressing herself using speech. She learned to use both manual signs and a communication board with graphic signs. The girl preferred the manual signs but used the board in situations where the manual signs did not suffice (Culp, 1989).

Manual signs

With regard to the signs that have been used in the teaching of deaf children, there is little evidence to suggest that one sign language or system is easier or more difficult to learn than another. All sign languages have some signs that are easy to perform and others that are more difficult. The sign systems that follow speech contain the inflections of the spoken language and, if these are included, the signs may become rather complex. Natural sign languages also have inflections. The sign system's degree of difficulty is less dependent on the sign system used than it is on the extent to which inflections are used. In the early stages of teaching the use of inflections is unnecessary.

For individuals with dyspraxia (difficulty in performing voluntary actions) or other forms of motor disability, it is advantageous if the signs are simple to perform. In the vast majority of experiments with manual signs, sign systems that were originally designed for deaf children have been used. When necessary, the signs were simplified so that people with motor disorders would find them easier to perform (compare Grove, 1990). This has worked well.

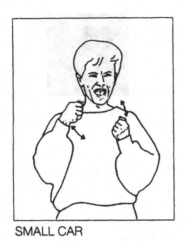
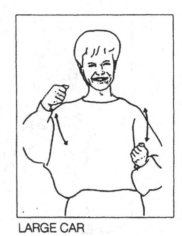

SMALL CAR   LARGE CAR

Graphic signs

Language comprehension is an important consideration when choosing a graphic sign system. Blissymbols, for example, place greater demands on language comprehension than PIC signs. These sign systems are also usually aimed at different groups, i.e. they are intended for people with varying degrees of language comprehension.

There has been considerable discussion about the characteristics of graphic sign systems and how easy they are to learn (Clark, 1984; Fuller and Lloyd, 1987; Schlosser, 1997a, 1997b). Experiments have predominantly shown that, for people without communication disorders, Rebus signs are easier to learn than Blissymbols (Clark, 1981). Drawings are easier to learn than Blissymbols (Hurlbut, Iwata and Green, 1982). Blissymbols, Rebus signs and Lexigrams are easier to learn than normal writing (Clark, 1981; Romski et al., 1984; Brady and McLean, 1995), but only if the individual is unable to spell. By using normal writing, the individual who is able to spell has access to an unlimited number of words without needing to remember every single one.

It would thus seem as though there is a certain hierarchy in terms of how difficult the various sign systems are to learn. However, it is not certain that the relative ease of learning is the same for all who use the systems. There are, for example, no comparisons of the use of PIC signs and Premack's word bricks in the teaching of learning-disabled people. Many of the graphic systems are very similar, and those who claim that one system is better than another often base this on supposition, or make the claim because they have participated in the creation of that particular system. For example, it is conceivable that it is better to use a white silhouette on a black background, as is the case with PIC signs, than it is to use

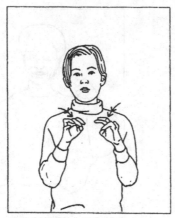

FINISHED

normal line drawings, such as those found in PCS and Picsymbols. However, this still has to be demonstrated.

It is also not the case that the vocabularies of the sign systems are tailor-made for each user. They represent limitations with regard to the signs that can be learned. Even though a good deal of work has gone into choosing the signs that make up an individual system, the vocabulary should nevertheless be regarded as a suggestion. The user's requirements should determine which signs should appear on the communication board and, if a word that is required does not exist, a new graphic sign should be made. To emphasize the sign's linguistic function, it may never-theless be helpful if the home-made sign resembles the graphic sign system that the individual uses. There is, for example, no PIC sign for 'finished'. FINISHED has often proved to be a useful manual sign, and one may therefore make a graphic sign consisting of a white silhouette on a black background for people who otherwise use PIC signs. As Lexigrams are also white on black, one of these could possibly be used. With regard to names of people, places, etc., it is often practical to use photographs.

There is no reason why different graphic sign systems should not be mixed. There is nothing magical about them which makes it necessary to stick to just one system. There is a limited number of PIC signs, and it may be necessary to supplement them with PCS signs. Sometimes the user may have a preference for one of the forms. This makes the choice easy. PCS and PIC signs will also gradually become too limited for many users, and Blissymbols may be placed among PIC and PCS signs as a link in the devel-opmental chain. Blissymbols generally have a wider use than PCS and PIC signs, and therefore make a more efficient and useful instrument for the user. At the same time, Blissymbols place greater demands on, and build on, the communicative skills that the user has acquired through the use of PIC, PCS or another pictographically oriented system.

Tangible signs

For people who are not visually impaired, the most commonly used tangible signs are probably objects and models of objects. They are typically chosen among objects in the individual's environment and their meaning tends to be idiosyncratic (compare Bloom, 1990). The use of objects is often impractical. In addition, young children may have greater difficulty in understanding that an object symbolizes something other than a graphic representation itself (DeLoache, Miller and Pierroutsakos, 1998). To avoid confusion with ordinary objects, one of the aims is usually to change to graphic or manual signs as soon as possible. If the continued use of tangible signs is needed, a system is preferable, and the only system available is Premack's word bricks. People with visual impairment will need signs that may be discriminated by feel without visual support (Mathy-Laikko et al., 1989). There is at present no coherent system.

Chapter 3
Communication aids

The term 'communication aid' is commonly used to denote aids that help users express themselves. Hearing aids are regarded as an aid to the senses, whereas glasses or spectacles are not considered an aid in the same way. Neither of these resources is considered to be a communication aid, although both undoubtedly contribute to improving communication between individuals.

Communication aids have been in use for a long time, and range from 'manual' boards and aids employing simple technology with, for example, lights and pointers that move, to aids based on advanced computer technology using monitors and artificial speech (see Fishman, 1987; Goosens', Crain and Elder, 1992; Quist and Lloyd, 1997a, 1997b). Communication aids, and the way in which they are used, have received special attention since communication aids employing computer-based technology came into use.

Access to communication aids is usually most important for motor-impaired people, but many individuals with autism, language disorder and learning disability, who are not motor impaired, may also benefit greatly from their use. Communication aids should be transportable so that they are accessible in a variety of situations. Until quite recently, high-technology aids in particular were fairly heavy or bulky and therefore difficult to carry around (compare Romski and Sevcik, 1996). Some also required an external power supply or frequent charging. Motor-impaired people who are relatively immobile may find it easier to use such aids than more mobile motor-impaired individuals. Users of electric wheelchairs may plug the aid into the wheelchair battery. Relatively heavy, battery-driven communication aids may be easy to transport with the help of a wheelchair, but are of little help to users if they have to be carried. Individuals who do not need wheelchairs will therefore tend to use more traditional pointing boards or books with graphic signs or pictures.

Traditional aids

Traditional aids are generally boards or trays with letters, words, graphic signs or pictures (Figure 11). In some cases, the board may contain only numbers or another form of *code* that refers to a list of words (glossary). A number code, or its equivalent, gives users the means of expressing a greater number of graphic sign words or sentences than they would otherwise be able to reach.

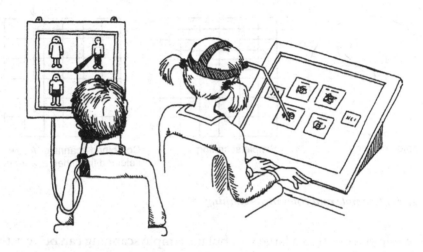

Figure 11. *Examples of traditional aids.*

The aids are operated with the help of direct selection and automatic or directed scanning:

- *Direct selection* means that the users indicate directly what they want to say. The pointing may be done with a finger, foot, a pointing-stick attached to the head, a beam of light, the eyes, etc. Direct selection may also involve moving the graphic sign that is selected to a particular position on a board or a screen.
- *Automatic scanning* implies that a light, a pointer or something similar moves. The user activates some form of switch when the light or pointer is in the desired position.
- *Directed scanning* is usually performed when the user applies two or more switches. One or more switches are used to move a beam of light, pointer, etc. around the board and another switch is used to make the selection.

Directed and automatic scanning can be either simple or combined:

- *Simple scanning* describes the process whereby all the signs on the board are scanned in rotation (Figure 12).
- *Combined scanning* implies that each dimension is scanned separately. This may, for example, mean that the individuals select a row first, and then select the sign in the row that they want to indicate. There are, however, several ways of organizing the scanning (Figure 12).

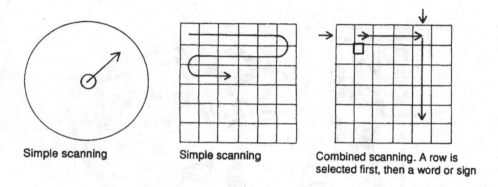

Simple scanning   Simple scanning   Combined scanning. A row is selected first, then a word or sign

Figure 12. *Simple and combined scanning.*

When the user has a large vocabulary, simple scanning can be very time-consuming. Combined scanning is quicker and more effective. With small children and learning-disabled individuals, it is natural to begin with simple scanning and progress to combined scanning when the simple scanning has been mastered. There are also dependent and independent forms of scanning:

- *Independent scanning* means that the user directs or stops the scanning pointer, e.g. a light, without help from anyone else.
- *Dependent scanning* means that another person points systematically at the board and the user informs the helper when she or he is pointing at the desired row, letter, word or graphic sign by uttering a sound, blinking, etc.

Direct selection requires that the individual has relatively good motor co-ordination and reach. Directed scanning demands that the user is able to carry out repeated movements, whereas automatic scanning requires that the user can co-ordinate his or her own movements with the movements of a light, pointer, etc. A person is more sensitive than a technical aid. Dependent scanning can therefore be a good way of initi-ating the development of more varied communication with children who are dependent on scanning, but who are at present incapable of mastering an independent scanning technique. In situations where it is impossible to find a movement that the individual can utilize, dependent scanning is also useful. A change in facial expression or posture may well be enough if the communication partner knows the user well. The general objective, however, should always be that the scanning gradually becomes as independent as possible.

Traditional communication aids, i.e. manual and low-technology aids, are used a lot and fill important functions for many users. However, they do have a number of weaknesses. Using a letter board is time-consuming if the listener does not guess the words and sentences correctly before the user has finished spelling. It may take several minutes for the user to point at the letters that make up a single word or wait for an automatic scanning device to move to the desired graphic sign or letter. When the user produces long utterances, communication may break down, frequently because the listener has difficulty in retaining the words spoken earlier while simultaneously registering the letters in the next word. It may also be difficult to concentrate on what the user is doing for an extended period. In ordinary conversation, the listener may divert his or her gaze without this causing problems in following what has been said. In a conversation with someone who uses traditional aids, a little inattentive-ness can lead to bad guesswork and frustration, and the user's utterance may be either not understood or misunderstood.

High-technology aids

The new generation of high-technology aids often consists of dedicated devices based on computer technology. However, after the introduction of relatively inexpensive laptop computers with long-life batteries, it has become more common to use special programs on a personal computer (PC). It is not possible to use programs specially designed for one type of machine on another system. Apple and IBM-compatible computers use different operating systems and this may limit the selection of programs. However, at present, many suitable programs are available for both Apple and IBM-compatible machines.

Ordinary PCs are designed for many types of use, and the fact that they are so widespread is also a significant factor in the development of computerized communication functions. This applies especially to their use in nursery schools, schools and at work, or as a 'workstation' at home on which to write essays, letters, orders, tax returns, poetry, etc. Many individuals who use graphic signs have never written a letter by themselves, and a computer with graphic signs can provide them with a whole new realm of opportunities. This applies not only to intellectually competent individuals. Learning-disabled people with some writing skills (ordinary writing or graphic signs) can enjoy sending letters with birthday greetings, messages, etc.

Ken was a 12-year-old boy with cerebral palsy and a moderate degree of learning disability. He was unable to speak, but had a good understanding of spoken language. He used a few manual signs and a communication board with 25 Rebus signs. He was unable to write. When he was given the opportunity to use a computer with a concept keyboard, it took no time at all before he began writing letters, especially to his girlfriend (Figure 13).

For a user of graphic signs to operate a PC, there must be a computer program available for the sign system being used. There are relatively few computer programs available that use sign systems, although programs that employ the most commonly used sign systems – Blissymbols, PIC and PCS – are available for Apple and IBM-compatible computers. However, not all these programs are user-friendly. In particular, individuals with autism or learning disability, including those with a good command of the sign system in question, may have difficulty in using the programs.

Children with severe motor impairment are often not provided with a high-technology aid if the motor impairment hinders their independent use of it. However, communication aids with large vocabularies used in dependent mode tend not to be used much because they are so slow in use. Instead of turning pages, parents and other adults revert to the pre-aid strategy of guessing (von Tetzchner and Martinsen, 1996). A communication aid based on computer technology allows faster sign selection also in dependent mode, and it is important that children get such aids even if their communication partners have to operate them.

In addition to their use as communication aids, computers can be programmed to function as environmental controls, i.e. they may be used to open doors, turn the radio, television and lights on and off, turn pages in a book, etc. This may give the user increased *autonomy*. Computers can also be used for educational purposes and for playing games. Games that can be controlled with switches can have a special significance for children with severe motor disorders. *Aided play* provides opportunities for independent activity, and gives disabled children and their caregivers a common interest to talk about. In addition, games can help train skills that may be used later in communicative situations. For example, the computer program 'Where is Blob' is a variation on the game of hide-and-seek, where the child can make a partially hidden animal appear by

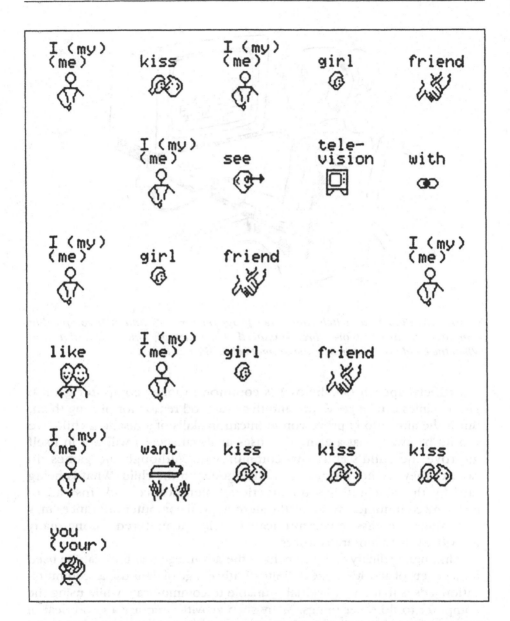

Figure 13. *A letter written by a learning-disabled boy (Osguthorpe and Chang, 1987).*

activating a switch. Once this has been learned, the child can choose between several animals by pressing the switch when a star shines above the animal that he or she wishes to make appear (Figure 14). It is easy to see how this game – and the scanning skills – can encourage functional language acquisition.

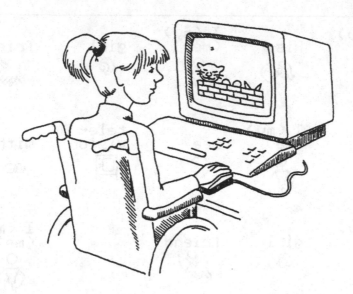

Figure 14. *Blob is a switch-controlled program for BBC and IBM-compatible computers. A star moves over three animals that are partially hidden behind a wall. When the child presses a switch, the animal below the star appears.*

Artificial speech (see below) is common in many computer games. These games can be good fun, and this is a good reason for playing them. But if the aim is to improve communication skills of a disabled child, we should be aware that a game that uses artificial speech will not in itself improve the child's ability to communicate. Although the games do 'speak', they are not engaged in a dialogue with the child. What is being said by the machine has no functional significance and, instead of fostering communicative skills, the stereotypical computer utterances may encourage the passive communicative style encountered among many individuals with motor disorders.

Although ordinary computers have the advantage that they can be used for a variety of activities, one definite disadvantage of their use as communication aids is that the individual is unable to communicate while using the computer to do other things. Many such activities require a good deal of communication. It is therefore important that the individual has a means of communicating while doing these other things. This emphasizes the limitations of aids that have too many functions, and shows how essential it is to have a specialized communication aid, even though this would be more limited in function or vocabulary than an ordinary computer (Figure 15).

As with the traditional aids, high-technology communication aids are based on direct selection and scanning. However, they are more flexible.

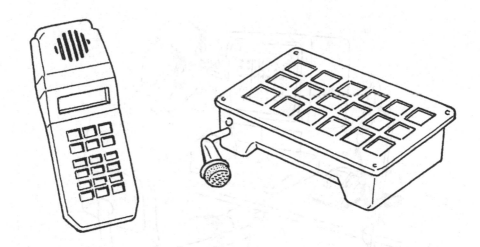

Figure 15. *Examples of electronic aids.*

For example, using a computer makes it easy to scroll through pages and gain access to a large vocabulary. If the output is graphic, what is being said will not disappear when no longer indicated, but remain on screen until it is erased or replaced by new utterances. High-technology aids therefore place fewer demands on the listener's attention. This may make the user and the listener less tense and improve the communicative situation. It will also be easier for the conversational partner to observe non-verbal behaviour, such as facial expressions and posture, without losing the gist of the conversation.

A number of high-technology aids that are based on orthographic writing make use of abbreviations or prediction:

- *Abbreviations* mean that the user needs to write only a couple of letters and then press the space bar or another key in order to spell out the whole word or expression. For example, the user writes pls, and please will appear on the screen. Abbreviations fill the same function as the combination of letters, words and sentences on manual letter boards. The user may also be able to select a 'word list' after writing one or more letters. Commonly used words that begin with the letters that the user has written will then appear on screen, and the user will be able to select the desired word (Figure 16).
- *Prediction* means that the machine makes suggestions as to what the next word or the rest of the word the user is writing will be. If the suggestion is wrong, the user merely continues writing. If the suggestion is correct, he or she can carry on to the next word by typing a full stop, pressing the space bar, etc. The suggestions are based on the

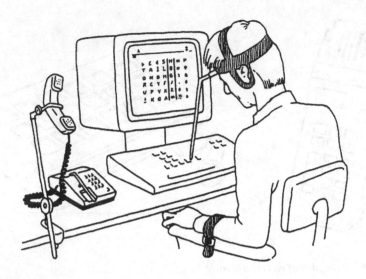

Figure 16. *MAC-Apple is a switch-controlled program. It can also be used to communicate via the telephone.*

words that the user has previously used. The machine remembers which words are used, and suggests the word that is most commonly used and that begins with the letter selected by the user. For example, after f the machine might suggest family, after fr from and after fri Friday. If Friday is the word the user was thinking of, the typing or selection of the letters has been halved. In some programs, several alternatives will appear, and the user may either choose one of these or continue typing.

Abbreviations and prediction can be useful, but both systems are dependent on the words being fairly long and used sufficiently frequently of the system to save time. Time is saved on the number of letters indicated by pressing keys or otherwise, and it has been shown that some of the prediction systems save between 40 and 60 per cent of the number of keystrokes (Newell et al., 1992; Venkatagiri, 1993). Prediction also implies a higher perceptual and cognitive load (Koester and Levine, 1996). Individuals who type quickly will be interrupted in their writing if they have to follow closely what is happening on the screen. For those who type slowly but are quick to follow what is happening on the screen, however, a considerable amount of time can be saved.

Prediction may also serve as a writing prosthesis and educational tool for children with writing disorders, a condition that is also common among non-speaking people with good comprehension of spoken language (Newell, Booth and Beattie, 1991; von Tetzchner, Rogne and Lilleeng, 1997).

The most advanced forms of prediction – presently at an experimental stage – include not only suggestions for words based on parts of it, but also pragmatic functions and selection of words according to the conversational setting and emotional state of the user (Alm and Newell, 1996).

A special form of coding system termed 'semantic compacting' has gained popularity and is used in many high-technology aids, usually called Minspeak (Baker, 1982, 1986). It is a coding system for words and sentences, which are spoken with the aid of synthetic or digitized speech (see below). By activating keys in different orders, different words and sentences can be produced. For example, if the *MILK* + *HOT* are activated, the machine may say *'I want hot milk'*, but *'The milk is too hot'* if the combination *HOT* + *MILK* is used. A combination may also lead to the articulation of a single word. Advanced communication aids have several settings or themes, and the word or sentence that is spoken depends on both the setting or theme that is chosen and the order in which the keys are activated. In 'café mode', the combination mentioned above may elicit *'cappuccino'*. Which key combination will correspond to which sentence is determined in advance. Minspeak is not dependent on any specific graphic sign system. In fact, Baker (1986) argues in favour of signs that are unique to the individual because he believes that one's own associations are easier codes to remember than graphic signs constructed by others. However, recently a dedicated graphic system has been developed (Minsymbols). It may also be an advantage to use an ordinary sign system because, if the batteries run down or the machine develops a fault, it would be easier to use it without the coded sentences. Minspeak is widely used in the USA and is becoming more popular in the UK and Australia. Because, until recently, it has been based on English synthetic speech systems, its use in other parts of the world has been limited.

Artificial speech

The most important technological developments in high-technology communication aids lie in the use of artificial speech. There are two forms of artificial speech: synthetic and digitized (Venkatagiri and Ramabadran, 1995).

*   *Synthetic speech* comprises a set of rules for the transferral of combinations of letters to speech (text-to-speech). These rules differ depending on the language spoken, and every country must therefore have its own system. English synthetic speech is the system most commonly used in communication aids.

An aid that uses synthetic speech is able to say everything that the user writes, but the user must be able to spell and write reasonably quickly for the communication to work. Of course, it is possible that another person writes and stores words and phrases, but then the flexibility is lost. Synthetic speech may, however, function well in combination with abbreviations, word lists and predictive systems. Synthetic speech is therefore especially useful for people with good linguistic skills, because it opens up the use of a flexible language and an unlimited vocabulary.

Synthetic speech is more difficult to understand than natural speech but, with regular use, one becomes accustomed to it, just as one might to another regional accent (McNaughton et al., 1994; Venkatagari, 1994). However, as with natural speech, non-native speakers may have greater difficulty in comprehension and be more susceptible to noisy surroundings (Reynolds, Bond and Fucci, 1996). The intelligibility of synthetic speech varies between producers (Raghavendra and Allen, 1993; Scherz and Beer, 1995) and from language to language. In particular, English synthetic speech is of high quality as a result of the competition between several producers.

At present, synthetic speech gives the user few opportunities to vary it and create a distinctive voice, in particular for languages other than English. Some systems have a male and female voice, as well as a child's voice, but owing to technical reasons the male voice is somewhat more distinct and easier to understand than the female and child's voices.

• *Digitized speech* is speech that is recorded by people with the aid of a sound sampler and stored in the memory of a computer or other computerized device, e.g. a talking aid. A sound sampler is a device that converts sound waves (an analogue signal) to numbers (a digital signal). The speech is stored in this digital form. Digitized speech is similar to a recording made by a tape-recorder, but there is no need to spool backwards or forwards in order to find the word that one wishes to say. Digitized speech is therefore better suited than tape-recordings for use in talking aids. Digitized speech is not language dependent.

Quite a number of aids based on digitized speech are available and, as a result of the general technological development, prices have come down. The advantages of digitized speech are good quality and the possibility of recording a voice that suits the user in terms of dialect, age, sex, etc. The disadvantage of digitized speech is limited vocabulary: each word must be recorded. A sentence may be strung together by selecting several single words but, to have sentence intonation, the whole sentence must be recorded as one entity.

The employment of artificial speech has positive social consequences because conversation becomes more normal. The users do not have to wait to make eye contact with the listener, or ring a bell, etc. They can interrupt and begin speaking in the same way as the other participants in the conversation, hear immediately what they have said and whether the word selected is the right one, and they can correct any mistakes. Another important advantage is that artificial speech makes it easier for users of communication aids to communicate with one another without a normally speaking person serving as interpreter and mediator.

Telecommunication aids

Practically all language teaching has been directed at face-to-face communication. In society in general, telecommunication is playing an increasingly greater role, and new services are being established. Both stationary and mobile telephones play an important role in the maintenance of social networks and the co-ordination of activities. This is especially true in the activities of young people.

The technological developments in the 1990s led to general use of advanced telecommunication services such as electronic mail and the Internet. In addition, new technology has made telecommunication possible for a number of people who previously did not have access to it (von Tetzchner, 1991; Roe, 1995). Speech-impaired people are able to speak on the telephone using synthetic speech, or transfer text and graphic signs with the aid of a PC or text-telephone (see Figure 16). There are aids that make it unnecessary to lift the receiver, dial the number automatically, etc. Videotelephones, which enable the transferral of live images over the telephone network, are already generally available, although still at a high price. Videotelephones make it possible to communicate over great distances using manual signs. For learning-disabled individuals, it may be crucial for their understanding of telecommunication equipment that they are able to see the person with whom they are communicating. A shared visual focus may also facilitate their understanding and production of messages (Brodin and von Tetzchner, 1996).

Paradoxically enough, those groups who are not particularly mobile and who have difficulty visiting others also have had the least opportunity to use telecommunication equipment. As access to telecommunications improves, individuals with language and communication disorders may have more opportunities to take part in a wider social network. This is especially important for learning-disabled people because many of the larger institutions are being closed down in favour of smaller communities. This means that the former residents of those institutions will live further apart and need to use telecommunication to organize their coffee meetings and other joint activities. In the professional literature, little thought has been given to how the social networks that have been built up over the years spent living in one institution are to be maintained, and how the creation of new social networks should be facilitated for those residents who arrive in a small community without having first lived in a large institution. Most learning-disabled people have ordinary relationships with other people. They have close friends, with whom they will perhaps live, and other friends and acquaintances whom they would like to see now and again.

When organizing situations with communicative interactions, it is also important to take into account the needs that individuals have for telecommunication devices and the opportunities that they represent. These can be extremely important for many, especially young people who have left home or are away from their family for long periods of time.

Pointing

Direct selection is often based on touching, pressing buttons or keyboards, etc., or one or another form of pointing. Pointing does not necessarily imply that an outstretched forefinger is used. Many individuals with motor impairment are unable to extend their forefinger, or to use it to point at all. It is important not to be formalistic, but instead to accept the form of pointing that the user can manage.

> Peter is a 30-year-old severely disabled man. He often experienced problems making himself understood because the staff at his school insisted that he use his forefinger to point at the communication board. It was far easier for him to use the innermost joint of his thumb, something that was accepted at home. By their inflexibility, the school hindered Peter's language acquisition and caused him unnecessary frustration.

For people who are unable to use their hands to point, there are a number of other ways in which they can point. The feet can be a good alternative, likewise a head stick or a lamp that sends out a beam of light (Figure 17).

For some learning-disabled and autistic individuals with sufficient manual skills, it may be easier to learn to move graphic signs to a designated location (they may be kept in place with Velcro). Many computer-based aids have this as part of the screen layout. It may be easier both for the individuals to understand the function of the graphic sign, and for the conversation partner to see what they are communicating. Some individuals point very fast and may fail to adjust their pointing to the visual

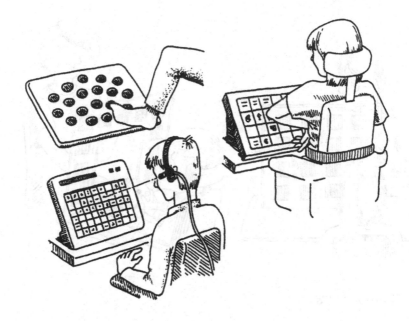

Figure 17. *Different forms of pointing.*

attention of the other person. It may be especially beneficial for promoting multi-sign utterances because the signs remain visible until the sentence is completed (see p. 260). In the *Picture Exchange Communication System* (Bondy and Frost, 1998), the graphic sign is given to the communication partner.

There are a large number of different forms of *eye-pointing* for those who have insufficient control over their body or head. There are special coding systems designed for eye-pointing (ETRAN), but eye-pointing may also be used in the same way as other forms of pointing (Figure 18). In addition, there are communication aids that register the direction in which the eye is looking, and that write or say the letter, word or graphic sign that the user is looking at if he or she does so for longer than, for example, 3 seconds. These forms of eye-pointing are, however, very tiring to use.

Eye-pointing is usually the form of pointing that one turns to as a last resort, despite the fact that this form of pointing is a natural part of the communication repertoire of many disabled children. However, there is a difference between having this as the only form of expression and using it to point at objects in the environment. Pointing and other ways of indicating objects, people and locations outside the communication board may be part of an aided language strategy. When a child lacks a

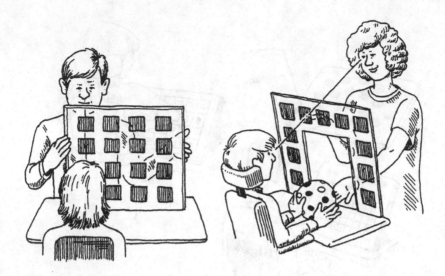

Figure 18. *Eye-pointing.*

useful sign, indicating an object or person may be a way to overcome this. It may also save time if such items are more readily available than the graphic sign, which may take more time to select. Pointing to an object may even be considered symbolic communication if the object is used to name or represent a category, an activity or a larger context. For example, an 8-year-old child, sitting next to the door of his room, looked at this door to express 'I'. This strategy, which is a kind of trope, was faster than going through the pages of his communication aid to indicate *I* (von Tetzchner and Martinsen, 1996). Moreover, it is easier to follow eye movement over longer rather than shorter distances.

When eye gaze is used to point at some kind of board, the conversational partner must be located so that he or she is able to follow the user's gaze, thus dictating how successful the communicative situation will be. Furthermore, the eyes have so many other functions that it is an advantage if another form of pointing can be used. If the user is able to use a hand or foot, it may be easier for the conversational partner to see the pointing. For people who are unable to use their hands or point in other ways, as is often the case with people with severe cerebral palsy, eye-pointing can nevertheless be an effective way for them to indicate their ideas, wishes and other messages.

Keyboards

The most common way of using a computer is by means of a keyboard. Many communication aids also use ordinary keyboards with letter keys, and in some circumstances extra keys for special functions as well. For people who are unable to reach very far, there are miniaturised keyboards and, for individuals whose aim is fairly inaccurate, there are keyboards with larger keys and more space between each key (Figure 19).

From the time computers began to be used as communication aids, special forms of keyboards called *concept keyboards* have been used. A concept keyboard is made up of areas that may be pressed. There are also concept keyboards where the different areas are scanned and one or more of the areas are lit up. The number of areas that can be pressed may vary, but 128 is the usual number. However, several areas may be combined to produce a larger area where all the keys within that one area share the same function. The size of the *functional* fields is therefore not fixed, but depends instead on the program in use. If all the keys have the same function, there will be only one functional field. A concept keyboard with 128 keys may thus have between 1 and 128 functional fields. By giving several keys the same function, it is easy to adjust the concept keyboard to an individual's motor and linguistic abilities. The keys are covered with a sheet of paper on which the functional fields are marked off. These may consist of letters, words, graphic signs, pictures, etc. (Figure 20).

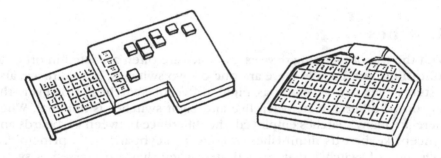

Figure 19. *Examples of keyboards with different designs.*

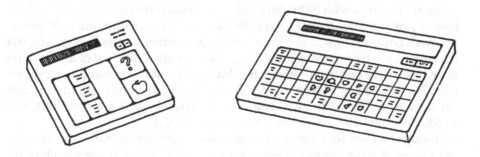

Figure 20. *Concept keyboards.*

On both ordinary computer keyboards and concept keyboards, it is possible to regulate the sensitivity of the keys. Normally a letter or graphic sign will be repeated if the key is held down, but this function can be turned off so that the pressure on the key must be released before that key is activated again. It is also possible to extend the time that the key may be held down before it is reactivated, so that the letter or sign is repeated only after the key has been pressed for, say, 2 seconds. The operation of a computer often requires that the operator is able to press two keys at the same time. This is difficult or impossible for individuals with poor coordination skills, and for those who are able to use only one hand or a head stick. There are therefore special programs that enable the user to press one key after the other to perform a function that normally requires two keys to be depressed simultaneously.

The most recent technological addition is touch-sensitive screens. With this technology, the keyboard and the screen are blended. This means that the surface of the 'keys' (touch-sensitive areas) can be changed as easily as a computer screen page (sometimes called 'dynamic displays'). This is a great advantage for individuals who have difficulties understanding the relationship between keyboard action and what is happening on the screen.

Switches

With the use of scanning devices, switches are often activated in order to control the aid. Usually there are one or two switches, but there are also systems that use as many as eight different switches. However, the functional difference between five and eight switches is minimal. When there are many switches employed, the difference between keyboards and concept keyboards diminishes. A concept keyboard is, in principle, a collection of switches that are activated when they are pressed. A switch may be controlled with the hand, arm, foot, head, eyes, etc. There are switches that require little pressure and those that can be treated roughly; they may be large or small, shaped like a normal light switch, have a 'tongue' through which the hand slips, or consist of a frame that a hand or foot is pushed into. Switches may be activated by sucking and blowing, or by small contractions of the muscles. Some switches consist of a tube that contains a drop of mercury, which reacts to small positional changes. If the user has better control of his or her limbs, a joystick or something similar can also be used as a switch. (For an overview of switches and instructions on how to make your own, see York, Nietupski and Hamre-Nietupski, 1985; Fishman, 1987; Goosens' and Crain, 1992.)

Using the eyes to activate switches places greater demands on the user than normal eye-pointing. When the eyes are used to activate switches, it is often because it has not been possible for the user to achieve control of the switches in any other way.

There are two main types of eye switches. The first type consists of a pair of glasses that transmit weak infrared rays to the eye. The rays react to colour changes between the white of the eye and the coloured area (iris). Moving the eye will therefore produce the same effect as another type of switch being turned on. The second type of eye switch consists of electrical sensors, which are attached behind the eyes. These detect electrical activity in the nerve when impulses from the brain make the eyes move. When the brain sends a message to the eyes telling them to move left and right, the effect is the same as that of flicking a switch or two.

The choice of switches can determine how well an aid will be mastered. There are many different types of switches, but adjusting the switch is often still the most difficult and time-consuming part of adapting a communication aid for use by individuals with extensive motor disorders. It is very common to start with the hand, because this seems most 'natural', and go on to try other parts of the body after having trained for a long time without results. Experience shows that 80 per cent of users have best control of their heads and will most effectively learn to use a head switch first. The hand or foot will often be the first choice for switch number two. Although it is desirable that the individual is able to use his or her hand, it is more important to make a start by using the aid and avoiding frustration. In cases where hand functions are doubtful, the best strategy is to begin by using the head to activate the switch. If the individual later proves to have good hand control, it is possible to change to a hand-controlled switch.

Professionals often try to find *the one* switch that functions well for the disabled person. However, this switch may be difficult for the user to master and such switches should not be used unnecessarily. The user may tire quickly and concentrate more on activating the switch than on the process of communicating. Although head switches may be a good start, extended use may cause strain to the neck muscles and dizziness. The user's general condition may also vary from day to day and this may influence the ability to use switches and thus communication in general. To reduce strain on the muscles, it is therefore important that communication aid users have switches that may be activated in somewhat different ways.

Choosing a communication aid

Whether the communication aid is to be used on its own or in combination with manual signs, the aim is to find one or several aids that best fill

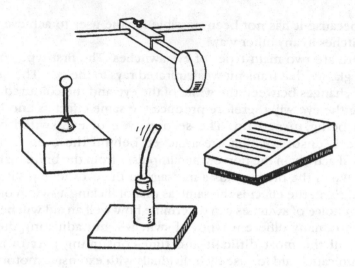

Figure 21. *Examples of switches and joysticks.*

the individual's current communication needs and those in the not-too-distant future. The communication aids should give the individual the chance to develop. This means that one aid may not always be sufficient. It is also important that the individual feels comfortable using them. It is important that other modes of communication should be attempted if the use of communication aids does not prove successful (Smith-Lewis, 1994).

It is usual to begin by assessing the individual's communication needs, to list the aids that are suitable and, with the help of elimination, to find the aid that best suits these needs. However, the communication needs will only partially determine the type of communication aid. Most individuals would like to be able to communicate with both people who can and those who cannot read (adults and children) in different settings. The need to be able to write electronic and non-electric letters, essays, reports, etc. will vary, and the need for a workstation for written work should, to a certain extent, be considered independently of the need for face-to-face communication. However, the individual's ability to use normal writing will be important for the choice of aid because spelling skills give access to synthetic speech and an unlimited vocabulary.

There should be a distinction between the selection of a graphic sign system and the selection of an aid. The assessment of the individual's communication and the environment in which he or she lives (see Chapter 5) will often have greater significance for the choice of sign system than for the choice of aid. The choice of aid will depend on the individual's physical, cognitive and linguistic abilities, the physical design of the aid, how it is to be transported and used, and how easy it is to learn to use. In Scotland and the mountains, for example, equipment must function under extremes of temperature and in rain and snow. For a user on holiday in Spain, a communication aid has to be able to withstand direct sunlight and extremely high temperatures. The priorities that often have to be made when choosing an aid reflect the fact that aid development is still in its infancy. These priorities will limit the communication, both for intellectually competent people and for learning-disabled individuals.

One main problem with communication aids is that they are generally designed for use by older children and adults. No communication aids are especially designed for use by children at an age when they generally learn to speak. This means that it is difficult to make provisions for non-vocal 'babbling' and the early development of language skills among children who grow up with aided communication.

Mobility

Mobility is an important factor for everyone who uses communication aids. The overall aim should be for an individual to have access to as large a vocabulary as possible at any given time. People who use electric wheelchairs will be able to use fairly large and heavy aids. For children and individuals who are able to walk, but are unsteady on their feet, it is essential that the communication aid is not too heavy or bulky. A book containing graphic signs or writing, or a thin board with signs or writing on both sides, may be the best choice for this group, depending on the size of their vocabulary. A miniature doll's suitcase may also be practical. The problem of transporting aids may make it necessary to have several. A child may have a laptop computer with a large vocabulary, synthetic speech and the possibility of printing while at home and in the classroom, and use a pointing board or a small, lightweight aid with digitized or synthetic speech in the schoolyard and outdoors.

The fact that an aid must be used in many different situations means that users will not always be seated in a chair or wheelchair. It may be necessary or easier for them to use the aid when lying down, and it should be possible to alter the aid for such use (Figure 22).

Direct selection and scanning

It is the individual's ability to use the limbs that determines devices and strategies for indicating letters, words, sentences and graphic signs. If the user has the necessary skills, direct selection is quicker and easier than scanning, although scanning may be individually configured to speed up the process (Lesher, Moulton and Higginbotham, 1998). Scanning may be carried out using one or more switches and the more switches that are used the less difference there is between direct selection and scanning.

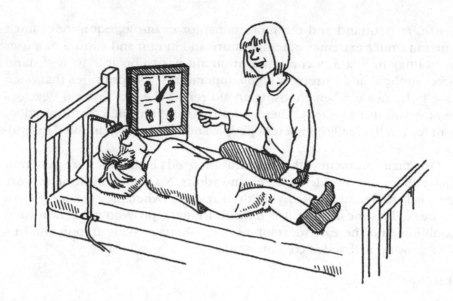

Figure 22. *Communication aids can also be used from a prone position.*

The difference between using a joystick and direct selection can in fact be fairly small. A joystick has the advantage that it can be adjusted to the individual's motor function by increasing resistance in order to stabilize it, so that the amount of force exerted makes no difference. However, a joystick places fairly large demands on motor control and sense of direction. Scanning may take more cognitive resources than direct selection (Ratcliff, 1994; Horn and Jones, 1996).

The choice of direct selection and scanning is determined by the individual's reach, accuracy when pointing, speed, ability to perform several controlled movements successively and activation strength.

Reach and accuracy

With the exception of eye-pointing, direct selection assumes that the individual is able to reach a sufficient number of graphic signs or letters. For example, people with muscular diseases often have an extremely limited reach. This can be remedied by using such technical aids as a miniaturized keyboard. Scanning with switches or a joystick is another way of increasing the individual's functional reach. The beam of light, the pointing stick, etc. function as an extension of the individual's own direct pointing.

Direct selection also assumes a certain degree of accuracy. Many people with cerebral palsy have no difficulty in reaching things, but they need rather large graphic signs or letters because motor impairment makes it difficult for them to indicate the signs so that they are clearly understood. Accuracy will also determine the choice of switch type and the distance between switches. A low degree of accuracy will necessitate large fields for the switches and a lot of space between them.

Speed

Communicating with aids always takes longer than natural speech, and the aim should always be that the communication is as quick as possible. Although scanning is a slow method, direct selection is an even slower process for some individuals, and can be more exhausting as well. If it takes a long time from the time that a movement is started to its completion, scanning may be an alternative because the individual can use the time spent scanning to begin his or her own movement. The individual's speed will also determine the scanning rate of the aid, i.e. how quickly the indicator moves from one sign to another.

Repeated movements

Directed scanning can be quicker than automatic scanning, provided that the individual is able to carry out several movements in rapid succession. Some people spend a long time preparing themselves whereas others are able to carry out several movements in quick succession. Some individuals have problems in stopping after pressing a key the correct number of times. In such cases, automatic scanning may be more functional. With technical aids, it is possible to program delays and prevent the user from double-keying by allowing the switch to react only after a certain period of time has passed.

Activation strength

When the graphic signs or text is pointed at, no demands are made on activation strength. If the individual has to activate switches, press keys or use a concept keyboard in order to display letters or signs on a screen or produce synthetic speech, this requires a certain amount of strength on the part of the user. The various types of keyboards and switches place different demands on activation strength. For a number of communication aids, the strength required is fairly small, whereas others require a considerable amount of strength. For aids that use a keyboard or switches, the individual's activation strength will play an important role in the choice of aid, switch and keyboard.

Manual and electronic aids

In discussions of principles for choosing communication aids, a distinction is often made between the need for a manual and that for an electronic aid. This distinction is not particularly productive, however. It is important to find one or more aids that can enable the individual to communicate. Whether or not an electronic aid is used is determined by many different circumstances. A large vocabulary may require an aid based on computer technology. Use of independent scanning will always imply some form of technical device.

It is sometimes claimed that, in order to be able to use a technically advanced communication aid, the individual must first have mastered a manual communication aid. There is little basis for this viewpoint. Rather, there is reason to believe that the individual who has learned to use an electronic aid can also use a manual board with direct selection or dependent scanning if the need should arise, for example, in the case of technical faults or problems with the power supply.

Artificial speech

Artificial speech has chiefly been used in aids for intellectually competent older children, adolescents and adults. Being able to hear the word spoken at the same time as they select a graphic sign or picture may, however, also be of considerable importance for small children and people with learning disability. The language comprehension of the individual is used fully, and understanding of the activity that is taking place may be improved. For individuals with visual impairment, artificial speech may provide them with crucial cues. The possibility of comparing one's own 'speech' with what others say can facilitate the acquisition of new words. Artificial speech may therefore be more important for individuals in the early stages of language development than for those who have already developed some communication skills. Several studies have demonstrated positive effects of using communication devices with artificial speech output for severely learning-disabled children (Romski and Sevcik, 1996; Schepis, Reid and Behrman, 1996), and that they may prefer such a device over a manual communication board (Soto et al., 1993).

For individuals with limited language comprehension, it is especially vital that the aid is easy to use, i.e. that a long period of training is unnecessary for the aid to have a functional use. This is not the same as saying that the aid should be technically simple. An aid utilizing artificial speech may be simpler to learn than a manual board because the relationship between the user's actions and the consequences of those actions is made clear. Kobacker and Todaro (1992) attribute the success of the intervention with a 6-year-old autistic girl to the fact that her first communication aid had voice output.

Price

Many of the newer electronic aids are still quite expensive. This is not an argument against using them, however, although the usefulness of such aids should be in keeping with their price. Some of them may have limited communicative benefit. For a child who communicates quickly and easily with Blissymbols on a manual board, an aid that employs digitized speech does not necessarily mean an improvement in communication if that aid is more difficult to carry around. On the other hand, if a child has not yet learned to read, an aid employing synthetic speech may be essential in facilitating the acquisition of reading skills (see p. 237). If reading disorders can be prevented in children without speech, price is hardly an issue.

Some characteristics of aided communication

To be a good conversational partner and provide adequate teaching of how to use communication aids, it is vital to know about the special characteristics of aided communication, i.e. how conversations with communication aids usually take place. There are many differences in conversations between people who speak naturally and those where one individual (or, on rare occasions, both) uses a communication aid. There are great differences between users and the type of aid, but one thing that they have in common is that production in aided communication differs from, and takes longer than, the articulation of normal speech, and that the conversational partner has other functions in addition to formulating his or her messages and negotiating the meaning (compare Kraat, 1985). It is important that interventionists and communication partners are aware of these characteristics and try to reduce their potential negative influence on communicative interactions.

Articulation

People who speak naturally do not normally think about how they should pronounce the words that they are speaking. They do not think about how they move their tongue or mouth, or how they make their vocal cords vibrate. Apart from those occasions when they are using an unfamiliar word or speaking a foreign language, pronunciation is an automatic process. Only occasionally do they stop and search for the word that best expresses what they wish to say.

Operating a communication aid may be regarded as the functional equivalent of pronouncing sounds, but, for individuals using communication aids, the physical formulation is not normally an automatic process. It is a conscious activity that takes a considerable portion of the attention and cognitive effort used to formulate what is to be said. Reduced motor control and involuntary movements can also lead to the user making mistakes. Imprecise movements may make understanding difficult for the listener if the letter, word or sign is not presented on a screen or in synthetic speech. The result may be misunderstandings, breakdowns in communication and frustration. In addition, attention is drawn away from what is actually being said.

Time

The time spent producing the utterance is probably the most important difference between natural and aided communication. Even if the communication aid is operated fast, the number of words or graphic signs produced per minute will be considerably lower than for natural speech. The low speed means that it takes longer to express what one wants to say. It places other demands on the listener (see below) and may hinder users in taking part in many communicative situations.

The time it takes to relay a simple message is illustrated in the example below. George, aged 7 years, communicated with eye-pointing and dependent scanning. His communication aid was a book containing 845 PIC signs, drawings and photographs. He and his father were going to start playing, but the father saw from George's expression that something was wrong.

F: *Here*? [Turning pages, asking for each page.]
G: *BODY*.
F: *Body. Body*? [Turns pages.]
G: [Vocalises and gets tense in the body.]
F: *Hm*? *Was it not the body*? *What was it*? *Was it this one*?
G: 'No.' [Eye movements.]
F: *This one*? [Points at *CLOTHES*.]
G: 'Yes.' [Eye movements.]
F: *Clothes*. [Indicates domain. The father turns the pages to the clothes pages.]
    And here?
G: 'Yes.' [Eye movement.]
F: *What*?
G: *SWEATER*. [Gaze.]
F: *Is it something with the sweater*?
G: 'Yes.' [Eye movement.]
F: *What*?
G: 'Yes.' [Eye movement, probably prompts guessing.]
F: *Are the sleeves too long*?
G: 'Yes.' [Eye movement.]
F: *Oh, they are. Yes*.

It took George 2 minutes to ask his father to pull up his sleeve (von Tetzchner and Martinsen, 1996). In the next example, the message took even longer to produce. Bob had 50 words on a communication board and could make a few gestures. The conversational partner (John) is a male nurse (Kraat, 1985, p. 81).

B: *HOME.*
J: *Home? What about home? Is it something to do with your sister?*
B: 'No.' [Shakes head]
B: *DAY-OF-THE-WEEK.*
J: *Sunday? Monday? Tuesday? . . . Saturday?*
B: 'Yes.' [Nods]
J: *Something to do with home and Saturday?*
B: *MAN.*
J: *A man? Is there a special man who's coming?*
B: 'No.' [Shakes head]
J: *Shall I find out who the man is?*
B: 'Yes!' [Nods emphatically]
J: *A relative? A friend? Someone at the hospital?*
B: 'Yes.' [Nods]
J: *Someone at the hospital. Let me see, a doctor, a therapist, a friend? Can you give me some more clues?*
B: [Looks at the top of John's head]
J: *Head. Part of the head. Brain. Does he work with his head?*
B: *COLOUR.*

This 'conversation' consisted of over 100 exchanges and lasted for 20 minutes before the nurse understood what Bob wanted to ask: 'Can Carl (a coloured security guard) drive me home on Saturday in the hospital van?' These conversations demonstrate that the conversational partner may be an important factor in how well aided speakers can express themselves.

As a result of the slow production rate, as well as other factors, the total amount of language produced by communication aid users is considerably lower than that produced by natural speakers. Beukelman and associates (1984) registered the number of words that four adult communication aid users produced during a period of 2 weeks. The number of words varied between 269 and 728 per day. Similar numbers are not available for children, but interviews with Norwegian parents and professionals indicate that the number of words and graphic signs produced with communication aids may be even lower for children. This is in stark contrast to normally speaking children who, at an age between 3 and 12 years, may produce 20 000–30 000 words in a day (Wagner, 1985). In addition to other aspects, children who use communication aids have fewer and more limited opportunities for learning to express themselves than normally speaking children.

The role of the conversational partner

In ordinary conversations, the conversational partners are equal. Both can formulate what they wish to say and, although negotiation of meaning is an inherent part of conversations, normally speaking people are not usually dependent on help from the other person in order to express themselves. Users of communication aids experience a totally different situation. As in the examples above, they may need a *message formulator* to produce what they want to say on the basis of incomplete and fragmented single words and sentences produced with orthographic script or graphic signs. In fact, producing what George and Bob wanted to say in the examples above came out as the result of co-operative efforts between them and their communication partners, George's father and John. After 100 conversational turns, John had yet to say anything of his own: he had merely interpreted what Bob had said.

The amount of time that aided communication takes may make the listener, in order to save time, guess what the user wants to say. In the example above, with George telling his father about the sleeve, the guess-work was beneficial. The communicative goal was achieved much quicker than if George had had to indicate a complete sentence, which would have been possible for him. For Bob, John's systematic guessing was necessary for him to get the message across. However, studies have also shown how speaking communication partners with the double role of interpreter and communication partner sometimes show little sensitivity to the messages produced with the aid, e.g. they fail to acknowledge or comment on them, and impose their own views or false interpretations on the communication aid user (Kraat, 1985; Light, 1988; Collins, 1996). If the listener guesses wrongly, the utterance may take more time instead of less, or even lead to complete communication breakdown, as in this dialogue from Silverman, Kates and McNaughton (1978, p. 407).

B: *When's the holiday?*
J: [Points at the communication board containing Blissymbols] *MONTH O*.
B: *Month O? I don't get you, Joey.*
B: *Try to form a sentence with it.* -
J: [Pounds three times on the letter] *O. O. O.*
B: *Does the month begin with an O?*
J: 'Yes.'

B: *October?*

J: 'Yes.'

B: So. A holiday in October. Uh, let's see. Oh, I know. Thanksgiving [Canadian]. *Do you like Turkey as much as I do?*

J: [Points at the board] H̲.

B: *H? I don't understand. What does H have to do with Thanksgiving?*

J: [Does not answer]

B: *Do you know why we celebrate Thanksgiving? About the pilgrims and Plymouth Rock and all of that?*

J: [Expresses frustration]

The non-speaking person in the dialogue above, Joey, was known to have a good comprehension of spoken language. Still, the speaking partner, Bill, did not seem to take seriously what Joey said (H was for Halloween) and instead continued to guess from his own perspective. Moreover, he took on a dominant 'school-teacher' role. The communicative consequences were devastating.

In conversations between aided and natural speakers, particular attention has therefore to be given to the strategies used by the communication partners in communicative interchanges. A major concern is that communication partners may restrict the expressive output of aid users and in other ways influence the content of the communication. For example, although sensitive guessing may be a useful strategy for speeding up the turns of aided communicators, guessing may also limit the person's ability to get his or her message across or slow down the communication even more. It is also important to be conscious of the fact that communication partners often function as general helpers and may be unaware of how they influence the communication (von Tetzchner and Martinsen, 1996).

It should be noted that the problems described here are not in the disabled person *or* in the conversational partner, but in their relationship. For the disabled partner, the possibility for expression is reduced, and for the speaking partner the possibility of receiving what the disabled partner intends to communicate is negatively influenced. This complementarity creates a relationship with an uneven distribution of power, a condition that warrants ethical consideration. A moral requirement for *autonomy*, i.e. an equal footing or right to expression, places an ethical imperative on the more competent communication partner to strive to overcome the asymmetrical relationship and help the disabled person create authentic messages (von Tetzchner and Jensen, 1999).

Chapter 4
Children, adolescents and adults in need of augmentative and alternative communication

There are a large number of people in need of augmentative and alternative communication. Even if one includes only individuals with developmental problems – with whom this book is primarily concerned – the number of people in the USA who are unable to speak is estimated to be around 900 000 (Blackstone and Painter, 1985). Comparing population sizes, this would suggest that there are about 225 000 people of all ages in the UK who are without functional speech as a result of developmental disorders.

Burd and associates (1988) found that 0.12 per cent of hearing children, adolescents and adults aged 5–21 years had 15 or fewer intelligible words. Excluding people with hearing impairment, the size of the population whose 'speech is inadequate to meet all communication needs' has been estimated to be at least 0.12 per cent (Bloomberg and Johnson, 1990). In a survey carried out in Washington State in the USA, Matas and associates (1985) discovered that 0.3–0.6 per cent of children of school age were unable to produce speech that was sufficiently understandable for them to use as their main form of communication. This accounted for only 3.5–6.0 per cent of the children in special education and did not take into account children with less extensive speech disorders. If it is assumed that 0.5 per cent of British children between the ages of 1 and 19 are unable to produce sufficiently comprehensible speech for it to be their main form of communication; this amounts to 75 000 children and adolescents.

Three functional groups

Individuals who need augmentative and alternative communication fall into three main groups, depending on the function that the alternative communication system will fulfil, i.e. the extent to which they need a means of expression, a supportive language or an alternative language. All three groups are characterized by either not having started to speak at the usual time or having lost their speech skills at an early age as the result of disease or injury. This makes it difficult for these groups to communicate with other people. The biggest differences among the groups, and the basis for a distinction, are the varying degrees of language comprehension displayed and the ability to learn to understand and use language in the future.

The expressive language group

Children and adults who belong to the expressive language group have a large gap between their understanding of other people's speech and their ability to express themselves through spoken language. Some members of this group are children with cerebral palsy who do not have sufficient control of the organs of speech to articulate speech sounds intelligibly (anarthria). Their language comprehension may, however, be adequate. In addition, they often have motor impairments that affect all or most of their movements, making graphic sign systems the obvious choice. However, normal intelligence is not necessary for inclusion in the expressive language group. Individuals with learning disability or language disorder may also have a significant gap between language comprehension and expression, with age scores of say 3-4 years, and fit the expressive language group best. This is not uncommon in children with Down's syndrome.

For individuals who belong to this group, the purpose of alternative communication intervention is to provide a communication form that will become their *permanent* means of expression, i.e. a means of communication for use in all kinds of situations and for life. Comprehension is not usually a significant goal of the intervention, except to compensate for a reduction in natural learning situations. The main focus is the relationship between the spoken language used in the environment and the alternative language form used by individuals to express themselves. However, intervention may include teaching comprehension of simple and complex graphic signs (e.g. Picture Communication Symbols [PCS], Pictogram Ideogram Communication [PIC] and Blissymbols) and traditional orthographic reading. If manual signing is used, unless the child is living in a signing environment (e.g. with deaf parents), sign comprehension is usually included in the teaching.

The supportive language group

The supportive language group may be divided into two subgroups. For the first subgroup, *the developmental group*, intervention with an alternative form of communication is for the most part a step towards the development of speech. This subgroup is similar to the alternative language group except for the fact that they tend to have less pervasive disorders and do not need an alternative communication form as a permanent tool. The alternative communication is not intended to be a replacement for speech – neither for the individuals nor for others who communicate with them. Its chief function is to encourage comprehension and expressive use of speech, to function as a 'scaffold' for the development of a normal mastery of speech. The most obvious use of an alternative communication form as a supportive language is with children who are expected to start to speak, but whose language development is very delayed. Children with developmental dysphasia belong to this group, as do many children with learning disability (compare von Tetzchner, 1984a; Launonen, 1996; Romski and Sevcik, 1996). There are also children who are unable to speak for a limited period as a result of an operation on the larynx (English and Prutting, 1975; Adamson and Dunbar, 1991). The general focus of the intervention for this subgroup is to make clear the relationship between speech and the alternative language form, as well as solving social problems related to their limited speech. Comprehension of spoken language varies within this group and therefore also to what extent comprehension training will be included in the intervention.

The other subgroup, *the situational group*, is made up of children, adolescents and adults who have learned to speak, but who have difficulty in making themselves understood. This subgroup resembles the expressive language group most closely, but those in it do not have an alternative communication system as their main form of communication. The degree to which they are able to make themselves understood through speech varies with how well people know them, the topic of the situation and noise conditions. For example, discussing experiences shared with the listener, individuals in this group may easily make themselves understood whereas descriptions of a film that the listener is not familiar with may not be understood. A child who is well understood in a small classroom may be almost unintelligible in a train or on a street with normal traffic. In such situations and with unfamiliar people, individuals in the situational subgroup may need to produce manual signs or letters, or to point at graphic signs, written words or graphemes corresponding to the speech sounds not understood by the communication partner. For this group, intervention should focus on conditions that help the individual learn when he or she needs to augment speech, how to monitor the comprehension of the communication partner, and how to use appropriate means and strategies in different situations. People with severe articulation disorders may belong to this group.

Using an alternative communication system as a supportive language with which to accelerate the use and understanding of speech is easiest when the individual has been diagnosed and there is a good grasp of how speech usually develops among children with this diagnosis. In most cases, however, conditions will not be this clear to start with. This is especially true of children with Down's syndrome. In this group, there are children who develop very good speech, children who develop speech that is difficult to understand, and children who develop no or very little speech (Launonen, 1996, 1998). We may hope, and perhaps believe, that the child will learn to speak, but only time will show whether this will be the case.

The incidence of social and psychiatric problems is far greater among children with language disorders than among children in general (Ingram, 1959; Baker and Cantwell, 1982; Cohen, Davine and Meloche-Kelly, 1989). Language disorders often cause conflicts in the family, and the difficulties and frustration produced may create an exceptionally difficult family situation. One should therefore aim at providing the children in the supportive language subgroup with a temporary linguistic instrument, which may reduce the negative effects produced by language disorders.

The alternative language group

For individuals who belong to the alternative language group, the alternative communication form is the language that they will use for the rest of their lives. This is also the language form that other people will generally need to use in order to communicate with them. The alternative language group is characterized by using little or no speech for communication. The aim is therefore the use of an alternative form of communication as their native language. Intervention comprises both comprehension and production, and a principal goal is to establish conditions in which the child may learn to understand and use the alternative language form without needing spoken language, an environment in which the alternative language form is truly functional.

Autistic and severely learning-disabled individuals, among others, belong to this group (compare Romski and Sevcik, 1993; Peterson et al., 1995). Individuals with *auditive agnosia* or 'language deafness' will also be found. The diagnosis 'auditive agnosia' encompasses children or adults who appear to have special problems in interpreting sounds as meaningful linguistic elements. They have normal hearing in the sense that they can signal when they have registered a sound, but they are unable to distinguish between speech sounds and, in severe cases, between, for example, a child crying and a foghorn (Luchsinger and Arnold, 1965).

Distinguishing between the groups

The main reason for distinguishing expressive, supportive and alternative language groups is that children with language and communication disorders may follow different developmental paths to their final competence. There are different objectives for implementing alternative and augmentative communication training and the intervention will differ in each of the groups. Objectives should be formulated on the basis of each individual, and the division into the three groups may be helpful in their formulation. Romski and Sevcik (1996) make a distinction between children showing a *beginning learning pattern* and those showing an *advanced learning pattern*. This may give the impression that they denote children at different stages in a developmental sequence, whereas the main difference between these two groups is comprehension of spoken language. Children with limited comprehension of spoken language may not learn to understand spoken language, but may make significant gains in communicative competence in non-speech modes, provided that these modes are taught independently of speech and spoken language instructions. A child showing a 'beginning achievement pattern' may not be at the start of the same path as a child showing an 'advanced achievement pattern', and they may not simply need different quantities of the same intervention. A 'beginning' child may in fact be on a wrong path – meaning that the optimal path is not supported because his or her limited comprehension of spoken language has not been taken sufficiently into consideration.

The division into three groups does not imply that it is always easy to determine to what group a given individual belongs. It is particularly difficult to distinguish between people in the supportive and those in the alternative language group. This is well illustrated by the experience gained from teaching manual signs to learning-disabled and autistic people in recent years. Success has been achieved in teaching signs to people aged 40–50 years who had not learned to speak despite years of traditional speech training, but who have started to speak as a result of the signing. For some of these people, speech has gradually become their main form of communication. Before this it was reasonable to assume that they were incapable of learning to speak.

The most common groups in need of augmentative and alternative communication

Among individuals belonging to these three groups, there are different clinical groups; in addition, the same clinical groups can be represented in more than one of these three language groups. Some individuals with cerebral palsy need a communication aid in order to be able to express themselves at all; others need support for speech that is difficult to understand, or they may require only an aid for a short period of time. Some autistic people begin speaking after having used manual and/or graphic signs. Others never learn to understand or use speech, but are able to understand and use some manual and/or graphic signs.

Motor impairment

First and foremost are the children and adults with cerebral palsy, who have motor disorders that render them unable to use speech to communicate. This group includes people who have insufficient control of the speech organs (tongue, mouth, throat, etc.) to be able to articulate language sounds normally (anarthria, dysarthria). They may be paralysed or have spasms that make it difficult for them to control their articulation properly, which will make it difficult for people who do not know them well to understand what they are saying (Hardy, 1983; Capute and Accardo, 1991).

Motor disorders that affect only speech are rare. The vast majority of people who have a motor speech impairment also have other impaired motor functions: they may experience varying degrees of reduced co-ordination of the arm and hand movements; many are dependent on wheelchairs or crutches.

About 1 in 1000 children between the ages of 4 and 16 have combined language and motor disorders (Lagergren, 1981). The incidence increases in adolescence, mainly as a result of traffic injuries and other accidents that cause brain damage. Around half of these children have no functional speech and are totally dependent on a communication aid. Motor-impaired children with some functional speech may also have a need for permanent or temporary aids as supportive forms of communication.

In the UK, where around 700 000–900 000 children are born every year, 500–600 of them will be born with a motor disability and will need a form of alternative communication. The type and extent of the motor impairment will have a direct effect on which form of communication the children will be able to use. For most, some type of communication aid will be required.

For children who grow up with motor disorders, both the difficulties that they experience in moving and speaking and the influence from their environment may contribute to their development of a passive style. The children often place great demands on their parents. Training, feeding and washing take much of their time, and there are few activities that the children and their parents can take part in together. Even when the children are small, their parents consider them to be happiest when they are passive. 'She's as quiet as an angel' and 'She is so good' are typical remarks made by mothers about their small children with cerebral palsy (Shere and Kastenbaum, 1966).

Smiles, crying and vocalization are cues for adults' reactions to children, and they play an important role in early interaction. Children with motor impairments may not be able to smile or vocalize, and their crying may be deviant compared with that of other children. Signals produced by these children are therefore unclear and fairly inconsistent, and it is easy for their parents to misunderstand them. The same applies to their movements. The children's reflexes and involuntary movements may affect their attempts to react to both people and events that occur in their environment (Morris, 1981). For example, the sideways movement of the head, which is associated with the tonic neck reflex, may make adults construe the child's interest in, and attempts at, investigation as a lack of interest or rejection of a person or object (Bottorf and DePape, 1982). These children are often regarded as more alert and interested when they are tense than when their muscle tone is low (Burkhart, 1987). However, high muscle tone leads to reduced motor control and makes interaction more difficult.

Even crying can be less functional among children with motor impairments than among other children. Parents usually react to their child's crying and interpret it as an expression for different needs, depending on such circumstances as how long it is since the child ate, had a nappy change, etc. Among children with motor disorders, crying is often caused by matters beyond the parents' control, e.g. muscular pains resulting from increased muscular tension, or pains in internal organs caused by curvature of the spine. It may be difficult or impossible to calm the child down, and the parents may become frustrated and feel inadequate. Long-term and frequent bouts of crying can be a source of constant irritation for the parents. If all this is taken into consideration, it is hardly surprising that the parents feel that their children are happy when they are passive.

Over-interpretation, i.e. a tendency on the part of the caregiver to act as though a child is communicating something specific before it can be assumed that the child is really communicating, may be an important force in the child's development (Ryan, 1974; Lock, 1980). When caregivers react to children's activities in this way, they create conditions in which the children may learn to communicate. Over-interpretation is dependent, however, on the child acting in a manner that the parents can construe as communicative. Children who display few such 'legible' activities (Martinsen, 1980), and this applies to children with motor disorders among others, often have a poorer language environment, i.e. an environment in which people react to them less than they would to normally developing children (Ryan, 1977). Comprehension of spoken language may also be reduced, even though the neurological basis for language acquisition has not been affected. Children with extensive motor disorders lose a significant part of the natural language 'teaching' that other children have. Children in the prelingual period cry, laugh, take hold of and reach out for objects, make gurgling noises that may resemble words, etc. These are activities to which parents and other adults react and then speak to the children; this leads indirectly to language learning. After the children have begun to speak, they develop their language in a similar way by taking part in conversations. They receive comments about what they themselves say and do, and answers to questions about objects and activities in which they are interested. Children with motor disorders lose out on many of these experiences, and this may lead to reduced language comprehension and less knowledge about the environment.

The children's motor impairments place considerable restrictions on their personal development. There are activities in which they cannot participate and many areas where they gain only limited experience. Part of this limitation is not caused primarily by the motor impairment, however, but by the fact that, as a result of negative experiences, they believe that they are unable to do anything. Later on, they will no longer try to do things of which they could have been capable. They learn that they are dependent on others because others do things for them that they could have managed alone. At the same time, they may experience themselves as an inconvenience and a hindrance and that adults are most content when they are passive. The adults' attitude to the children, which the children then to a great extent assume themselves (compare Madge and Fassam, 1982), therefore plays a significant role in forming their life and opportunities for personal growth.

A passive communicative style becomes a general characteristic as the children grow older, and there is reason to believe that the foundation of this is already laid at an early stage. Many children with motor disorders who have experienced affirmation and denial as their only form of communication – a kind of 'twenty questions' with, say, eyes up for 'yes' and down for 'no' – have been given new opportunities with the advent of the new generation of high-technology communication aids. However, it appears that, although they have mastered their communication aid and are able to answer all sorts of questions, they do not initiate conversations, even when it appears that they have something to say. For children who have grown up with answers to questions as their only communicative strategy, it is difficult to learn to use language in new ways. It is therefore important to find communicative expressions that the children can make use of in order to take the initiative, so that they do not learn that they must wait until others have asked them a question before they can say anything.

The level of language comprehension varies considerably among children and adults with speech problems caused by motor disorders. Many of the people in this group have normal comprehension of spoken language and belong to the expressive language group, but there are also people with multiple impairments and language disorders resulting from brain damage. For some, an alternative communication system will be the form of communication that they understand best. Thus, among those with motor disorders, there will also be people who belong to what we have called the supportive language group and the alternative language group.

Developmental language disorders

In general, children speak their first words between the age of 10 and 13 months, and on average they begin using two-word sentences by the time they reach 18 months. About 3 per cent of all children have not started to speak by the time they have reached 2 years, and 4 per cent have not said three words with coherent meaning by the time they are 3 (Fundudis, Kolvin and Garside, 1979). The incidence of a serious degree of developmental language disorders is 7–8 in 10 000 (Ingram, 1975).

Children who are considerably more retarded in their language development than in other areas are usually regarded as having specific language disorders. In practice, most of those who are given this diagnosis score within the normal range on non-verbal intelligence tests.

The group is multifarious and contains many variations in terms of special characteristics and the degree of problems. Different subgroups may be identified on the basis of their scores on intelligence tests such as the Wechsler Intelligence Scales for Children (WISC). There are also subgroups that are characterized by different background factors, i.e. they have different histories of development and different forms of associated disorders (Ottem, Sletmo and Bollingmo, 1991; Locke, 1994; Lees and Urwin, 1997).

Most children with developmental language disorders, regardless of the subgroup to which they belong, gradually begin to speak, even though their speech, generally throughout the preschool period, will be poorly articulated. This makes it difficult to understand the children, especially for people other than the parents, who often understand them better. When the children reach school age, most have begun to speak sufficiently clearly that even those who do not know them will understand them. As a result of their retarded language development, however, the children will have a smaller vocabulary and often less knowledge of their environment than their peers. The extent to which this happens will vary according to the children's functional level in other areas. Reduced knowledge is characteristic of most children with moderate or more serious developmental language disorders, at least until they are well into their school years.

An important subgroup appears to be children with *dyspraxic traits*, i.e. children who have difficulty in performing voluntary acts, especially those that require co-ordinated movement. These children have problems in carrying out practical acts in a large variety of activities, although not to the same extreme degree as girls with Rett's syndrome (see below).

Another important subgroup of children with developmental language disorders is made up of children with the so-called *language disorder syndrome* or 'cluttering' (Luchsinger and Arnold, 1965; Weis, 1967). This language disorder syndrome appears to be a genetically influenced language disorder occurring relatively frequently in families. It is characterized by delayed onset of speech, difficulty in articulating words, and problems with syntax and inflections. In addition, the children show difficulty in perceiving and discriminating between language sounds, clumsiness in carrying out complex movements and amusicality. The problems of articulation consist of the rate of speech increasing at the end of the word or utterance, and consonantal sounds being pronounced 'carelessly', as though the child had a stone in his or her mouth. This poor articulation means that, in the first years after the child has learned to speak, it is difficult for people other than those who know the child well to understand what he or she is saying. The problems are particularly evident when the child becomes excited. Most of these children speak clearly by the time they start school and are understood except when they are especially excited. The problems with syntax appear when the children omit a word or change the word order of a sentence. If they receive only ordinary reading instruction, they often develop reading and writing difficulties.

In conversations with other children or adults, both children with language disorder syndrome and those with developmental language disorders may find that they are not understood. The difficulties experienced by people in understanding them result in meaningless answers being given, such as *yes, no* or *hmm*, to the children's communicative efforts, no matter what they say; thus, the children may not receive an appropriate answer to their questions (Schjølberg, 1984). Also, adults often solve the problem of not being able to understand by taking control of the interaction with the child, giving more commands and asking fewer questions (Bondurant, Romeo and Kretschmer, 1983). This reduces the pressure on the adults to understand what the children are saying, but at the same time deprives the children of the chance to control the interaction based on their own interests. In addition to the fact that the children lose out on interactions typically enjoyed by other children, articulatory disorders may reduce the children's participation in ordinary social interactions. These interactions are a natural form of learning for children and important for the acquisition of language, concepts and general knowledge about society.

The problems that adults and other children encounter when they are with children who have language disorders may lead to the latter withdrawing from the interaction. Many preschool children with developmental language disorders are shy and timid in the company of others, with both adults whom they do not know and other children. When they start school, they often have problems getting along with other children. In extreme cases, this may lead to selective mutism, i.e. the children do not speak outside their home, even after they have begun to speak clearly. Others may be bothersome and aggressive (Rutter, Mawhood and Howlin, 1992; Bishop, 1994).

It is likely that the problems experienced by these children are an indirect result of the difficulties experienced in making themselves understood. Most social situations require speech. When they meet new people, the children are asked such questions as 'What is your name?' and 'How old are you?', and must thus reveal their impaired language skills. In some cases, children with poor articulation find speaking 'clearly' and understandably to be such a strain that it also becomes more difficult for them to do other things. The specific speech disorder may then spread and become a more extensive problem – a kind of acquired dyspraxia.

Children with developmental language disorders are not usually taught an alternative communication system in order to provide them with a native language. They typically belong to the supportive language group, and are clear examples that augmentative communication is a support in the development of speech. It is most common to use manual signs, but other forms of communication have also been used (Hughes, 1974–75). Relatively little systematic research has been carried out into the use of manual signing in this group, but positive results have been reported in case studies (Caparulo and Cohen, 1977; von Tetzchner, 1984a).

The effect that signing may have on the children's conversational partners is almost as important as the effect of learning on the children. It can be easy for adults either to overestimate or to underestimate how much children understand. If the children use manual or graphic signs as they speak, it will be easier for adults to understand and reply in a meaningful way. For the children, this means that the interaction with adults may become more meaningful and pleasurable. At the same time, it may be easier for adults to comment on what the children are doing, and tell them about objects and activities that are happening as they would with other children. This increases the probability that the children will learn names of objects, how events are discussed, how objects are used, social rules, etc. These are important foundations for language development (Nelson, 1996). If sign teaching is successful, one consequence may be that the children are less likely to have a poor vocabulary and concept development.

A third aim of sign intervention is to increase children's social control. Even after the children have begun to speak clearly and make themselves understood, there may be many social and interactional rules that they have not learned, with which their peers are familiar. Improving the children's ability to make themselves understood and increasing their participation in good social interaction may make them less shy and timid, and thus help them to enjoy improved social interaction with their peers and with adults whom they do not know well.

Learning disability

Learning disability is not a professional diagnosis, but rather an *administrative* category. Traditionally, the term covered all children who, it was felt, were unable to benefit from normal schooling and therefore ought to attend special schools. Today 'learning disability' is used as a collective term for a whole range of different conditions with wholly different causes. Common to these, however, is the fact that the learning ability of those concerned, and their chances of coping in society, are more or less restricted and that the condition is visible at an early stage. (Many terms have been applied to this group: general or mental retardation, intellectual impairment, etc. 'Learning disability' is the preferred term in this book because it denotes the main characteristic of people belonging to this group, i.e. a reduced ability to learn, without implying that it is a delay that may be compensated for later or that the individuals function as younger, normally developed individuals.)

It is usual to distinguish between different degrees of learning disability on the basis of scores on intelligence tests. An intelligence quotient (IQ) of between 69 and 50 is considered a mild degree, an IQ between 49 and 35 as a moderate degree, an IQ between 34 and 20 as a severe degree and an IQ below 20 as a profound degree of learning disability. People who would score 70 or below on intelligence tests comprise 2–3 per cent of the population (World Health Organization, 1993). However, it is essential to remember that an IQ does not say much about an individual. The group of learning-disabled people contains wholly different individuals with very different developmental backgrounds. The score attained on the intelligence test conceals these differences to a far greater extent than it reveals them. Even what may be called the ability to learn varies considerably among people with the 'same' level of intelligence. It is especially difficult to predict linguistic skills on the basis of the score attained on an intelligence test. For people who achieve a score of more than 40–50, there is no connection between IQ and the milestones in language development, i.e. the time at which they begin to speak and the time that they produce their first word combinations. Among people who achieve an IQ score lower than 40–50, it is difficult both practically and theoretically to distinguish between poor language and communicative ability and other cognitive functions. Performance on intelligence tests are, among other things, dependent on the fact that the test instructions have been understood. Among those who have the poorest linguistic and communicative competence, this condition is difficult to fulfil. Poor linguistic skills also prevent people from learning other skills that are measured in intelligence tests. One will therefore find a clear statistical correlation between the obtained IQ score and linguistic skills among people with moderate and severe degrees of learning disability. Even though a smaller proportion of severely and profoundly disabled individuals develop language than those who function rather better, individuals belonging to the weakest group also develop language.

There are a number of subgroups of learning disability. In some instances, the aetiology of the impairment is known, but in about half the cases the cause is unknown. There is a high frequency of multiple impairment. In a large Norwegian institution, 30 per cent of the inhabitants had non-correctable visual impairments. Of these, 7 per cent were totally blind and 11–12 per cent were functionally blind, i.e. there was nothing at fault with the eye itself, but rather in the regions of the brain that are concerned with visual perception (Spetalen S, personal communication, 1990). In addition, even lesser visual problems may have greater consequences for learning-disabled people than they have for others. Among those who have the most severe learning disability, compensating for the loss of sight is often problematic because spectacles are easily broken and contact lenses may cause injury. Hearing impairments are also more frequent among learning-disabled people. For example, in a survey in the UK 8 per cent of learning-disabled children in institutions were deaf. In the same survey, 14 per cent were found to be so motor impaired that they were unable to move on their own (Kirman, 1985).

As a result of the great differences in functional levels and the high incidence of sensory and motor impairments, all uses of alternative communication are relevant for the learning-disabled group. Some will belong to the expressive language group and others to the supportive or alternative language group.

People with Down's syndrome constitute 20 per cent of the learning-disabled population; this is the largest and best-documented single group (compare Nadel, 1988; Cicchetti and Beeghly, 1990) and will therefore be used to illustrate the collective category 'learning disability'. However, it is important to emphasize the great differences that may be found both between and within the subgroups of learning disability.

Children with Down's syndrome often have a need for a supportive language, but some of them belong to the alternative language group.

Smith and von Tetzchner (1986) investigated ten 3-year-old children with Down's syndrome. On the basis of the information given by the children's parents, it was found that the children used an average of 45 words. The number of words used by each child varied between 0 and 250 words. At the age of 5 years, only one of the children had a mean length of utterance of more than 1.5 words, which implies that most of the utterances produced by the other children were one-word utterances.

Compared with normally developed children, children with Down's syndrome have a significantly delayed language development. Their acquisition of spoken language is related to their development in other areas, and the extent to which they are able, or permitted, to interact with their caregivers. The children's participation in social interaction with others, and thus their opportunities for natural language and concept learning, is affected by the fact that they spend more time processing and reacting to impressions than other children, and that they often have such a low level of activity that most of the interaction is controlled by adults (compare Ryan, 1977).

In principle, the objective of intervention with an alternative communication form in children with Down's syndrome – as in children with developmental language disorders – is to accelerate the acquisition of speech and increase the quality of interaction in the period before they start to speak. At the same time, an alternative language will be secured for those who develop little or no speech, or whose speech is difficult to understand. The similarity with children who have developmental language disorders is emphasized by the fact that the articulation of children with Down's syndrome is often very difficult to understand.

The most common form of alternative communication for children with Down's syndrome is manual signs. In recent years, manual sign intervention has been carried out in several countries, and the great majority of reports have been positive (le Prevost, 1983; Johansson, 1987; Launonen, 1996, 1998). In a Norwegian study, the manual signs of eight learning-disabled children were systematically registered (Rostad, 1989). Four of these children had Down's syndrome. It was noted how old each child was when the intervention was started, at the acquisition of each new sign, when he or she began to speak, and when each new word was first spoken. The four children with Down's syndrome learned both manual signs and spoken words during the course of the intervention (Figure 23). All of them learned signs first. The acquisition of manual signs and spoken words was slow to begin with but gradually became more rapid. Progress was noted first in the use of signs. Gradually, the children began to learn more words than signs, and the number of new signs they learned levelled off and decreased. This regularity in the increase of words in relation to

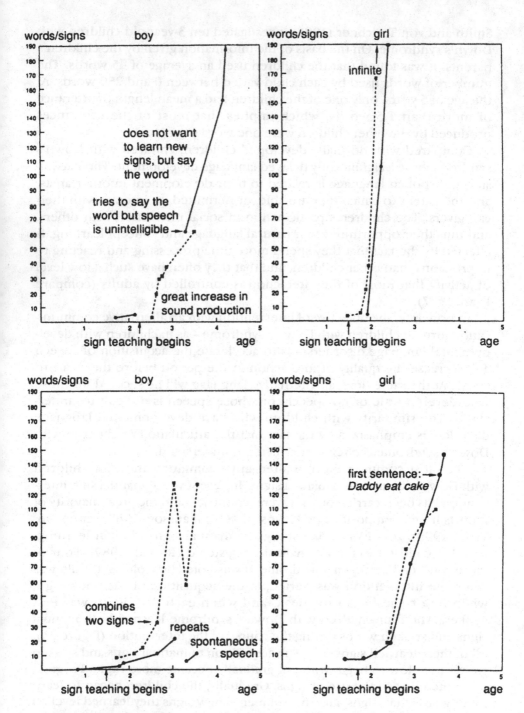

Figure 23. *Sign development among four children with Down's syndrome (Rostad, 1989).* ■ Manual signs, ● Spoken word

the use of manual signs, together with the fairly large age difference in terms of when the sign training began, suggest that the training had a positive – perhaps directly catalytic – effect on the development of speech.

In a large study of children with Down's syndrome in Helsinki, Launonen (1996, 1998) found that a group of children who had received comprehensive services, including manual sign intervention, from the first year of life had a significantly bigger average vocabulary of *spoken* words at the age of 4 than children who received the same services without manual signing. In addition to their spoken words, the signing group had substantial sign vocabularies, making their total expressive vocabulary much larger. When the children were 8 years old, the non-signing group showed significantly more behavioural problems. Hence, enhanced communication seems to promote a more harmonious personal development.

It should be noted, however, that teaching the use of manual signs did not have the same effect on all the learning-disabled children in the Norwegian survey. For one of the four children in Rostad's study who did not have Down's syndrome, the development took a different course. This child did not benefit from the manual sign intervention, but gradually learned to say many words. This highlights the fact that there is no single form of intervention that suits everyone.

Autism

In most cases the onset of the autistic syndrome will occur before the child has reached 2 years. The description of the disorder will vary according to age. The three main characteristics of autism are extensive language and communication disorders, difficulty in relating to others and abnormal reactions to the environment.

The incidence of autism varies somewhat according to how strictly the diagnostic criteria are interpreted. If the classic criteria are taken strictly, then the incidence is 1 in 10 000. On the basis of the most common interpretation of the criteria, the incidence is approximately 2–5 in 10 000, or 10–20 in 10 000 if broader definitions are used. The diagnostic criteria of ICD-10 are listed in Table 2 (WHO, 1993). At least twice as many boys as girls have autism. The causes of the syndrome are not known but there are clear indications that the difficulties have a biological basis. It is believed that there are several causes of autism (Lord and Rutter, 1994; Howlin, 1997).

Poor communication and language is a characteristic of autism, and about 50 per cent of autistic adults have no functional speech. Autistic infants and children typically have poor mastery of gestures. They may use them for goal-directed and instrumental purposes, e.g. leading a person

Table 2. *ICD-10 diagnostic criteria for childhood autism (World Health Organization, 1993)*

A.   Abnormal or impaired development is evident before the age of 3 years in at least one of the following areas:

    (1)   receptive or expressive language as used in social communication
    (2)   the development of selective social attachments or of reciprocal social interaction
    (3)   functional or symbolic play

B.   A total of at least six symptoms from (1), (2) and (3) must be present, with at least two from (1) and at least one from (2) and (3):

    (1)   Qualitative abnormalities in reciprocal social interaction are manifest in at least two of the following areas:

        (a) failure adequately to use eye-to-eye gaze, facial expression, body posture and gesture to regulate social interaction
        (b) failure to develop (in a manner appropriate to mental age, and despite ample opportunities) peer relationships that involve a mutual sharing of interests, activities and emotions
        (c) lack of socioemotional reciprocity as shown by an impaired or deviant response to other people's emotions; or lack of modulation of behaviour according to social context; or weak integration of social, emotional, and communicative behaviours
        (d) lack of spontaneous seeking to share enjoyment, interests or achievements with other people (e.g. a lack of showing, bringing or pointing out to other people objects of interest to the individual)

    (2)   Qualitative abnormalities in communication are manifest in at least one of the following areas:

        (a) a delay in, or total lack of, development of spoken language that is *not* accompanied by an attempt to compensate through the use of gesture or mime as an alternative mode of communication (often preceded by a lack of communicative babbling)
        (b) relative failure to initiate or sustain conversational interchange (at whatever level of language skills is present), in which there is reciprocal responsiveness to the communications of the other person
        (c) stereotyped and repetitive use of language or idiosyncratic use of words or phrases
        (d) lack of varied spontaneous make-believe or (when young) social imitative play

    (3)   Restricted, repetitive and stereotyped patterns of behaviour, interests and activities are manifest in at least one of the following areas:

Table 2. *Continued*

(a) an encompassing preoccupation with one or more stereotyped and restricted patterns of interest that are abnormal in content or focus; or one or more interests that are abnormal in their intensity and circumscribed nature though not in their content or focus
(b) apparently compulsive adherence to specific, non-functional routines or rituals
(c) stereotyped and repetitive motor mannerisms that involve either hand or finger flapping or twisting, or complex whole body movements
(d) preoccupations with part-objects or non-functional elements of play materials (such as their odour, the feel of their surface, or the noise or vibration that they generate)

---

by the hand to obtain something, but they do not seem to try to influence the adult's attention (Sarriá, Gómez and Tamarit, 1996; Stone et al., 1997). This makes it difficult to establish joint attention and create shared context. For children with autism, relevance may in fact be their largest problem, even if they learn to speak. Their problem may not be primarily one of human relationships, but a social one of sharing context.

Among those who learn to speak, linguistic development is often delayed and language skills extremely varied. Some autistic people use neither signs nor speech and have almost no understanding of language. Others can speak and understand a lot. Still others gradually build up a large vocabulary, use seemingly normal syntax, and are able to express thoughts, feelings and needs. The vast majority of those who do begin to speak display, to start with, a high degree of echolalia, i.e. the reiteration of words and phrases out of context. They rarely initiate contact with other people. Even those autistic people who function best often speak in 'monologues', without taking heed of the listener, and they often take what other people have said quite literally.

There are also great differences in terms of non-verbal skills. Some autistic people have an even skill profile, whereas others are more skilled in some areas than in others. In surveys in which large groups of autistic children and adolescents have been followed up into adulthood, it appears that there is a relationship between the functional level and the extent to which the autistic individual began to use language in the preschool period. The degree of meaningful speech that occurs before an autistic individual has reached the age of 6 has proved to be the best indicator of later functional levels, both linguistically and non-linguistically. In a Norwegian survey of 64 autistic children and adolescents, there was little progress evident in the quality of language from preschool age to early adulthood. The few exceptions to this rule were among children who had been given systematic manual sign teaching (Kvale, Martinsen and Schjølberg, 1992).

The unusual reactions to other people are closely linked to the exten-sive communicative and language problems experienced by autistic people. Autistic babies and infants have fewer of the normal behavioural forms on which early communication between children and adults is based, and their parents feel that it is difficult for them to achieve contact with their child. The children seem uninterested, do not appear to react when they are being played with or tended to, do not like to cuddle, are difficult to calm down when they cry and often appear content when left alone. In infancy, they often dislike being lifted up and do not usually mould their bodies to the body of the person who is carrying them, as children normally do. Many autistic people like bodily contact, whereas others shriek, become tense and seem afraid when they are touched. Eye contact with autistic people is often missing. Some autistic people will merely cast a fleeting glance at the face of the person with whom they are interacting, others will stare and scrutinise the face at close quarters. When in groups with other children or adolescents, they appear to show little interest in what the others are doing, and seldom learn by imitating others (Prior and Ozonoff, 1998).

'Unusual reactions to the surroundings' includes a long list of peculiar-ities that occur in varying degrees within the group. Among those charac-teristics that are most commonly mentioned are negative reactions when fixed routines are broken and surroundings change. Many autistic people react to changes with displays of anger or anxiety.

Most autistic people are only rarely self-occupied. They have a limited range of activities, and can carry on performing those same activities for long periods of the day over months and years. 'Unusual reactions to their surroundings' is also an expression of the fact that autistic children are generally interested in different activities from most children. In particu-lar, many of them are interested in objects that revolve or can be twirled and in flashing lights. Normal toys are usually of no interest. Typical examples of favourite activities are wandering aimlessly, twirling and spinning things round such as a whirligig, filling a basin with water, leafing through books, turning lights on and off, tapping objects and listening to music. Closely linked to this are the stereotyped acts that characterize the group. These include sitting and rocking, 'flipping' with their fingers or objects that they are holding, 'filtering' light through their fingers, twining hair, waving arms, banging the head against objects, and twisting their body, arms or hands into unusual positions.

Many autistic people react abnormally to external stimuli. Some autistic children do not seem to react to voices, and may be suspected of being deaf. Even among well-functioning autistic children, adolescents and adults, it can be difficult to know whether they are listening when being spoken to and interested in what is being said. Some autistic people are oversensitive to sounds. Normal sounds are troublesome and sometimes painful, especially in periods where the autistic individual is under a lot of pressure. Some autistic individuals have no visible reaction to pain, which has led to speculation that they have a reduced sense of pain. Children who show no signs of feeling pain early in life do, however, show this when their general functional level improves. Other autistic children and adults are oversensitive to touch and abnormally sensitive to visual stimuli. With the exception of autistic people who also have visual defects or reduced sight or hearing, however, no specific sensory deviations have been found. The deviations seem rather to be linked to perceptual processing (Hermelin and O'Connor, 1970; Grandin, 1989).

Considering the relatively poor prognosis that autistic children have in terms of developing language, it is natural to give them intervention including alternative communication. As it is assumed from the outset that over 50 per cent of autistic children will never begin to speak and in addition lack language comprehension, it is a warranted starting assumption that a graphic or manual communication system will become their main form of communication – an alternative native language. On the basis of their abilities, many autistic children belong to the alternative language group, although for a large proportion of them the alternative communication form will be a supportive language to augment their spoken language.

Autistic people can use different forms of alternative communication. Manual signs, different graphic systems, script and pictures have all been used. Until recently, manual signs have been the most common (Kiernan, Reid and Jones 1982; von Tetzchner and Jensen, 1996). In Norway, most autistic children who have not learned to speak receive training in the use of manual signs. It has become common systematically to introduce autistic children to manual signs as soon as they have been diagnosed, despite the fact that it is too early to expect these children to have started to speak.

Experiences from teaching autistic children to use manual signs are unequivocally positive, including those where sign training was implemented to improve the speech of children who can speak (e.g. Schaeffer, Musil and Kollinzas, 1980; von Tetzchner, 1984b; Bonvillian and Blackburn, 1991). Not all sign teaching has led to the acquisition of many manual signs, but almost all the autistic people receiving this training have at least learned some signs, often in a short space of time. Among autistic individuals who have profited most from sign teaching, after several years of training, one may find the spontaneous use of long sentences of manual signs, and – among some exceptional individuals – a vocabulary of several

hundred signs. It seems realistic to assume that even those autistic individuals who have the lowest functioning will be able to acquire between five
and ten manual signs during 1 year's intervention. This may seem like a
modest objective, but even such a limited improvement in the autistic
individual's capacity for self-expression and understanding of others can
have a great significance for everyday well-being, provide opportunities to
learn necessary social and practical skills, and improve the general quality
of life.

In spite of the documented positive effects of manual signing, it has
become less fashionable in the USA, Canada and many other countries.
Technical aids and graphic signs have taken over. This limits the variety of
strategies that are applied and hence opportunities for learning for autistic
individuals.

Autistic people in all age groups are very different from one another,
and the diagnosis autism comprises a multifarious group. There is great
variation in verbal and non-verbal skills among both children and adults,
and even the most striking characteristics of this group – such as the fact
that they are preoccupied with special things, react negatively to change,
are sensitive to sound, etc. – are not apparent in all autistic individuals.
Intervention for autistic people cannot therefore follow one path, but
must be individually planned.

Rett's syndrome

Children who have multiple impairments and profound communication
disorders are at risk of being left out and not offered communication intervention. This group is represented here by girls and women with Rett's
syndrome, a severe neurological disorder that mainly affects girls. Their
development is seemingly normal until the age of 6–18 months, but in
retrospect it may appear as though they were also more passive than other
infants before the disease became apparent. After the age of 6–18 months,
they begin to lose previously acquired skills. The circumference of the
head is normal at birth but growth slows, and the circumference will
eventually be less than normal. Epilepsy is common and may appear at any
age. Rett's syndrome has recently been linked with malfunctioning of
MeCP2, a regulating gene on the X chromosome (Amir et al., 1999), but
further research is needed before a gene test can be used to determine
whether a girl has Rett's syndrome. It is therefore the course of development that determines the diagnosis, and it can be difficult to give a reliable
diagnosis before the girl has reached the age of 3–4 years (Hagberg, 1995;
Kerr, 1995). Four stages of development have been suggested (Table 3).
The stages may differ in length, however, and the course of development
varies considerably. Not all the characteristics occur to the same extent
among all girls (Hagberg, 1997).

Table 3. *The four clinical stages of classic Rett's syndrome (from Hagberg, 1997)*

Stage I: *early onset stagnation*
Onset from 5 months of age
Early postural and developmental delay; developmental pattern still not significantly abnormal; dissociated development; 'bottom-shufflers'
Duration: weeks to months

Stage II: *developmental regression*
Onset 1–3 or 4 years
Loss of acquired skills: communication, finger, babble/words, active playing; mental deficiency appears; occasionally 'in another world'; eye contact preserved; breathing problems yet modest; seizures in only 15 per cent
Duration: weeks to months, possibly 1 year

Stage III: *pseudostationary period*
Onset after passing stage II
'Wake up' period: some communicative restitution; prominent hand apraxia/dyspraxia; apparently preserved ambulant ability; inapparent, slow neuro-motor regression
Duration: years to decades

Stage IV: *late motor deterioration stage*
Onset after passing stage III
Subgroup A: previous walkers now non-ambulant, when ambulation ceases
Subgroup B: never ambulant; no clear border between stages III and IV
Complete wheelchair dependency; severe disability: wasting and distal distortions
Duration: decades

The prevalence of Rett's syndrome is typically about 1 in 20 000 of the population, i.e. it occurs in 1 in every 10 000 girls (Hagberg and Hagberg, 1997; Skjeldal et al., 1997). Initially, a diagnosis of Rett's syndrome was based on strict adherence to the traditional criteria (Trevathan and Moser, 1988). However, after attention had been brought to the characteristics of Rett's syndrome, cases were presented that did not fulfil all the necessary criteria, but that still seemed to be more similar to Rett's syndrome than to other known conditions. Several variants have been described, which, in addition to the classic type, seem to be part of the same syndrome or set of symptomatology (Hagberg and Skjeldal, 1994).

During the course of the disease, hand control deteriorates. Fine motor skills worsen and gradually the girls are no longer able to, for example, use a pincer grip to pick things up. One result of the girls' steadily deteriorating control over their hands is that they lose the ability to play with and manipulate objects. They may clutch at things with a 'pawing' movement and grasp objects with their whole hand. It becomes difficult for them to

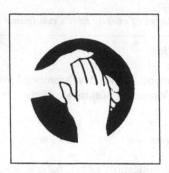

get hold of things and they drop them easily, so that they have increasing problems occupying themselves and doing things on their own initiative; they therefore become more dependent on others.

Most of the girls – although not all – develop a special hand stereotypy, in which the hands are rubbed in sort of 'hand-washing movements' that are sometimes performed for most of the day. Many girls may also sit and open and close their hands almost incessantly. Stereotypical hand-washing movements are not uncommon among children with learning disability or autism, but this does not occur to the extent that is typically found among girls with Rett's syndrome. The hand-washing movements have therefore become a 'trademark' for the girls.

Perhaps the most characteristic feature of Rett's syndrome is the girls' *dyspraxia* – the reduced ability to perform voluntary actions. The dyspraxia is apparent not only in the problems the girls have in learning new skills, but also in the implementation and carrying out of activities that they have already mastered. Even the act of beginning to walk or lifting a leg to walk up a flight of stairs can take a long time, and they may need help in getting started. Another characteristic of dyspraxia is that it increases with excitement so that, when motivation increases, the action becomes more difficult to perform. It is commonly noted that the girls function best in tranquil surroundings where they are under little pressure. Intervention is therefore aimed at helping the girls to perform actions, thereby lessening their frustration.

Girls with Rett's syndrome appear to be severely or profoundly learning disabled and the deceleration of head growth and low brain weights provide support for this impression (Armstrong, 1997; Percy, 1997). Attempts to assess cognitive functions have shown that females with Rett's syndrome – with no regard to age when tested – are rarely able to perform more advanced tasks than seen in normally developed 1-year-old children, and many of them obtain significantly lower age scores (compare Olsson and Rett, 1987, 1990; Garber and Veydt, 1990; Woodyatt and Ozanne, 1992, 1993). Interpretations of test results should, however, take into account that assessment of this group is extremely difficult and that it is not at all clear which categories are best suited to describing the development of cognitive functions in females with Rett's syndrome (Trevarthen, 1986; Van Acker, 1991). Most of the affected females almost totally lack functional hand use. Studies including assessment of cognitive skills have invariably applied tasks that implicate hand use, such as building block patterns, reaching for hidden objects, moving objects and other manipulative skills.

With the exception of those who have preserved speech, girls with Rett's syndrome almost never speak. Most of them have no use of words and are dependent on alternative communication means to express themselves. However, they can be observed to touch or look at objects, and move towards a person, an object or a particular location. Movements often appear random, but systematic observation may show that they are not (Sharpe, 1992). Alternative communication intervention may involve structured overinterpretation and/or structured total communication (see p. 136). The aim of these strategies is to help the girls gain control over their environment and provide them with possibilities for indicating intentions related to interests, needs and preferences. As a result of their difficulties in using their hands, manual signs are not suitable. Aided communication is therefore a natural choice, including objects, photographs or graphic signs, and a range of different intervention strategies. However, using communication aids is also not easy for them. Even a simple motor movement such as pointing may be difficult. If their attention is concentrated on the action, in this case pointing, this may exacerbate the dyspraxia. Instead, attention should be focused on the object at which the girl is pointing. Moreover, all strategy use must take into account their need for time to process and react to people and events in the environment (von Tetzchner, 1997b).

It is important that the communication aids chosen can be used even after the loss of motor skills is well advanced. For example, the girls are often able to use simple switches, which do not require fine motor skills, for a long while after they have lost most of the functional motor skills in the hand. Eye-pointing seems to be a useful alternative for those who are unable to point or whose hands perform incessant stereotypical movements. However, with eye-pointing, it is also important not to focus on the action. There are examples of apraxia appearing in the use of eye-pointing. Perhaps the reason why eye-pointing may work is precisely because usually no attempt is made to influence the gaze itself and draw the girl's attention to it. It is also vital to allow them time for visual and mental processing, even if this may be a long time (von Tetzchner, Jacobsen et al., 1996).

There are relatively few documented examples of girls with Rett's syndrome being taught alternative communication (Sigafoos, Laurie and Pennell, 1996; von Tetzchner, 1997b). It is our impression that such training traditionally has been rare, but it is becoming more common. The girls' understanding of language is absent or severely limited, and it should be noted that it is difficult for people with severe dyspraxia, who have great difficulty in expressing themselves, to show what they understand. There are some anecdotal accounts of girls laughing at the right moment, showing interest when a person is mentioned, etc. Isolated outbursts of spoken words or sentences have been described for some girls with Rett's syndrome, usually when they were febrile or excited about something.

> A girl with Rett's syndrome was in town with her father. They stood for a long time waiting at a pedestrian crossing for the 'red man' to change to green. Her father talked while the girl stared in fascination at the traffic light. During the evening meal that same evening the girl suddenly said *Red man* (Lindberg, 1987).

> A girl with Rett's syndrome had her grandfather to stay. When he came down to eat breakfast, she said clearly *Hi Grandad!* (Lindberg, 1987).

However, such incidents have no positive prognostic value and may not be taken as a sign of speech emerging (von Tetzchner, 1997b). Girls with Rett's syndrome have also reacted positively to the use of digitized speech.

> Dawn is a 7-year-old girl with Rett's syndrome. As part of her training in alternative communication, a communication aid with digitized speech, Alltalk, was tried out. Dawn had a picture of a glass of milk and a biscuit on her talking aid. When she pressed the pictures, the machine said 'chocolate milk' and 'biscuit'. Once she held her hand on the picture of milk while she was drinking and the machine continued saying *'chocolate milk'*, *'chocolate milk'*. Dawn laughed heartily. Despite the fact that she had only tried Alltalk a few times and it was difficult to press the pictures, Dawn was very interested and appeared very active when she was using it (von Tetzchner and Øien, 1989).

These observations may indicate that some girls with Rett's syndrome have more understanding of language than is generally thought. The limited results obtained from teaching them to express themselves seem to suggest that it is almost impossible to improve their understanding through use of communication aids. This means that some of this group, despite their limited understanding of language, may belong to the expressive language group. On the other hand, most girls with Rett's syndrome seem unable to direct the attention of another person and establish joint attention. Without this skill, language acquisition may be impossible or extremely difficult (see p. 123).

Some common problems

A number of problems often occur when teaching people with communication disorders. These problems are often related to the fact that learning takes time and can be difficult to transfer to new situations, and that many individuals trying to learn have become passive or dependent on others and may show behavioural disorders.

Learning takes time

One of the most common barriers in language intervention is that teaching can be extremely time-consuming. Some people with communication disorders may take years to learn even seemingly simple skills. This applies to a greater extent to some subgroups of learning-disabled and autistic children and adolescents, but is also true of some children with developmental language disorders.

Some professionals take the individual's progress or lack of progress as a measure of their own success. They may therefore set themselves unrealistic aims and be impatient about the results. This may result in the intervention ending too early and other methods being tried instead. It is important to assess one's own efforts, but this assumes that the efforts have been tried out long enough and that one has feasible short- and long-term aims.

The protracted time needed for intervention also has other consequences. One indirect consequence is that those who take the longest time to learn are also those who are most prone to breaks in continuity. They may have to change schools, or new teachers may be recruited who have insufficient knowledge of what the students know and can do, and are unaware of how the teaching has been organized. Breaks in continuity may lead to established skills not being reacted to and these may therefore be forgotten or 'unlearned'. New teachers may try to teach the communication-impaired individuals something that they already know, or teach them new ways of expressing things that they can already express. Discontinuities and changes in intervention routines may cause frustration and lead to behavioural problems, which in turn will make the learning situation even worse.

There are examples where years of intervention for autistic and learning-disabled people have been rendered worthless as the result of a change in, or loss of, an educational programme (Kollinzas, 1984). The negative consequences are further reinforced by the fact that there is a great danger that the skills acquired by those people who function at the lowest level will disappear altogether if intervention is not continued.

Generalization

A great problem encountered in intervention is that skills learned in a teaching situation are not transferred to other situations. This is a problem that affects a large number of people in need of augmentative and alternative communication, not only those who function poorly. Even when special emphasis has been placed on making conditions favourable for transfer of skills, the results have been unsatisfactory. When the problems of transferring knowledge to new situations are seen in relation to the fact that the intervention takes a long time, it is important that, as far as is practical, the teaching of language and communication takes place in natural situations where one can be sure that the skills being taught will be useful for the individual. This means that time must be spent assessing the environment and finding situations where communication is functional and suitable for teaching purposes. If teaching is planned in other situations, it is important that there is a plan for the transfer to new situations.

Learned passivity and dependence on others

In early language intervention, it is often necessary to help individuals to some degree. Although this help may be absolutely necessary, it also represents a problem. The individuals often become dependent on the help and will be unable to use their skills spontaneously.

The dependence associated with language intervention is related to the great degree of learned passivity and dependence on others found in all groups in need of augmentative and alternative communication. People who belong to the expressive language group share the characteristic that, in most situations and especially with regard to self-expression, they have been dependent on other people helping them. This antecedent creates habits and ways of adapting to communication that may be difficult to alter when one attempts to give communication-impaired people new means of expressing themselves.

People who belong to the supportive or alternative language group may develop a similar dependence on others. It is not uncommon for children who have delayed language development to ask their parents to speak for them when strangers approach them, even after their speech is understood by others. In cases where the children's mobility is not impaired, the lack of initiative to communicate is most apparent. For example, among autistic children who are unable to speak, the incidence of communicative episodes is extremely low in comparison with other children, and the lack is particularly communication initiated by the autistic children. For these groups as well, it is important that the communication does not become responsive – the individual answers only when spoken to by others or takes the 'initiative' after being urged to do so. Although not intentional, teaching may reinforce a child's dependence.

Behavioural disorders

It is often possible to demonstrate a relationship between limited communication skills and behavioural problems, and improvement in communication skills is typically accompanied by a reduction in such problems (Durand, 1993; Carr et al., 1994). One reason for this improvement may be that the individual has become more proficient in relaying wants and problems that would otherwise have led to frustration, despair and anger. Another reason may be that problem behaviours helped the individual get attention (a very positive and laudable achievement for a person with few social skills), which is necessary for directing another's behaviour in some way – to go out, to obtain something, to be comforted, etc.; this is more easily obtained using more conventional communicative acts. The frequency of problem behaviour may also increase temporarily in the early phases of communication intervention, e.g. in the form of very frequent initiatives and refusals to participate in certain activities. As the individual's conventional communication skills improve, negotiation also becomes easier, and behavioural regulation and self-regulation improve. The important point is that behavioural problems should never be regarded as an obstacle to communication and language intervention, but rather as a positive sign that the person has something to communicate, and that communication intervention is very much needed.

Chapter 5
Assessment

Children, adolescents and adults who need augmentative and alternative communication are from all ages and have very different skill levels. It is usual to begin by assessing the individual's communication 'needs'. However, it should be noted that most people have the same kinds of communication needs: they want to make themselves understood and understand others, to be able to communicate with different people (adults and children), in diverse settings and about a variety of topics in order to fulfil physical, emotional and social needs, follow interests and ideas, etc. The general objective when planning intervention for individuals with communication disorders is to make possible and promote development of communication and language. People, settings and topics will vary from individual to individual, and change over time, but one should be careful with calling these different 'needs', as if they expressed a well-defined characteristic of the person. Assessment of 'needs' is rather a matter of making priorities, of deciding which skills and settings may be feasible to attempt first.

The need for total intervention

The vast majority of people who need augmentative and alternative communication also require other forms of intervention. This is increasingly true the more pervasive the disability. Individuals with the most extensive and complex disabilities will require intervention and support throughout their lives. The primary objective should be that the sum of interventions provides the individual with the best possible quality of life.

The different forms of intervention are aimed at providing a quality of life that most people take for granted: a home of their own, a job – or at least meaningful employment – meaningful leisure time and pleasure in the company of others, especially family, but also friends. Individuals should also experience control and choice in their own life, and have a sense of self-respect.

People who need augmentative and alternative communication run the risk of losing all these qualities of life. Only when the total intervention is appropriate can these objectives be realized to some extent. Viewing the measures as one entity is the best guarantee for quality of life. Language and communication intervention which does not take into account the total life situation of the person concerned and fails to contribute to overall improvement is inadequate in terms of the individual's interests. It is probably also poor language and communication intervention.

Communication and language teaching should form an integral part of the total intervention, i.e. be co-ordinated with other intervention measures. This applies particularly to teaching of self-help, work activities and activities that lay the foundations for improved social contact with other people. The content of the teaching is chosen on the basis of a comprehensive assessment of what will be of most benefit to the individual.

What should be included in the total intervention, and how each element should be assessed on its own and in relation to the total intervention, is only outlined here. The various elements that make up a good total intervention must always be adapted to the limitations and possibilities of the individual and will also vary for each of the different groups in need of augmentative and alternative communication. The construction of *an individual habilitation plan* covering all aspects of the individual's life is the main tool in the assessment process. A plan for assessment, with assignment of responsibility, is one of the first tasks.

Assessment methods

Tests

Formal tests will have varying value in an assessment, depending on the group in question. This applies to both general intelligence tests and tests directed at more limited fields such as language comprehension, drawing skills and gross motor skills. Structured testing may provide information that is useful for determining the form and content of language and communication intervention, but it is still a good rule to ask how the test results will be used before a test is carried out.

A number of conditions limit the use of the ordinary tests among people who may need augmentative and alternative communication. Many individuals have disabilities that imply that the tests cannot be administered in the prescribed manner. This is true, for example, of people with extensive comprehension problems, motor disorders, or visual and hearing impairments. Most tests are based on the assumption that the individual can see, hear, understand instructions and speak, as well as move building bricks or other objects. Typical test items are answering questions or following instructions, drawing figures, or building patterns with building bricks and repeating sequences of numbers. Many of the tasks must be completed within a time limit.

Few tests are constructed with people with disabilities in mind. To use the tests with these groups, it is necessary to change the instructions, the method of presentation and often what kinds of replies are needed. Completing a test with adapted testing procedures of this kind implies, however, that the test's standard norms cannot be used and that the result cannot be interpreted in the usual way. The norms are based on the test being completed in the prescribed manner.

It may still be useful to administer tests. They have the advantage that one knows how normal children, adolescents and adults score on similar tasks, and over time one may gain experience of how a specific group usually accomplishes the tasks.

Age scores and standard scores

If the use of tests is to be of benefit, the test results must be used in a meaningful way. In many instances the results achieved are 'translated' to an *age score*. This may be a straightforward way of describing a child's functional level, but it often gives the wrong impression. For example, even though a 20-year-old man manages to solve the same tasks on a test as an average 3-year-old, his functioning will nevertheless differ considerably from that of 3-year-old children. It is better to use *standard scores*, which indicate how an individual accomplishes a given task in relation to others of the same age. The advantage of standard scores is that they bring out the variations in a specific age group. An age score gives the average of the age level.

Standard scores are based on a distribution curve where the average is 0 and a certain proportion of the scores fall within each standard score (Figure 24). For example, 68 per cent of the scores will be between +1 standard score and −1 standard score, and this is often termed the 'normal area'. However, there should be a departure of more than 2 standard scores from the average before one may speak of a significant deviation. In most intelligence tests, the standard score is about 15 points, so that an IQ of 70 is 2 standard scores below 100, which is the average performance of all people of a given age. An IQ of 70 is also usually considered the borderline for learning disability.

There are many examples of the misleading nature of age scores. The scores on Reynell's language test level out at the age of 4 years, so that small differences in raw scores may give large differences in age scores (Reynell, 1985). If a 6-year-old obtains a raw score of 13 on the subtest

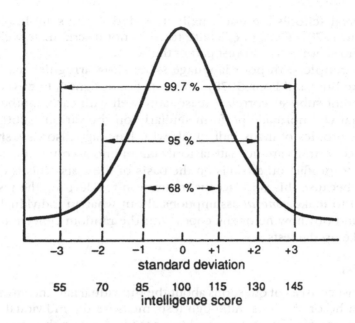

Figure 24. *Normal distributional curve with standard scores and scores for a normal intelligence test.*

'Verbal expression' in the Illinois Test of Psycholinguistic Ability (ITPA: Kirk, McCarthy and Kirk, 1968), this will give a standard score of –1. This means that the child's skills lie within the normal area, but in the lower region. The raw score is equivalent to the average performance obtained by children of 4 years and 3 months (4;3), which is also the age score, but the subtest consists of tasks where the frequency of solution changes little between 4 and 6 years. It may be a shock for the parents of a child aged 6 to learn that he or she is on the same level as a 4-year-old. It may give a more correct picture of the child's skills to say that he or she is somewhat slow in the ability to express him- or herself, but within the limits of what is regarded as normal for the age group.

Test profiles

Some tests provide little information about the individual skills in which one is interested when planning intervention for individuals with language disorders. In many intelligence tests, most people with poor language skills will obtain similarly poor results, because the tests are designed to distinguish between people who belong to a normal population, not to give information about people with special disabilities. When tests are devised and their scores standardized, individuals in institutions and special schools are not usually included in the sample (compare Undheim, 1978). Thus, intelligence tests do not discriminate well among those who score on the lowest part of the scale.

Most people with poor language skills show irregular test profiles (compare Burr and Rohr, 1978). The tests are designed, however, so that the different subtests correlate reasonably well with each another, i.e. an individual will normally perform similarly on the various subtests. The irregular profiles of many individuals with language disorders show that the test conditions are not satisfactorily taken into account. It is therefore difficult to predict other skills on the basis of the tests. This is critical in test use because this is in fact the motivation for devising the tests. Tests are used to make *general* assumptions about what an individual can do, not to find out how he or she copes with the random collection of tasks that make up the tests.

Checklists

A checklist consists of questions about the individual and the environment in which he or she lives. Although tests measure the individual's performance in standard situations, checklists are filled out on the basis of observations or interviews with people who know the individual well. Some checklists are intended to describe skills (Sparrow, Balla and Cicchetti, 1984; Kiernan and Reid, 1987), others are meant to facilitate diagnosis (Rimland, 1971; Schopler et al., 1980).

It is often practical to use checklists to assess everyday skills. *The Vineland Adaptive Behaviour Scale* (Sparrow, Balla and Cicchetti, 1984) is often used and gives a comprehensive picture of the individual's level of skills in various areas. Checklists pose questions about different skills at a relatively detailed level, and cover such areas as self-help skills, social skills, behavioural problems and communication. Concrete questions about everyday functioning are asked, including activities such as dressing, eating, going to the toilet, etc. The best checklists contain many questions about each particular domain, so that it is possible to draw up profiles. What checklists are often lacking, however, are questions about the type and amount of help that are required, i.e. how much help the person must have in order to carry out a specific activity and in which situations it is mastered. This is information that will be needed by the person who is planning the intervention.

For many autistic and learning-disabled people, the ways in which they differ from their peers are so obvious that the norms and questions about the size of these differences are of little significance. The aim is first and foremost to discover which skills the person has, and to build on these in subsequent interventions.

Information from those in contact with the individual

Information from parents and other people who know the individual well is collected through conversations and interviews, and in many ways represents a continuation of the checklists. However, this information is more detailed and of more direct relevance for the person and his or her environment than similar information obtained from the checklists, which contain standard questions. The information acquired from those in contact with the individual is not only useful in ascertaining the skills that he or she possesses, it also provides details about their own opinions of the individual and what he or she is able to do.

Systematic observation

Regardless of the type of disability, systematic observation is always an important part of the assessment. It is important to observe the person in different situations and activities, in the company of others or alone.

Video

In recent years, video recordings have played an increasing role in the documentation of interaction and communication skills of disabled people. As they do not disappear, video recordings can always be viewed again. Information that crops up at a later stage or circumstances not noticed immediately can be checked. Several people may view a video together and look at specific sequences several times. Video recordings also make it easier to document progress in children who are slow developers.

Video recordings are a good starting point for discussions with parents and other people in close contact with the individual. They can say whether the behaviour demonstrated in the video is typical, and can confirm or invalidate assumptions about what the person can and cannot do, and typically does. By analysing video recordings, innovative ideas for new forms of intervention and communication situations may spring to mind.

The use of compact discs makes it possible to write habilitation plans and other reports that include information in the form of both small video recordings and text.

Experimental teaching

The first assessment does not always give clear answers to the question of which intervention strategies will be best suited to the individual. Experimental teaching may be required before a decision is made about how to continue. Such teaching is similar to *dynamic assessment* and is part of the assessment. The objective is to find out whether a particular task is within the individual's *zone of proximal development*, i.e. whether the individual can learn from the task. The zone of proximal development is the problem-solving that lies between what the individual can do independently and what he or she can do together with a more competent person. If the task is too easy, it is within the individual's independent mastery and does not add any new knowledge. If the individual does not understand the nature of the task, it is outside the zone and will not advance the child's knowledge. Thus, new knowledge is developed through social collaboration (Vygotsky, 1962).

Basic information

When initiating assessment, the focus should be given to principal issues to find out what is required in order to get started. Among these issues is the question of the objectives of the language and communication intervention, e.g. whether the person is likely to need the alternative communication form as an expressive means, as a support in order to develop speech or as an alternative form of language. Although it is often not possible to answer this question, it helps to focus on what is fundamental to the communication intervention. In addition, information is required about such central areas as social functioning, activity level, comprehension of everyday situations, self-help skills, the general level of knowledge and behavioural problems.

Once these steps have been completed, the assessment should follow a plan and be effected stepwise. The first step is to outline the plan and the information that forms its basis. The need for more precise information will increase as the problems gradually become clearer. Evaluations of interventions that are implemented are a significant part of a continuous assessment.

It is important that the assessment does not delay implementation of intervention measures, if there is already enough information available for these to be effected. It is often the case that intervention is postponed because part of the assessment takes too long. For example, with children with motor disorders it often appears as if the child is assumed to have other disorders, and language intervention might be postponed until the child has demonstrated an understanding of language. The communication aid is thus used to reveal skills instead of contributing to their development.

To start with, it is easy to ask about too much. This may lead to extra work and can sometimes make co-operation difficult. In particular, there are many parents who have experienced professionals asking for detailed information that has never been used. It is also not uncommon for time to be spent carrying out routine tests and investigations, which do not have a clear use as a basis for intervention.

Overview of the day

Before beginning language and communication intervention, it is necessary to have an overview of the activities in which the person already participates. An overview of this kind is the quickest way of gaining insight into the individual's total intervention, and it gives a suggestion of the individual's strong and weak sides, and the kind of life that he or she has. The overview also provides information when intervention is already taking place. In this way, new intervention measures can be planned so that they do not disturb current positive activities and enhance the totality. The overview should include all hours of the day and be so fine-meshed that most activities occurring during the course of the day are clearly discernible.

A *day clock* is a useful aid for presenting and structuring the information. This consists of fields that are filled in with activities pertaining to the individual (Figure 25). The information is collected through interviews with parents, professionals and others, depending on who is responsible for the activities at different times.

When filling in a day clock, it is necessary to ask about a *typical* day. It is a good idea to begin by asking about the previous day. If this was not a typical day, one should ask about the last day that was suitably typical. The day clock can be divided into 15-minute intervals. Information is required about what the individual was doing and who was with him or her at every 15-minute interval. Notes should be made about any variation. It is also useful to ask whether any problems usually occur in each of the situations, whether communication occurs and, if so, the type and manner of communication. It is a good idea to make two day clocks – one for normal weekdays and one for normal weekends. When planning communication intervention, one should produce separate day clocks for communication. These contain the times of the teaching situations, situations in which the individual regularly communicates and those in which he or she sometimes communicates. In this way, it will become apparent when the person is not communicating.

A good day clock gives a picture of existing intervention measures, the person's activity level, activities that occur regularly and any problematic behaviour. This will include an overview of the total intervention, including daytime measures (nursery school, school, work or work training), leisure activities and various forms of relief services. In addition, comprehensive interviews provide information about self-help skills, self-occupancy and communicative skills. When this information is pieced together with the routine tasks carried out by the family and other people in contact with the individual, one may get a picture of how the existing total intervention appears to work.

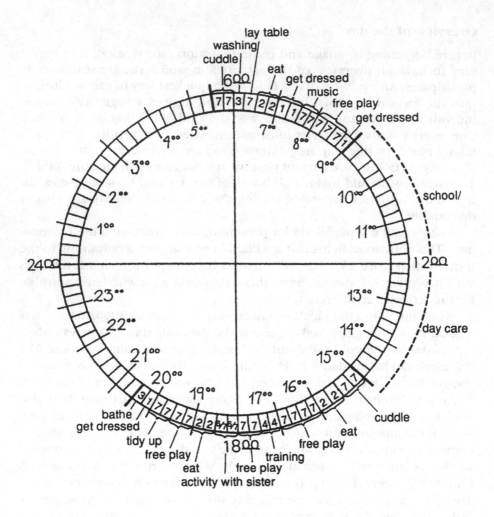

Situation	Code	Number	Time
Dressing/training	1	4	1
Eating	2	6	1.5
Washing/bathing	3	2	0.5
Training	4	2	0.5
Occupied alone	5	0	0
Occupied with children	6	2	0.5
Occupied with adults	7	20 (2)	5

Figure 25. *Day clock for a 12-year-old autistic boy.*

The day clock is used to find times that are suitable for communication teaching and other measures. As new activities are introduced, these are included in the day clock so that it always shows how the individual's day is organised. Comparisons of day clocks from different times provide a picture of how the intervention is proceeding. Thus, day clocks may play an important role in the ongoing evaluation of the intervention.

General skills

Interest in objects, activities and events

A basic principle that applies to intervention with augmentative and alternative communication is that all people wish to communicate, but not everyone is able to do so. It has often been said that motivation on the part of the individual is a prerequisite for the implementation of teaching, but this raises the question of what it means not to be motivated. A lack of 'motivation' generally signals that the person appears negative and unwilling. There is no reason to take this as an expression of a general reluctance to communicate, but rather as an expression of the fact that it is frustrating not being able to do so. Experience also shows that people become less reluctant and negative when they have acquired some communicative competence.

Although everyone has a fundamental desire to communicate, they do not necessarily have a desire to communicate about anything and everything. If the intervention is to be successful, it is imperative that what is being taught is communication about things, activities and events about which the person is aware and interested in communicating. Assessment with regard to language intervention should therefore begin with an evaluation of the individual's interests. Only then can intervention become meaningful from the perspective of the learner.

In some cases it can be difficult to find activities that are interesting for the individual. When this is the case, measures must be taken to improve the situation. In such instances, teaching should begin by creating interest and awareness.

Attention and initiation of communicative contact with others

Among people in need of augmentative and alternative communication, attention and initiation of communicative contact with others vary. This applies both within and between the main groups. The initiation of contact can be so unusual that only people who know the individual can understand it. This can lead to the individual being strongly selective in terms of the people with whom he or she decides to initiate contact.

Within a 'pure' expressive language group, the ability to initiate contact with others may be deficient and perhaps non-existent. Some people do not have the physical abilities to do anything that may be construed as a communicative initiative. The problem may also result from the fact that they have learned only to answer others, not to take the initiative themselves – a form of learned dependence.

There is great variation among individuals in the supportive language group, but in this group many individuals also seldom initiate contact with others. The problems may be caused by both learned dependency and the systematic unlearning of initiating contact through bad experiences. Many children in this group are shy and timid when they meet strangers, or may appear bothersome and aggressive. They may develop an aversion to speaking or, in extreme cases, selective mutism, where they speak only to their close family or significant others (Cline and Baldwin, 1993).

It is in the alternative language group, however, that the most severe problems are found, in terms of both attention and initiation of communicative contact with others. This is probably related to the fact that they generally have the poorest linguistic, communicative and social skills. They may not be able to understand eye gaze, eye-pointing and other cues for seeking the attention of other people, or to use such behaviours to direct the attention of others. One distinctive subgroup in this respect consists of children and adults with autism syndrome, whose problems in relating to other people are a diagnostic criterion. Initiation of contact and attention to others vary considerably within the group, however, and depend on the situation.

Self-help skills

Self-help skills include the ability to care for oneself, dress, wash, cook, etc. With the exception of very young children and people with severe motor impairments, most people in need of augmentative and alternative communication possess some self-help skills. These skills comprise a significant part of the individual's self-determination, and are of fundamental importance if the individual is to have good living conditions. Self-help skills are generally discussed in interviews with people who know the individual, but it may also be useful to make observations of one's own. All three main groups have in common the fact that people around them often believe that they can do less than they are actually capable of doing.

In language and communication intervention, it is important to take into account the need for self-help skills and, if possible, increase and facilitate the training of these. As far as possible, language and communication training should be adapted to self-help training so that both forms of training are improved.

Self-occupancy

The extent to which individuals are able to occupy themselves determines how the intervention is arranged. Many families and other people in close contact with the individuals find that their inability to occupy themselves poses a considerable strain. Language and communication intervention may increase the degree of self-occupancy. As far as an improved ability for self-expression may provide the individual with a better chance of determining what he or she wants to do, good language and communication intervention may also improve the individual's initiative skills and reduce learned dependency on others.

Motor skills

The individual's motor skills are crucial for the choice of communication system and possible aids. Hand movements are assessed in order to determine whether or not the individual is able to produce intelligible manual signs, i.e. to vary hand shape, place and manner of sign articulation in such a way that it is possible for a communication partner to distinguish individual signs (compare Klima and Bellugi, 1979; Grove, 1990).

It is clear that people with obvious motor disabilities are unable to use manual signs, but others may also have difficulty in performing manual signs. However, it is important to distinguish between difficulties in producing manual signs as a result of motor disorders and problems in following an instruction. For example, it may be difficult for a learning-disabled child to understand the idea of imitating a hand form. In the case of children with no obvious physical motor impairments, it can be practical to take the performance of everyday skills as a starting point. The way in which these activities are carried out will also give cues as to how, if necessary, the signs can be simplified so that the individual is able perform them (Figure 26). It should be noted that many severely motor-impaired individuals use some signs or gestures and, even if the number must be small, they may play an important part in the communication, and it is important to ensure that they are actually understood by people in the environment.

For individuals who will be using aided communication, assessment of motor function is aimed at finding sitting positions and methods for pointing or activating keys and switches. People with extensive motor disorders rely on a stable sitting position in order to use their motor skills. It is therefore important to find the sitting positions that best facilitate the use of communication aids and other technical devices. If it has been decided that the individual will have to use a communication aid, it is imperative that the best possible method of pointing or activating keys and switches is found. This is often a difficult and time-consuming task, but it

Figure 26. *Everyday activities that can be used to assess motor skills (from Dennis et al., 1982).*

Hand form	pull trousers up/down	pull shirt up/down	squeeze oranges for juice	palm on table, pick up pencil in fingers	put on sock	squeeze toothpaste onto toothbrush	hold brush handle when brushing hair	crumple paper	wipe table with cloth or sponge	turn key	pick up book from table edge
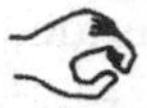 1 squeeze	x	x	x	x							
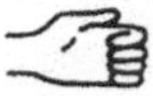 2 palmar						x	x	x			
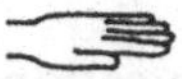 3 thumb adduction									x	x	x
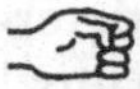 4 midposition of the forearm											
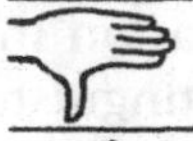 5 thumb abduction											
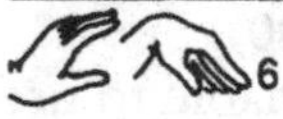 6 wrist movements						x					
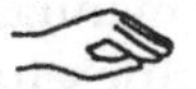 7 opposed grasp						x					
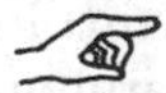 8 pointing radial finger											
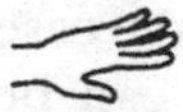 9 release											
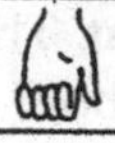 10 full supination											
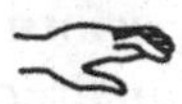 11 crossed finger											
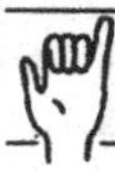 12 pointing ulnar finger											

Movement

1 unilateral			x		x						
2 bilateral mirror	x				x						
3 unilateral across midline									x		
4 bilateral/one base–one mover						x					
5 bilateral two movers											
6 bilateral crossing midline											

self-feed using fingers/drink with cup	self-feed using utensils	turn steering wheel	hold sandwich or finger foods	hold jar of jam and twist lid	turn knobs/dials	comb hair	brush teeth	stir (contents in stable bowl)	pouring from container into glass held by other hand	button/unbutton	open and close zip on jacket	dial phone number	play instrument with keyboard	use finger puppet	wring wash cloth	tear paper	remove glove from fingers	retrieve object from pocket	throw ball up in air and catch
	x	x																	
			x	x	x	x	x												
						x	x	x											
										x	x	x	x	x					
												x	x						
																	x	x	
																			x
																	x		
x	x																		
x	x							x											
										x									
		x								x					x	x			

is essential if individuals with severe motor impairment are to be able to express themselves in the best possible way. There are some computer programs that are designed to assess motor functions, and there are also games and other programs that are designed to train individuals in the use of switches.

Vision and hearing

Visual and auditory disorders are more common among all the three main groups than in the population in general. It is therefore important to have information about the individual's vision and hearing when a communication system is chosen and intervention is planned. It is also vital that any problems in visual and auditory perception are made known to all the assessors, so that behaviour and test results can be appropriately interpreted. However, it is often difficult to test the sight and hearing of many of the individuals in need of augmentative and alternative communication.

There are 'objective' tests for both sight and hearing, i.e. examinations that do not require co-operation on the part of the individual being examined. It is possible to examine whether the eye and ear are intact and in working order, and to register whether stimulation of the visual and auditory organs reaches the brain. The last type of examination may not be a reliable test for children with brain damage (compare Rosenblum et al., 1980).

A seemingly intact sensory organ is no guarantee that perception is normal. Many learning-disabled and autistic people appear to have disturbances of perception that are caused by brain damage. As a rule, these do not lead to deafness or blindness in the normal sense, because the person reacts to changes in stimulation, but the sensory impressions will not be processed and perceived normally. Objective examinations must therefore be supplemented by observations of how the individual seems to use vision and hearing in everyday activities and in familiar and less familiar settings.

Diagnosis

There are several good reasons for emphasizing the necessity of an accurate diagnosis, even when this has no direct bearing on planning the intervention. In some cases, the diagnosis is essential in order to provide the necessary medical treatment, but intervention is rarely a *direct* result of the diagnosis. Quite frequently, the measures that are implemented are general in the sense that they are provided for children and adults who belong to very different diagnostic groups.

The most important reason for procuring a diagnosis is that a diagnosis is often a means of securing the necessary intervention. The diagnostic label makes it easier to get support for the urgency of the intervention. For parents and others in close contact with the individual, the diagnosis can be necessary for obtaining realistic and tangible information about the individual's disorder(s). Information of this kind is also often provided by parents of children with similar disorders, through organizations and courses. Parents of disabled children arrange their own courses and also participate in courses that are open for both professionals and parents. The diagnosis provides contact with all these various sources of information.

A correct and accurate diagnosis is also necessary in order to make a prognosis, i.e. what may be expected based on previous experience. This applies to both professionals and the individual's family.

There are many examples of a correct diagnosis of children and adults with language disorders helping to produce more suitable forms of intervention and improving the planning of such measures for future needs. For example, a girl may prove to have Rett's syndrome rather than autism, as was previously assumed. This implies that the intervention will differ in a number of areas. For example, the diagnosis may well lead to a move away from manual sign teaching, based on the knowledge that the girl's motor skills are likely to deteriorate, to a communication board that the girl can use as long as she is able to point with her hands or eyes. Pressure may also be reduced and a calm environment created because it is known that girls with Rett's syndrome function best in such conditions.

The family's need for support, relief and help

The families of individuals who need augmentative and alternative communication generally experience a great deal of strain. The degree of strain, and which pressures are greatest, will depend on which group the child belongs to. Parents of children with severe motor disorders are normally subjected to a great deal of physical tension. Normal care and nursing are often time-consuming and require the individual to be lifted and moved frequently. For parents of autistic children, the pressures of always having to be present in order to prevent the child from injuring him- or herself, or running away or damaging things are often the greatest. What most families of children in need of augmentative and alternative communication have in common is that everyday tasks become considerably more time-consuming than for others, that contact with other family members and friends is reduced, and that they are concerned about the future.

The strains imply that the family has both a need for and a right to a reasonable amount of relief service. How great this need is and how the relief should be organized will vary. The help must also be viewed in relation to the family's organization and other duties. In many instances, day care for disabled children lasts only a short while during the middle of the day, and there may be a need for some sort of help to cover the period from the end of day care until the parents arrive home from work. The strain on the family may also be financial. It is an integral part of the total intervention to ensure that the families are given the economic help and support that they need and are entitled to, and that they are informed of their rights.

The ability to cope with these pressures differs from family to family. In families where several individuals need much care and help (young children, sick or elderly family members), it is essential that resources are distributed. Some people are not as strong as others, and it is unreasonable to demand that everyone is as resourceful and robust as ideal parents. Experience shows that, in many instances, effective interventionary measures are not implemented because they place too great a strain on families that are given insufficient relief and help. A good relief system makes it easier to implement other measures.

The relief should depend not only on the immediate needs. Many families have a desire to fend for themselves and claim that they have little need for help, but over time the strain may nevertheless be too great. By ensuring that the family always has a reasonable amount of relief, they will also be more able to cope with pressures that arise later on. The relief is also directed not only at the other family members. Being away from the family sometimes may promote self-reliance and autonomy in older disabled children.

Language and communication

Use

Most individuals who are to start learning an alternative communication system have little or no speech. The exception to this is children and adults who, because of motor disorders, have such unintelligible speech that it is not functional in communication except with those who know them well. An assessment of the individual's use of language and communication before intervention has started is therefore usually concentrated on forms of communication other than speech.

The form of communication initially used by children and adults in need of augmentative and alternative communication varies considerably. For children with severe motor disorders, the use of communication will in some cases be limited to looking at things in which they are interested, more or less articulated vocalization as an expression of wishes and interests, crying and other signs of excitement. Sometimes the strongest expression of interest is a change in muscle tone – the child's body stiffens and stops making small movements.

Other children and adults with motor disorders and relatively good language comprehension can often say 'yes' and 'no' by looking up and down, blinking, nodding and shaking their heads, or by moving their heads in other ways. If children and adults with developmental disorders communicate in such a way, even while an assessment is being made for the most appropriate first communication aid, this means that they will receive the communication aid too late because they have already developed a considerable amount of language comprehension.

Children who belong to the alternative language group may also have very different forms of communication, although a number of ways of communicating are common to many. The most usual form is that the child approaches an adult, takes hold of his or her hand and leads him or her to a place where there is something that the child wants, or where a particular activity is usually carried out. This may, for example, be the refrigerator where a bottle of orange juice is usually kept. In instances of this kind, communication typically takes place in a succession of events. After the child and the adult have arrived at the refrigerator, the adult will open the refrigerator door and the child will reach out for the bottle of orange juice, perhaps at the same time as he says *uh*, *uh*, or makes other sounds.

Children who belong to the alternative language group may also use locations as part of their communication. There are children who sit down under the table when they want to go to the toilet, stand by the door to the kitchen when they are hungry, or sit down by their boots when they want to go out. These activities may also be interpreted as communicative signals, but they may be difficult for adults and professionals to perceive in the midst of all their other daily tasks.

> Kathryn is an autistic 9-year-old girl. She is unable to speak. When her father drives the car into the garage, she often goes to the door and pulls at the door handle while she looks at her mother and makes a sound. In this way, Kathryn gives voice to the fact that she wants to go for a drive with her father.

Many individuals with communication and language problems display behavioural problems, which may be reduced through communication intervention (see also p. 89). Carr and Durand (1987) regard such behaviour as 'primitive attempts' at communicating, with the aim of either obtaining attention or escaping a demanding or unpleasant situation. In their view, the behaviour may be translated as 'Look at me' or 'Please, do not make me do this', and thus seem to imply that the intention of the problem behaviour is to direct the attention and action of another person. However, the behaviour may be associated only with a particular state of affairs. If the behaviour is not directed towards a person, it cannot be regarded as truly communicative, even if a professional interprets it in this way.

Still, possible 'communicative' consequences of problem behaviour should always be part of the assessment. Escape may be a possible motive in a boring or demanding situation where the person lacks overview and, for example, does not know how long the situation is going to last; attributing problem behaviour to an inherent motive of getting attention is, however, probably too simplistic. If a person seeks attention from another, attention itself is rarely the final goal. Just being looked at is seldom what an individual is trying to achieve. 'Gaining attention' is a rather empty category. Securing attention is usually only the first step in a communicative action. The individual may want safety, a cup of coffee, to go for a walk, to be comforted because of pain, etc. In fact, one reason why problem behaviour may be linked with attention is that gaining attention, but failing to relay the actual wish or idea, increases frustration. Thus, the objective of the assessment is to find out what the individual wants to express something about, and what the implicit or explicit message is. This is not constant, but varies from situation to situation. Information about problem behaviour may thus be used to gain insight into the variation in the person's interests, pleasures and fears.

Children who have normal motor functions but who have not developed speech use gestures in very different ways. Most children with specific language disorders begin to use pointing as a form of communication. Autistic children, on the other hand, typically have poor mastery of gestures. It is still important to assess the way that they use gestures and other forms of directive behaviours (compare Phillips et al., 1995). There are children who use pointing only when they have been specially taught to do so. Some children in the supportive language group and the alternative language group use idiosyncratic gestures that resemble words.

> Geoffrey is an 11-year-old autistic boy. He beats the table with his fist to say 'Daddy' (Steindal K, personal communication, 1990).

Idiosyncratic communication of this type is found not only among people with language and communication disorders. Similar communication is characteristic of the initial stages of speech development among children who develop language normally, and is usually called *vocables* (Ferguson, 1978). A vocable is defined as an articulation that has a fixed, recognizable acoustic form and a clearly defined use. Vocables have, however, no acoustic similarities with the conventional words. *Vroomvroom* may, for example, be used about toy cars and tractors, and *uvuvuv* about birds, aeroplanes, flies and other flying objects. Both vocables and the equivalent gestures or utterances that are used by children with language disorders have a use that does not correspond directly to specific words in the spoken language. The fact that children do not use the words in the same way as adults is, however, a general feature of their language, and is linked not only to the use of vocables. A 1-year-old child may use *bow-wow* when speaking of dogs, cars and other machines (over-extension), or say *dog* only when his father points at a picture of a dog on his bib (under-extension).

The most important source of information about the child's various types of communication is parents and others who are in daily contact with the child. This is a direct result of the fact that the communication often has a low frequency – this means that usually only those people who are in close contact with the child have practical opportunities to know the form and extent of the communication. A special problem for children with language disorders is that their idiosyncratic communication, which is the communication form they have that most resembles words, is often not recognized as 'proper' communication by teachers and other professionals. Parents also relate that they have been directly distrusted when they told others about how they interpreted their children's idiosyncratic communication.

When the assessment takes place after intervention, with initiation of one or several alternative communication systems, the use of these systems is an integral part of the assessment. The assessment should include how each manual, graphic and tangible sign is used (conceptual mapping), mean length of utterance, grammatical structures and pragmatic functions (see Chapters 10 and 11). Norms for alternative language development are lacking. The aim is therefore not to establish some kind of 'alternative language level', but to understand the complexity of the communication used by the person and to establish functional criteria for deciding the following steps in the intervention.

Comprehension

People in the environment of those who use alternative language systems usually use spoken language, and the strategies used by many interventionists are explicitly or implicitly based on assumptions about the individual's comprehension of spoken language. These assumptions may be false and hence the strategies applied inappropriate. To know what the individual is able to understand about what is said around him or her, and whether he or she will benefit from a particular set of intervention strategies, assessment of comprehension of spoken language, as well as other communication forms, is crucial. It can, however, be difficult to get a clear picture of what a person with pervasive language problems is able to understand. There are many examples where children and adults have been credited with a considerable understanding of speech, although careful observation has revealed that it was not the words they understood, but rather the gestures accompanying the speech, or special conditions in the situation.

> Martin is a 3-year-old autistic boy. He is very fond of going for walks, but does not react to the spoken message *Come on, let's go for a walk!* unless the nursery school teacher is simultaneously holding up his jacket or wearing her own coat (Steindal K, personal communication, 1990).

People with very extensive motor disorders may almost totally lack ordinary means of showing that they understand. Some have for years been underestimated in terms of what they understood of both speech and what was going on around them. The underestimation has meant that these individuals have not been given the stimulation and the development opportunities that they should have had.

> Joe Deacon lived in an institution for learning-disabled people. He was considered to have no language until the age of 24. At that time a learning-disabled inhabitant arrived who managed to interpret the sounds Joe made. Joe's abilities had to be totally reassessed. Later, the two friends allied themselves with two other inhabitants, a learning-disabled man who was able to use a typewriter and a motor-disabled wheelchair user who could spell. With the help of his friends, Joe wrote his autobiography – *Tongue Tied* (Deacon, 1974).

Less dramatic forms of underestimation occur frequently (compare Fuller, Newcombe and Ounsted, 1983). It is difficult to use normal systematic observation with this group because the events that are most interesting tend to occur rather infrequently. The observations would have to be so prolonged that it would be impractical to carry them out. However, systematic observation can be used advantageously when intervention is started, if it is carried out by those who are usually with the individual. The observations will then provide extra information about the individual's skills and form the basis for evaluation of the intervention.

Individuals' abilities to express themselves will to a certain extent also determine the methods that can be used to assess comprehension. If the individual can speak or write, and appears to have a reasonable vocabulary for self-expression, a good impression of language comprehension may be obtained by asking various questions. It is much more difficult to assess comprehension when the individual has fewer words with which to show understanding. A person who can look up for 'yes' and down for 'no' will be able to answer questions from the ITPA such as *Can boys eat*? or *Can tomatoes telegraph*? On the other hand, the person would not be able to complete another subtest from the ITPA, in which the task is to fill in sentences such as *Mountains are high, valleys are . . . .*

For people who belong to the expressive language group, and others whom one knows have a good understanding of spoken language, tests can be useful tools if the person has the necessary motor functions for carrying them out. A number of tests or test items place considerable demands on motor skills. For example, in Reynell's language scales, the child has to carry out instructions such as *Put the doll on the chair* and *Put all the pigs behind the brown horse*. Other tests are mainly based on pointing, but for many people with motor disabilities even pointing can be difficult to do, so that another person can safely say to which of several alternatives the person was pointing. If pointing in itself requires substantial cognitive effort, this may reduce the number of correct replies. Some tests are specially adapted to children with motor disabilities, such as computer-based language comprehension tests which may be operated with switches (von Tetzchner, 1987). It is important that assessment is not based on vocabulary alone, as such instruments tend to yield higher age scores than measures based on the comprehension of syntax and morphology (Whedall and Jeffree, 1974; Facon, Bollengier and Grubar, 1993).

However, the best information comes in the form of tangible reports from people who are in close contact with the person. These people have the advantage of a wealth of experience gained from being with that person. It is also these people, and particularly parents, who have laid the foundations for both their usage and understanding of language. The way in which these children and adolescents demonstrate understanding can be very unusual and difficult for other people to discover. Nor are the parents and significant others always aware of the cues that they use, although systematic interviews can provide important information about the basis of the individual's comprehension. This information is used in the planning of the intervention.

It is particularly important to take one's time when speaking with the family and others in close contact with the individual. As a starting point, ask such questions as: *Think of something you are quite certain that you can say to John or make him understand in another way. What is it John does that makes you sure that he has understood you*? Questions of this kind can be asked in many different ways, and we should choose our words in accordance with the person who we are asking.

Parents and other people in contact with the child will usually begin by answering too generally. They may say things like: *I can tell just by looking at him*. It is therefore important that the answers given are as specific as possible. General characterizations of the individual's language comprehension may well be correct, but may nevertheless be an insufficient basis for intervention. Follow-up questions are necessary. These may take the form of: *Yes, of course. But please describe it for me. What does he do? What does he look like when he's doing it? What is it he always understands? What is it he seems to understand only now and again?*

If the interviewer is patient, people in close contact with disabled people will almost always be able to answer such questions. It is our experience that this is also true of those in close contact with the lowest-functioning individuals. However, many parents experience that professionals are centred most on reducing parents' expectations for their child's future development. Disagreement about the level of functioning may make it difficult to collaborate about an intervention that must be adapted according to assumptions about the child's functioning.

A certain degree of over-interpretation is positive. However, the aim of the assessment is to obtain the most correct picture possible of the individual's language comprehension. Overestimation means that the language intervention is not adapted as well as it could be. It is especially easy to overestimate the language comprehension of a person who understands something of what is being said. For example, in a teaching or test situation, one might say *Point at the red ball*, whereby the person points correctly. On the basis of this observation, one may assume that the individual understands *everything* that is said. In addition, one may also make the assumption that the person comprehends words understood in a given situation in other unrelated situations. Often this is not the case. More extensive observation may reveal that an individual understands only one or a few critical words in the sentence and that he or she has learned to point in that particular situation.

> Martin is a 3-year-old autistic boy. He is fond of orange juice, and usually comes running when his mother shouts *Come and have some orange juice*. His mother was told to shout out in the same way as usual, but to sit still without moving. She was quite surprised to find that Martin did not react, but carried on twirling a toy. A short while later she stood up, walked towards the kitchen table where the bottle of orange juice was standing and repeated the words. Martin came running immediately (Steindal K, personal communication, 1990).

Understanding what is going on in communicative situations depends not only on what is being expressed in sign or speech. Many conditions contribute to the understanding of a situation and give cues as to what is being signed or said. The rattling of pots and pans in the kitchen may indicate that someone is cooking, holding a coat may indicate that someone is soon to leave the house, etc. In addition, what is being said, often accompanied by eye contact, pointing and other gestures, also contributes to the understanding of the situation, even if what is being said is not in itself understood.

Likewise, one may observe that some individuals show that they understand only when they are together with certain people. One should nevertheless be wary of concluding that the individual does not understand anything of what is being said. Many people in need of an alternative communication system have an understanding of single words or phrases that may depend on the situation.

The fact that an individual's understanding of speech is linked to the use of gestures or other types of non-verbal communication will, in many cases, not be apparent in interviews with those in close contact with the individual. The person who participates in the communicative situation will not normally be aware of this. Systematic observation of the communicative situation is therefore necessary when the information provided gives the impression that the communication is dependent on a situation or person. Documentation of such dependency can be a good starting point for further discussion about the intervention with parents and others in contact with the child.

Information about how the parents and others judge an individual's comprehension also has another function. It provides cues as to how people interpret the individual's comprehension and react to his or her means of expressing this understanding, and the extent to which they try to adapt their own communication so that the comprehension can be improved. This knowledge is useful when assessing the language environment and adapting it so that it encourages the best possible acquisition of linguistic and communicative skills.

When the assessment takes place after intervention with one or several alternative communication systems, the comprehension of these systems should be an integral part of the assessment. Some people understand spoken words alone, others only in combination with manual or graphic signs. Some understand manual and graphic signs alone, others need speech to support them as well. Some understand only manual and/or graphic signs in spite of years of simultaneous presentations of spoken words and manual and graphic signs. As with speech, assessment should be made up of the individual's interpretation of manual, graphic and tangible signs, as well as sentences and metaphoric use of sign combinations.

Evaluating the language intervention

There should be continual evaluation of the intervention on the basis of the explicit objectives. Regardless of how well one plans in advance, one cannot take for granted that development will proceed as assumed. It is therefore important that the evaluation is planned beforehand and is included as part of the intervention right from the start. Planned evaluations help clarify the teaching objectives and make it easier to see the relationship between the different aims of the intervention. As the evaluation is planned, the intervention does not have to be clearly inappropriate before it is adjusted or modified.

An evaluation should be as extensive as is practically possible. It should cover the specific aims that have been set for the language intervention, and also evaluate the generalized effects of the teaching in terms of the total life situation, i.e. whether the person shows fewer behavioural problems, is more social, participates in more activities, is more attentive during teaching sessions and in interaction with others, etc.

Specific goals

The evaluation of the language intervention should include information about the progress in terms of the specific teaching goals and the manual, graphic and tangible signs that have been taught. This means a registration of the use of signs and the development of other linguistic and communicative skills that are being taught. The specific goals can be the use of new signs, sentence construction, pragmatic functions or contact strategies, a higher level of linguistic activity, etc. To evaluate the effectiveness of the individual's language production, structured communication tasks may be useful (Møller and von Tetzchner, 1996).

The individual does not necessarily learn what has been stated as the intervention aim. Sometimes, the teaching situation has been such that the individual has learned another use from the one planned. This is not always negative.

> Giles is a learning-disabled boy aged 19 years. The intention was to teach him to use the conventional manual sign BREAD, but he quickly began to use this sign as a general call for help and to express that there was something he wanted. This usage of the sign was very functional for him and, instead of forcing him to use it 'correctly', the manual form of BREAD was redefined to mean 'help'. Everybody in his environment was informed about the idiosyncratic manual execution of HELP in Giles' vocabulary.

This example emphasizes how necessary it is not merely to register 'right' and 'wrong', but also to analyse the pattern of usage and understanding of each sign, and find possible fixed usages that were not intended by the teacher. If, in the example above, Giles' teacher had insisted that the sign retain the meaning she had tried to teach him, this would have taken away the communication he had acquired. By continu-

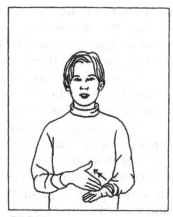

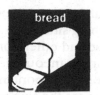

BREAD

ally evaluating the situation, it is possible to adapt to an unexpected development when this is most functional.

The evaluation report should also include the type and extent of help that are needed at any given time for the individual to accomplish a specific communicative act in the teaching situation. The teaching may be carried out in a number of ways, and reduction in the amount of help needed should always be a basic aim. In reports about sign intervention, it is common merely to indicate the number of signs that are being practised or are in use, often only in limited training situations. This may hide significant achievements by the learner. If the help level is included in the registration of sign use, the evaluation may show considerable progress, even if the individual has not begun to learn and use new signs, because the amount of help has been reduced. Inclusion of help level also directs the professionals' attention to the constructive process underlying communication and language learning.

Generalized effects

Other skills besides linguistic and communicative abilities should also be included in the evaluation, because different skills influence one another. New language skills bring with them new information about the surroundings, and the learning of concepts and social skills in the broadest sense (compare Konstantareas, Webster and Oxman, 1979). Likewise, the experience with, and understanding of, different activities is related to the individuals' ability to understand other people's communication and to express themselves. Successful language and communication intervention has great consequences for a large number of activities. In general, those aspects of the individual's general life situation that were included in the assessment before the intervention should also be included in the evaluation.

The evaluation of the intervention should contain not only reports about teaching situations, but also information about the use of language in the home and other non-educational settings. It is especially important that any spontaneous use of signs is registered. However, there are different forms of spontaneous use, e.g. spontaneous use may mean that the person uses the sign on request outside the teaching situation, or that the person takes the initiative and uses the sign without help. The reports should contain information about the type of help that may be given for what is called spontaneous use. Spontaneous use may also mean that the person uses signs to indicate things other than the ones practised in the teaching situation. These uses will perhaps be construed as wrong with regard to the intervention, but they may represent genuine attempts at communication. Thus, the evaluation should contain information about which objects, activities and events each sign is used to communicate, and whether the signs are used to communicate about other objects or activities from those within the teaching situation. One needs to know whether the individual uses the sign in a wider sense than is normal (overextension) or in a more restricted way, i.e. about a smaller set of activities and objects than usual (underextension).

A co-ordination of language and communication intervention with other intervention goals implies that the results of the language intervention can be seen only to a small extent in isolation. The evaluation must include those areas of life and functions that were the point of departure for choosing the specific intervention goals. For children and adults with motor disorders, this may entail an assessment of the extent to which the intervention has led to more conversations, and the extent to which the person has gained more control over the content of the conversations. The individual's semantic categories are likely to change over time, but information about this process is necessary in order to be able to guide the process towards more conventional use of the signs.

Information transfer when changing school, work and home

A large number of people who are taught alternative communication have a need for intervention that is not limited by time. For those people in the expressive language group with extensive motor disorders, new environments must be organized as they pass through new phases of life. Communication aids are being developed that create new possibilities, but they require the individuals and those around them to be given instruction and training in how to use them. In the alternative language group, the acquisition of new skills is often slow, and the need for intervention is likely to persist throughout life. This means that the intervention will take place in different environments as the individual changes school, work and residence. Children in the supportive language group who are given intervention with alternative communication forms for only a limited period of time may also change their school or home environment.

When a person with an adapted environment and organized teaching moves, it is crucial that there are routines for the transferral of information from those in charge of intervention and organization to those who are to assume responsibility. All too often these routines are lacking, which results in discontinuity in the teaching and loss or stagnation in the development of skills.

> Raymond is a learning-disabled 20-year-old man. He receives special education at a high school. He follows simple instructions, but he neither speaks nor uses any form of signs. According to his journal, he received intervention with manual signs from the age of 13. By the time he was transferred to another school at the age of 16, he had learned to use the signs EAT, WALK and TOILET, and was learning several new signs. When he was 18 he was transferred to a new school and, in the notes that were transferred with him, it said that 'he was in the process of learning to use manual signs'. At the age of 19 he changed school again. When Raymond changed school at the age of 20, the teacher sent with him a list of over 50 signs that the teacher had taught and comments as to how they were executed. There was no mention in the report, however, of Raymond using any of the signs spontaneously. Thus, after more than 6 years of teaching Raymond used no manual signs spontaneously (Kollinzas, 1984).

There is every reason to believe that Raymond's lack of signing skills is related to his changing schools and the discontinuity in teaching that he experienced. Kollinzas (1984) has devised a *communication record* for the registration of communication skills and teaching, which can be used

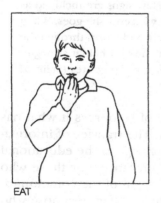
EAT

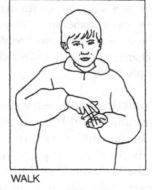
WALK

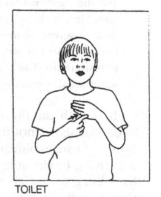
TOILET

for the transfer of this type of information (Figure 27). The record contains the information that *must* be included when the person changes training environment, i.e. the manual, graphic and tangible sign systems that are used, the gloss of the signs that are used or being taught, a description of how the person performs or points out the signs, and descriptions of the situations in which each sign occurs.

The communication record helps people in the new environment to develop realistic expectations of the individual and to organize the situation as well as possible. It also helps to uncover the need for training of people in the environment to which the person moves. It may be useful to have some guidance from the professionals who have worked with the individual before the move. External instructors and supervisors are often used in alternative communication intervention. The communication record makes it possible for the professionals who are taking over to assess whether it is desirable and possible to use the same external consultants for guidance and training in the new environment.

Some of the individuals with communication disorders who have acquired some linguistic skills may themselves be able to help in the training of new environments and new people who arrive in their environment.

Isabel is a 13-year-old girl with Down's syndrome. She uses approximately 70 manual signs spontaneously, and does not have comprehensible speech. Her teacher has made a folder with drawings of all the manual signs that she uses, and the signs' written glosses above the drawings. New signs are included as Isabel learns them. Isabel carries this book with her wherever she goes. When new personnel or helpers appear Isabel sits with them and works through the book. She shows how the signs are performed while the new helper struggles to learn them. This is a change of roles that Isabel clearly appreciates (Steindal K, personal communication, 1990).

It is both unethical practice and a poor use of resources if what has been learned is not maintained and built upon. The transfer of information that can minimize the negative effects of a change in the educational and living environment is therefore of great significance. For those who have been in charge of the intervention, the filling in of the communication record should be part of the planning of the transfer. For those who assume responsibility, it is part of the assessment of the individual.

COMMUNICATION RECORD

Name : Per Hansen   *Sign system*   *Code*
Age: 13;7   Pictogram   P
Instructor: Hans Larsen   Manual signs   H
Place: Vik school
Date: 2–10–88
Page: 2 of 4

Sign	System	Execution	Situation information
CHAIR	H	Normal	Performs the sign when the teacher shows the picture
TABLE	H	Normal	Performs the sign when the teacher shows the picture
KICK	P		Points himself in order to select the activity in the gymnasium
HORSE	H	Right hand between middle and ring finger	Executed alone when he knows he is going to ride
TOILET	H	Normal	Uses the sign spontaneously sometimes when he wants to go to the toilet. He is hand-guided to perform the sign when he is taken to the toilet
DOOR	H	Normal	Uses the sign spontaneously when he wants to go out
TELEVISION	P		Uses spontaneously at home when he wants to watch television
BOOTS	H	Indistinct	Not used spontaneously, the sign is hand-guided during dressing
SCARF	H	Indistinct	Not used spontaneously, the sign is hand-guided during dressing

Figure 27. *Communication record (based on Kollinzas, 1984).*

Defining areas of responsibility

In work with disabled individuals, experience has shown that the quality of the individual measures is to a large degree dependent on the presence and quality of other interventionary measures. Experience has also shown that it can be difficult to ensure coherence and continuity in the intervention measures. The measures that most generally cause problems are those administered by several help authorities, and to start with it is often unclear who has responsibility for the various areas. Experience shows

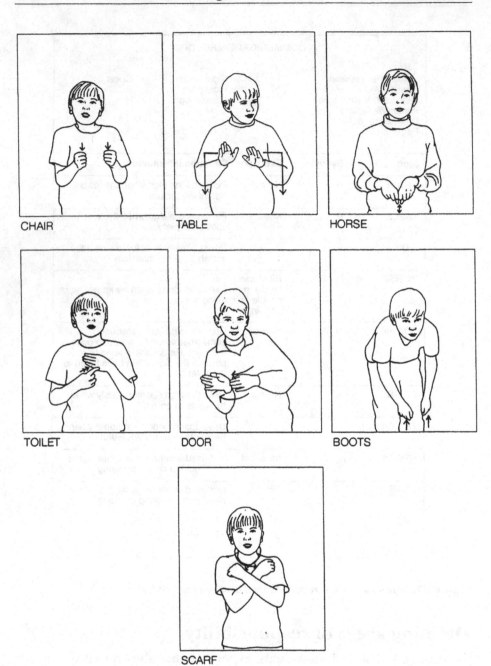

CHAIR   TABLE   HORSE

TOILET   DOOR   BOOTS

SCARF

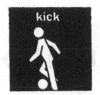

that, when things go wrong and the person does not get the necessary intervention, this is often the result of unclear areas of responsibility and a lack of co-ordination. This lack of co-ordination is even more clearly visible in long-term plans for intervention. The more extensive the disorder, the greater the need for both long-term and short-term planning in order to ensure that the measures that are given are in proportion to the present and future needs of the individual. It is therefore crucial that each measure is seen in terms of a total goal, and that an individual habilitation plan is drawn up, in which the areas of responsibility for the total intervention and the individual measures are clarified.

It has gradually been recognized that the need for co-ordination and planning is central in the care of disabled people. This means that the financial responsibility must be allocated, and likewise the responsibility for co-ordinating the various elements of the intervention and ensuring that they are seen in terms of a sensible long-term plan. There should be one person who knows all the measures well, and who can act as a care manager, and whom the family and the other professionals involved can contact. It is also useful to have routines for the implementation of new initiatives. When things go wrong, this is often because no one feels responsible for taking the initiative to implement the required modifications.

To fill this need, *responsibility groups* have gradually been established. The groups are multidisciplinary and which agencies participate depends on the intervention required. Parents take part in the group meetings, and together the group should have a complete overview of the intervention, be able to initiate new measures and distribute the various forms of responsibility.

Chapter 6
The teaching situation

Children and adults who are taught alternative forms of communication have been unable to acquire sufficient language and communicative skills in a normal environment. They are dependent on the environment being specially organized for them. Language intervention may be viewed as the construction of situations that may aid children's acquisition of language comprehension and use, i.e. situations in which they will come to have certain assumptions and expectations about people, actions and events, and be attentive to how vocal and non-vocal language forms are used by others and possibly themselves. Children learn language and communication through participation in social interchanges within such situations.

For the alternative language group and the supportive language group, the primary objective of this organization is to create communicative situations that are appropriate for teaching the alternative communication forms in such a manner that the individual can learn and use them in various settings. From an intervention point of view, a *communicative situation* may be defined as a setting in which at least one partner is attempting to relay some kind of information or taking part in another language act. This means that, in addition to the presence of two or more individuals, there must be a possibility of establishing joint attention or involvement around objects, persons, events, topics, etc. The ongoing activity and physical setting may provide clues to how speech and alternative language forms are used by others, by implicitly or explicitly directing the individual's attention towards certain aspects of the situation and ensuring uptake of relevant expressions from people in the environment. This may provide the individual with some of the knowledge that is needed to establish a representational frame or schema within which an utterance may be understood.

The expressive language group does not have the same need for language teaching as the other two groups. For people with good language comprehension, the main aim is to organize the environment so that it facilitates communication and the natural acquisition and use of language. In reality, this means providing manual signs or communication aids with the largest possible vocabulary that is accessible in all situations, and making it easier for others to understand what is being expressed. People in the expressive language group experience many situations during the course of a normal day, in which it is impossible for them to communicate with others. The aim of adapting potential communication settings is to remedy this and thereby enable the individual to experience increased participation in everyday activities. Direct teaching is most intensive for the youngest children in the expressive language group, although older children also need sign explanations and help to develop advanced strategies as they encounter more complex communicative challenges. Moreover, the teaching of reading and writing may need considerable effort at school and in the home for an extended period of time.

Joint attention

Communication is basically a matter of directing attention. The aim of communicative acts is to make another person aware of something. This may be something in the immediate surroundings (e.g. an object or an event), a wish for the other to do something (e.g. get something or go away) or an abstract idea (e.g. the theory of relativity). To direct the attention of the other, attention must somehow be shared. It is not sufficient that two or more individuals look at the same thing. In *joint attention*, the communication partners must also be aware of the fact that they share this focus (Tomasello, 1995). *Shared context* may be defined as awareness of some of the same aspects of the situation, and joint attention activities may be central in the acquisition and cultural shaping of this awareness. In typical language acquisition, eye gaze and deictic gestures usually play an important role as a means to establish the object or event of attention, and later this is also in combination with symbolic gestures and words or signs. Problems establishing both simple joint attention and a wider shared context may be a major obstacle to language learning.

Joint attention with more competent communication partners is a prerequisite for acquiring cultural knowledge, including language. In early language acquisition, whether typical or atypical, it is the adult partners who create *joint involvement episodes* and determine the relevance of objects, persons and actions (Schaffer, 1989). They do this by (over)interpreting the child's spontaneous expressions and using cues in the immediate setting and knowledge about the child, as well as by engaging the child in social activities in which the use of spoken language and alternative communication systems may be embedded. Adults explicitly name persons, objects and actions that are meaningful within the child's environment and the culture in general, make some language forms more pertinent than others, and embed the conversation in non-linguistic features, which may implicitly direct the child's attention towards relevant contextual aspects. They interpret whatever the child expresses within this frame, so that he or she implicitly learns the use of the language forms. The transition into language occurs when the child masters the words or signs that are used by adults to accompany routines and to refer to people, objects and actions. An essential requirement of such mastery is that the child learns to interpret the situation in which the words and signs occur in a similar manner to how an adult interprets it, i.e. the child and adult attend to some of the same aspects of the situation. A broader understanding of joint attention thus includes the participants' contextual frame which reflects their social and cultural knowledge. Children with severe language and communication disorders also bring to joint involvement episodes assumptions based on earlier linguistic and non-linguistic experiences with the same or similar people, activities and objects. As they get more communicatively and linguistically competent, these assumptions will gradually play a greater role in interactions.

This understanding of the language acquisition process implies that learning to understand and use spoken words and signs is not only a matter of mapping labels on to new or pre-established concepts, but to do so in a meaningful and contextually appropriate manner. The association between certain 'objects' or categories and, for example, manual or graphic signs is not the essence of language, but rather the fact that knowledge about such associations makes it possible to communicate about this type of object for a number of purposes. Language acquisition is often described as a process of de-contextualization, but the final result of the acquisition process is not that children become able to understand language out of context, but rather that they become able to comprehend and use the same words or signs in a variety of contexts – a culturalization process better described as *re-contextualization* (Goodwin and Duranti, 1992).

Designing the teaching situation

It is usually teachers and other professionals who define which settings, objects and actions are relevant to promoting alternative communication at pre-school or school, as well as in the home. When settings are chosen for intervention, their potential for establishing joint attention and creating communicative situations that allow for various language practices should be taken into consideration. Situations differ considerably, and knowledge about how different aspects of the situation may fulfil diverse supportive functions in language learning should also be taken into account when planning intervention. Particular settings represent opportunities for the individuals to use certain signs, and for normally speaking people to interpret them in a systematic manner and assist the disabled people in repairing the communication if they fail to make themselves understood. It should thus be possible for competent language users to direct the individual's attention towards relevant situ-ational cues, and they should themselves have sufficient cues for interpreting the individual's expressions in a consistent manner, and acknowledge whatever contribution he or she brings to the communicative setting.

It is usual to distinguish between *special training* and training in *natural situations*, also called *milieu teaching*. In special training the person who is being taught is taken out of the normal environment. Specific teaching procedures and goals have been formulated. The communication mode, the signs to be practised, the time and place for training, the people present and the material to be used are all planned in advance. When the teaching takes place in 'natural situations', it occurs in the environment in which the individual is usually found, and the teaching of specific signs is often linked to situations in which it is believed or known that the individual will have a use for them.

There is no clear dividing line between special training and training in natural situations. The degree of organization can vary considerably also when teaching takes place in the individual's normal environment. It is therefore appropriate to distinguish between *planned* and *spontaneous* teaching in natural situations. In planned teaching, a specific teaching goal has always been decided in advance. In addition to which signs or sign constructions will be taught, the time, location, material used and teacher may vary – but at least one of these has to be planned. If all aspects are planned, the only difference between planned teaching in natural situations and that in special training is that the teaching occurs in a location where the individual can usually be found. A training situation that is so meticulously planned that it significantly alters what the individual is used to can hardly be called a 'natural' situation.

Spontaneous teaching situations are characterized by minimal organization. It is generally a matter of being aware of the individual's use of specific signs, and perhaps of providing opportunities in which these signs can be used. In some cases the teaching goal – e.g. to teach the use of a specific sign – is decided beforehand, but training can also take place without this having been planned, merely because an opportunity suddenly presents itself.

At fixed times Jack is taken to a room in his nursery school that is used for individual training. Here he practises APPLE, BANANA and ORANGE. Two teachers take turns at teaching him. This is special teaching.

Three times a day Jack is allowed to choose between apple and banana or between apple and orange. The teaching takes place in the part of the nursery school where they usually eat, immediately before the normal meal. He is allowed to choose 10 small pieces of fruit so that he is not too full up before his meal. This is meticulously planned teaching in a natural environment.

Every day at 2pm, the children eat fruit in the nursery school. As Jack is learning to choose from apple, banana and orange, his teachers have made sure that the bowl of fruit contains only two types of fruit and that these two are apples and either bananas or oranges. This type of training may be regarded as one with a small degree of planning or as slightly planned spontaneous teaching.

The nursery school leaves a tray of fruit with apples, bananas and oranges on a table in the afternoon. If Jack tries to make a sign or approach someone in order to get fruit, the situation is an opportunity for him to use the signs. This is spontaneous learning.

There is no clash of interests between teaching in natural situations and that in special training. Whether one chooses to carry out teaching in specially planned situations in which the individual is not otherwise found depends on the teaching goal. An assessment of the individual's preferences, interests, needs and abilities determines this. In general, special training and teaching in natural situations occur at the same time. Planned teaching in the natural environment should be just as well prepared as special training. This implies, among other things, that specific teaching goals are formulated, and the motivation and attention of the learning individual are secured. At the same time, it is important to stress that skills learned are not automatically good or useful merely because the teaching has taken place in a normal environment. The signs that are practised should have an obvious utility value for the individual in question or for the surroundings.

In their *participation model*, Beukelman and Mirenda (1998) express concerns with regard to disabled individuals' access to and opportunity for participating in various social situations, and how the attitudes of

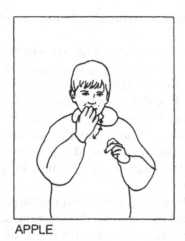

APPLE

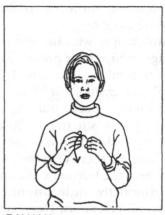

BANANA

people in the environment may be barriers to their use of existing skills. However, acquisition is not really part of the participation model. It seems to focus more on the environment's role as an aid to the individual's skills through communication partners' use of guessing and other conversational strategies, and less on the need for contextual instruction in intervention. There are barriers to access and participation and these are important to overcome, but participation does not in itself ensure optimal learning.

Planning for generalization

The ability to match a manual, graphic or tangible sign to a spoken word, or to an object or event, in a special situation may have limited value when disabled individuals need to express themselves in ordinary situations. *Generalization* of communicative skills is therefore a major objective of all interventions involving augmentative and alternative communication. Generalization means that the individual uses the signs *spontaneously* to describe new objects and events, in combinations with new words or signs, in new situations or with new people. *Spontaneous* use means that the individual uses the sign without being prompted to do so. Spontaneous use may occur in both teaching situations and new situations.

It is important to distinguish between generalization and *teaching extended use*. If the individual, having learned to use a sign in one specific situation, undergoes successful training in the use of the sign in relation to new objects and actions, combinations, situations or people, this is called extended use. The extended use is not in itself an expression of generalization, but it may be instrumental in laying the foundations for later generalization.

Many people who belong to the alternative language or supportive language groups have problems in transferring learning from the training situation to other situations. This is often called the 'problem of generalization'. For example, it is rare for autistic children who have learned to use a sign in a special training situation to begin to use this of their own accord in new situations. In addition, there are many individuals – especially in the alternative language group – who need a long time to learn. Both of these circumstances call for locating the training in situations where the learned skills are to be used.

Traditionally, little attention has been paid to generalization in language intervention. The main emphasis has been on the learning of the form itself, and it was assumed that generalization would more or less follow automatically once execution of the sign had been learned.

When language instruction is taking place in special training situations, it is essential that plans have been made in advance about how to solve the problem of transferring new skills to other situations. One of the most common methods is to include elements from those situations where the communication will be used, i.e. make the special training situation resemble the natural situation more closely. To do this effectively, it is important that before starting one has detailed knowledge of the situations to which the skills will be transferred. During planning of special training situations, it often becomes clear that it is just as expedient to start with planned teaching in the natural environment without preliminary special training. Thus, planning for the transferral of skills to natural situations ensures that special training is used only when there are strong arguments in favour of doing so.

Just as there are strategies for transferral from special training situations to natural situations, there must be strategies for making planned situ-ations less organized. During the planning of these strategies, it may also become evident that the natural situations can be accomplished with less organisation than was first assumed.

Training in extended use has also been used as a way of facilitating generalization. Less limitation of the teaching situations may lead to increased generalization. To promote the generalization to new objects, for example, it has been suggested that several different exemplars of the same class of objects should be used. This means that, when practising the sign CUP, one should use cups of different shapes, sizes and colours. Skills that are taught with only one teacher are often not transferred to other people. The generalization to new people may be facilitated if several people carry out the same teaching. Sometimes it may be sufficient for two

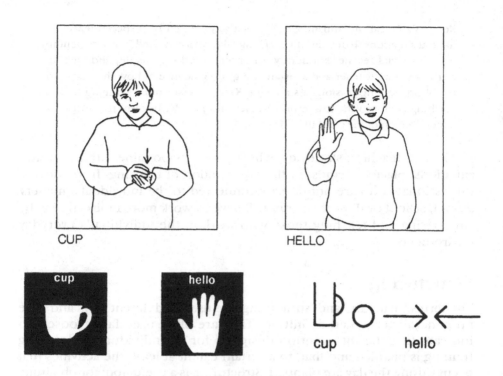

people to carry out the training so that the individual understands that the skill can be used in several different situations. Stokes, Baer and Jackson (1974), for example, trained learning-disabled children to say *hello*, but discovered that the children said *hello* only to the teacher who trained them. After two teachers began to take turns at teaching, the children began to say *hello* to the whole staff of 20 people.

Duration and location of the teaching sessions

When language and communication teaching is woven into and becomes an integral part of the ordinary activities, the duration of the teaching will dictate itself. With planned teaching in natural situations, the duration may vary, but the sessions should be short, preferably 5–10 minutes long, and be repeated several times each day. It is more important that the teaching is functional than that it be repeated many times. Special teaching situations should also be spread throughout the day. It is often practical to have individual sessions that last longer but not too long, so that the individual becomes bored or tired. Gradually, the teaching times can be varied, so that no unnecessary dependence on a particular time schedule is created.

Sometimes it is consideration for the professionals' schedule that makes teaching situations too planned or organized.

Kerry is a 5-year-old autistic girl. She is always taught by a special teacher in natural situations. However, the teaching takes place at fixed times, depending on the special teacher's itinerary. In order to reduce this dependence, the nursery school teacher and assistant are given guidance in how they can carry out short training sessions. As a result, Kerry receives more teaching and the teaching is more varied in terms of times and people. In turn, this will foster generalization of the skills that she learns.

Flexible teaching strategies, which, as far as possible, utilize natural situations, place demands on the organization of teaching. In particular, professionals who are not directly connected to the individual's nursery school, school or day-care centre will have to work more indirectly, i.e. by supervising and teaching those who work in the individual's everyday environment.

Structuring

The terms 'structure' and 'structuring' are used in different ways and have no generally accepted definition. They are often used fairly loosely to indicate that the intervention designed for an individual undergoing training is planned and that, to a certain extent at least, the activities that occur during the day are planned. Structuring is a useful tool for obtaining an overview of, and organizing, the day so that the activities play a part in promoting training in the use and understanding of language and communication. To be able to analyse the structure of a 24-hour period, it is necessary to distinguish between the various levels of structuring. In the following a distinction is made of *frame structure*, *situational structure* and *cues*.

Frame structure

Frame structure is the division into different *situations*, i.e. routines, events, activities, etc., that make up one day. Thus, a day always has a frame structure, whether or not it is planned. Producing an overview of a normal day for the learner means assessing the frame structure that exists before the intervention is implemented. An assessment of the frame structure provides a basis for obtaining a simple overview of how the activities are spread out during the course of the day, how long the different activities last and what proportion of the individual's waking day is planned. The assessment also gives information about how many of the different activities are repeated daily, and how fixed the daily itinerary is. This is basic information for the evaluation of the total intervention and the planning of language and communication teaching.

Weekdays may be more or less similar and the frame structure filled up to different degrees. The frame structure also includes the total intervention. It is therefore the total life situation and the need for teaching and function that should govern what is included in the future frame structure. An ordinary weekday should consist of teaching oriented towards the future, social intercourse, everyday routines, leisure activities and periods of relaxation.

What distinguishes a planned frame structure from a casual one is generally the range of fixed activities included in situations that are repeated at fixed intervals. The frame structure can be made more dense by filling in the periods of time in which nothing much happens in terms of new activities. A planned and dense frame structure can be a useful tool for language and communication teaching. This applies particularly to the alternative language group. For those who profit from a dense frame structure, the teaching should in principle be organized in 15-minute sessions, although some situations may last longer than this. This means that, for each 15-minute period throughout the day, a note should be made of what is going to happen, and the objective of each individual activity should be formulated. In reality the frame structure will not always be followed completely: some flexibility is needed to take into account unforeseen events and the family's need for variation.

For the expressive language group, assessment of frame structure usually has another function from that of planning the teaching. The lives of the people who belong to this group consist mostly of routines with little variation and flexibility. Daily routines, such as morning toilet and breakfast, can take a long time, and often the day consists of little other than the fixed activities. There is a lot free time and the individual is able to determine what will happen only to a limited extent. Many people with motor disorders are not very mobile and depend on a vehicle for mobility and a helper to accompany them. An assessment of the frame structure of children of school age will usually reveal a great need for help outside school hours. Such help with leisure-time activities and social intercourse with peers is often given little priority, and the result is that the children are at home for most of their leisure time. This hampers their chances of participating in social activities and developing independence and positive self-esteem.

When assessing the frame structure in the day of a disabled child, it may be a useful exercise to make a similar assessment of the frame structure in the day of a similarly aged child who lives in the same environment. A comparison of this kind will not only show the differences in their lives, but also provide ideas for activities that can be introduced for the disabled child.

Situational structure

The different situations that make up a frame structure also have their own built-in structure. This is what is called a situational structure. As the situations have varying degrees of organized content, it is possible to speak of varying degrees of structuring. In those situations with the least structuring, matters such as where the person will be, who will be present or which activities will take place are undecided. In those situations with the most structuring, everything is decided in advance and the situation also has a defined teaching goal.

A large degree of structuring will give an overview that enables one to be systematic. For those responsible for the teaching, a fixed and dense situational structure enables them to teach more effectively. The aim of the structuring is to make it easier to know what should be done in the situation, i.e. how one should react, create expectations for the individual in terms of what is going to happen, organize the communication and plan how to expand the language teaching.

Cues

Cues enable people to understand what another person is communicating. In principle, the number of possible cues is infinite, because communication may take place in so many individual ways and in different situations. In communication with people who are unable to speak, the cues that help comprehension may be activities that are carried out, objects in the surroundings, something that happens in the situation, cultural norms, knowledge about what the individual likes and usually does, etc.

> Angela is a 12-year-old girl with Rett's syndrome. When she heard her grandfather's voice from the room next door, she turned her gaze to a book. This was interpreted as a signal that she wanted her grandfather to read for her – a common occurrence. In this situation both the grandfather's voice and the fact that the girl looked at the book were cues that made such an interpretation reasonable.

In general, cues may be described in terms of people's tendency to react to behaviour as though it were communicative. It is the presence of cues to communication that makes people react to a given behaviour as though it were communication.

When cues have been described or planned in advance, they form part of the situational structure. The description of the cues to comprehension in a particular situation can thus be regarded as a third level of structuring. An assessment of the use of communication in an individual who is to learn an alternative communication form is largely an assessment of cues. In planning language and communication intervention, it may often be fruitful to ask how a teaching situation can be created by building cues into that situation. This means that, in addition to teaching the individual manual signs, for example, the situation is also arranged so that it contains elements that make the communication reasonable and understandable.

Initiating the intervention

For all children in need of augmentative and alternative communication, it is important that intervention is initiated as early as possible. The most important argument for this is that there appears to be a sensitive period for language acquisition – it is easier for children of pre-school age to learn language than it is for older children and adults. The same also applies to alternative communication.

The existence of a sensitive period is a probability for several reasons. Observations of small children show that they can quickly learn a foreign language without a trace of an accent, whereas older children and adults have difficulties in shedding their own accent. Brain damage may have different effects on language in children and adults (Taylor and Alden, 1997). For example, new-born babies who have had their left brain hemisphere removed – as is the case of Siamese twins joined together at the head – have learned to speak normally (Lenneberg, 1967). Children with a severe hearing impairment who are fitted with hearing aids so that they can perceive language sounds show fewer deviations from normal speech if they start using a hearing aid at a very early age (Fry, 1966). There are two main explanations of sensitive periods: first, that they are determined by maturational factors functioning as an independent timing device (e.g. Lenneberg, 1967; Locke, 1993) and, second, that earlier learning interferes with or makes later learning impossible (Elman et al., 1996).

Investigations of people with poorly developed language show that there appears to be an important dividing line around the age of 4–5 years in terms of speech acquisition. The proportion of people with learning disability who learn to speak does not seem to increase after this age. It is generally claimed that the chances of children developing speech are very poor if they have not begun to speak before the age of 5 years (Rutter, 1985). It should be stressed, however, that there are people who only start to speak later than this, and who have developed some speech without the use of augmentative communication. There are also examples of adolescents and adults without speech who have begun to speak later, after being taught alternative communication systems.

The effect of sign teaching on speech acquisition

The teaching of manual, graphic and tangible signs is often started at too late a stage. This is the result of a number of reasons, but the fear that teaching a child an alternative communication system may hinder the development of spoken language has been one significant reason. This fear has led people to defer augmentative and alternative communication intervention until traditional speech and language therapy has failed (e.g. Wells, 1981; Carr, 1988).

The discussion about the relationship between signs and speech has its origins in the education of deaf people, where this discussion over the last two centuries has had very emotional overtones (compare Lane, 1984). One stubborn myth has been that sign teaching can hinder the development of speech. There is no research to show that the acquisition of sign language has a negative effect on the development of speech. On the contrary, investigations show that manual signs have positive effects on speech. For example, hearing children of deaf parents develop both sign language and speech, and are thus fully bilingual (Prinz and Prinz, 1979, 1981).

A number of studies also demonstrate a positive relationship between manual and graphic sign intervention and speech. In a longitudinal study of children with Down's syndrome, Launonen (1996, 1998) found significantly more spoken words among the children who had manual sign intervention from infancy as part of the total intervention, than in a comparison group of children who had the same intervention without manual signs. Romski and Sevcik (1996) found increased speech intelligibility in learning-disabled children after the introduction of Lexigrams and communication aids with artificial voice output. According to a review by Bondy and Frost (1998), most of the 2- to 5-year-old children who were introduced to the *Picture Exchange Communication System* acquired spoken language, although this favourable result did not seem to include severely and profoundly learning-disabled children. Moreover, many communication-impaired people have undergone several years of speech and language therapy without appreciable results. Some of them have begun to speak after first learning to use manual or graphic signs (Casey, 1978; Romski, Sevcik and Pater, 1988). This gives firm support to the assumption that communication skills in different modalities influence and enhance one another.

The fact that speech and alternative forms of communication may support one another implies that alternative communication forms may be taught at an early stage without fear of negative consequences. This means that such intervention should be initiated as early as possible, i.e. as soon as the problems are apparent. In the case of children who are known to be at risk of not developing speech normally, intervention should be implemented *before* the problems become apparent, thereby preventing the negative effects of poor communication and encouraging the development of communicative skills.

Chapter 7
Teaching strategies

The need for the adaptation of intervention methods to suit individuals is universally recognized. In spite of this, many children and adults with different types of disorders receive the same type of intervention. In our opinion, the lack of a distinction between the intervention goals and the methods for individuals with different impairments poses a major problem in the field of augmentative and alternative communication. The object of this work is therefore not to give ready-made 'recipes'. Instead we wish to review the *principles* and methods of teaching alternative communication. Some of these principles and methods are based on theory, and some on our own experiences and those of others. The teaching aims and methods used should vary from individual to individual, and selection of these should be based on practical considerations. We would hope that a variety of methods is used, and that these are governed by principles and experience, adapted to the practical circumstances and in line with the total intervention.

There are various ways of teaching the use of manual, graphic and tangible signs. Most of these methods have been recognized and used for a long time. From time to time, however, new variations of recognized intervention strategies are presented, which give rise to trends and ideological debate. In this chapter, a number of different strategies are presented, some of which are very similar and some less so. The purpose of classifying the strategies is to bring out the fact that different strategies presuppose varying degrees of planning, structure and knowledge about the learner. The strategies do not preclude one another and can often be used in parallel. They have diverse strengths and weaknesses and will thus suit some disabled individuals better than others. The strategies presented in this chapter are most relevant to individuals with cognitive impairments.

Structured overinterpretation and total communication

Structured overinterpretation and structured total communication are two basic intervention strategies for people with limited language comprehension. Overinterpretation used as an intervention strategy takes advantage of what the individuals are capable of, and is based on their existing behaviours and signals. The aim of this strategy is to help severely and profoundly learning-disabled and autistic individuals to gain control over their environment through the *systematic* interpretation of behaviours as communicative by their significant others, to indicating that the intentions are related to interests, needs and preferences. Structured total communication implies the use of external means in the form of idiosyncratic or conventional manual, tangible and graphic signs. The aim is to provide individuals with possibilities for expressing their intentions. It is always a goal to move from structured overinterpretation to structured total communication as soon as possible.

Structured overinterpretation may help disabled individuals learn to express themselves if they have the potential for developing such skills. · However, for some profoundly disabled individuals, such as many girls and women with Rett's syndrome, neither overinterpretation nor other forms of intervention are likely to lead to spontaneous, self-initiated and independent communication. Even so, for both the females and their carers, systematic overinterpretation may still be of value and form a basis in the building up of an individual lifestyle. Structured overinterpretation as a *life form* may lead to a better overview of the physical and social environment, and a better understanding of what happens. For people in the environment, it may result in the accumulation of knowledge about how best to interpret the individuals and react to them in different situations. It may thus contribute to a responsive and predictable environment for the disabled individuals and, at the same time, to the establishment of a set of strategies that may be used by all significant others in their environment.

Implicit and explicit teaching

The distinction between implicit and explicit learning is fundamental in language intervention and directly related to the division of people in need of augmentative and alternative communication into three main groups (Martinsen and von Tetzchner, 1996). Implicit learning means 'that a person typically learns about the structure of a fairly complex stimulus environment, without intending to do so, in such a way that the resulting knowledge is difficult to express' (Berry and Dienes, 1993a, p. 2). Implicit teaching does not seek to make the individual aware of his or her own learning strategies. Explicit learning, on the other hand, means that the individual is aware of and able to verbalize the strategies used to acquire knowledge or skills. Explicit learning conditions imply taking a metaperspective. Thus, the skills underlying these learning forms are different.

The distinction between explicit and implicit learning conditions seems to parallel differences between strategies typically used in first and second language learning. First language learning is mainly implicit, whereas explicit teaching strategies seem to be best suited to second language learning (Berry and Dienes, 1993b; Dienes, 1993). For the expressive group, conditions often resemble second language teaching: the main focus of the intervention is the relationship between the spoken language used by communication partners, and the environment in general, and the expressive means of the disabled individual. As there is a large gap between comprehension and expression, spoken instructions may be used to explain the use of the alternative communication forms. Strategies will mainly be explicit, although they may result in implicit knowledge of language, and the application of the alternative communication system may in itself constitute an implicit learning situation. Explicit strategies attempt to utilize the asymmetry in knowledge of both speech and the alternative language form, which exists between the child and the teacher. In explicit learning, the ability to form hypotheses and follow certain strategies in problem-solving may be the most important skill.

At the other end of this dimension, the aim of the intervention for the alternative communication group is to develop a first language – a mother tongue. This necessitates implicit strategies, in which the individuals learn to change attention in accordance with the directions of others and to direct other people's attention. For people with autism, lack of attention to other people and difficulties connected with direction of attention are prominent features of their disorder. Metaphorically, implicit language learning may be described as exploration of new territories without knowing where one is going. Implicit teaching implies the use of strategies that develop skills that may increase in functional value and – for children with some comprehension of speech – make the relationships between language forms (speech and manual, tangible or graphic signs) and their use apparent to the child. This means that implicit teaching must be functional. A child belonging to the expressive group may be asked to point to the graphic sign corresponding to a particular spoken word, a strategy typical of second language teaching. The task will have little meaning for people who do not understand the spoken instruction. In spite of this, such instructions are also constantly used in intervention for people in the alternative group, although the possibility of following them may be based on skills that the individuals do not have. It may be noted, however, that, as the individual becomes more proficient in the use of an alternative communication system, this system may be utilized for explicit teaching by the teacher.

For children who belong to the supportive language group, emphasis may be on explicit or implicit teaching strategies, depending on their comprehension of spoken language and the communicative functions to be taught.

Comprehension and use of signs

In the following, a distinction is made between teaching directed at the individual's sign use and his or her comprehension of signs. In *comprehension training*, it is the conversational partners who address the learners. The individuals have to learn to understand manual, tangible or graphic signs, and either answer what has been expressed or perform an activity to show that they have understood. It is the conversational partners who point at graphic or tangible signs, or perform manual signs.

In the early stages of learning, most of the signs taught as part of comprehension training will be signal signs or command signs (Table 4). *Signal signs* indicate subsequent activities and events, and are used to give information to the learner. Signal signs may be performed by the teacher using either the individual's hands or the teacher's own hands to perform the manual sign or point at a graphic or tangible sign.

Table 4. *Three different uses of signs in intervention*

Signal signs
These signs are used to inform the disabled individual about subsequent activities and events. Manual signal signs are performed by the teacher with the individual's hands. If possible, the individual is helped to indicate a graphic. If this is not possible, the graphic sign is presented by the teacher. Tangible signs may be shown or given to the learner

Command signs
These signs are used by people in the environment to control the disabled person, to get the learner either to carry out an activity or to stop one. Command signs are pointed at or performed by the conversational partner

Expressive signs
These signs are produced by the individuals when they address another person as a means of achieving a particular goal, informing about a specific event, commenting on an activity, etc. During the teaching, the individual may be given help to perform manual signs or point at graphic and tangible signs, but only where necessary

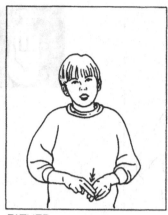
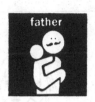

FATHER

Philip is 23 years old and learning-disabled. He lives in a community unit, where his father usually visits him on Saturdays. Before his father enters his room, one of the staff members makes the sign FATHER while simultaneously saying the word *father*.

The aim of teaching signal signs is to be able to inform disabled people, to help them say to themselves what will happen. FINISHED is a useful sign to tell that an activity or event is over.

Command signs are signs used by the conversational partner to get the learner either to carry out an activity or to stop one. These signs are pointed at or performed by the conversational partner. WAIT may be a particularly useful command sign.

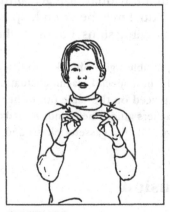

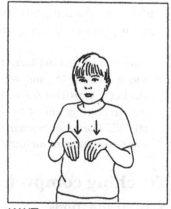

FINISHED   WAIT

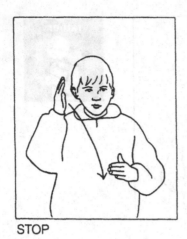

STOP

> David is an autistic boy aged 7 years. He can stand for long periods of time
> switching the light on and off. His teacher uses the sign STOP while saying *stop*
> emphatically in order to make David refrain from what he is doing.

The aim in teaching command signs is to control the person. The aim is
not for the individual to learn to use command signs, although they may also
prove functional for him or her. Signal signs and commands are not taught
expressively, but are seldomly used spontaneously by the individuals.

Expressive signs are manual, tangible and graphic signs, which are
indicated or made by the individuals when they address another person as
a means of achieving a particular goal, informing about a specific event,
commenting on an activity, etc. *Training use* implies the teaching of the
sign's functional use and to get the individual to initiate communication
with the conversational partner. The conversational partner must understand the signs and answer the individual or react to them appropriately.
During the teaching, the individual may be given help to perform manual
signs or point at graphic and tangible signs, but only where necessary.

> Mary is a 14-year-old learning-disabled girl. She likes to listen to dance music
> and is learning the sign MUSIC in a special teaching situation. There are two
> teachers. A cassette player is placed on the table out of her reach. When she
> tries to reach it, one of the teachers guides her hands to make the manual sign
> MUSIC. The other teacher gives her the cassette player and she is allowed to
> listen to one dance melody.

Teaching comprehension

Natural situations

Many individuals with profound language and communication disorders
have no overview of what their day will contain in terms of activities and

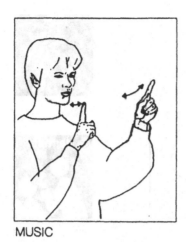

MUSIC

events. They are often taken passively from one activity to another by a teacher without being told what is going to happen. Nor do they take the initiative in starting an activity or showing whether or not they like what has been planned for them. Their reaction to this feeling of uncertainty about what is happening often results in anxiety or fear; they become passive or inactive or resist when someone wants them to take part in something new.

> Martin is a 3-year-old boy with autism. Every time he has to change activity in his nursery school and go to another room he lies down on the floor, kicking his legs and crying. It takes a long time to quieten him down. His day at nursery school is marked by these problems (Steindal K, personal communication, 1990).

One of the primary objectives of communication intervention with individuals who are unable to decide for themselves what they are going to do is that they should at the very least be told *what* is going to happen. One way of achieving this is to design a tight frame structure in which activities occur in the same place, at the same time and in the same order, and where routine activities are signalled with the help of signal signs. This approach may be called *signal-controlled frame structuring*.

Signal-controlled frame structuring is a form of comprehension training. The aim is that the individual will learn that the signs precede specific activities and events, i.e. that they function as signals. The signs are chosen so that they are easy for the learner to recognize, and they should be presented immediately before the activity begins. It is also useful if a signal sign is used to indicate when the activity is finished. In principle, signal signs may be anything: conventional manual signs performed with the individual's hands, graphic signs, objects that are used in the activities, etc. Using manual or graphic signs is the best

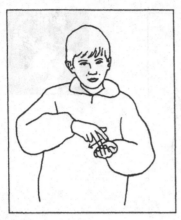

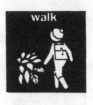

WALK

strategy because this will simultaneously lead to the acquisition of a communication system, but early signal signs are often objects that symbolize different activities. These signs may signal both positive and negative events.

John is a 10-year-old learning disabled boy who seems to like being taken out for walks in his wheelchair. Before he is taken out, he is guided to make the manual sign *WALK*.

Marie is a 17-year-old learning-disabled girl. She has very bad teeth and is often at the dentist. Before she visits the dentist, who is situated in the building next door, she is guided to indicate the PIC sign DENTIST.

Like many other people, Marie is afraid of visiting her dentist. If she is informed where she is going before each visit to the dentist, she will not be afraid of walking in the direction of the dentist's surgery on occasions when she is not going to visit the dentist. As she gradually begins to understand what the sign signals, she will begin to protest when a member of staff indicates DENTIST, but she will nevertheless go along – albeit reluctantly.

The clearest indication that a sign has begun to have a signal function is that the individual begins to anticipate what is going to happen. Among individuals with the most severe forms of impairment, this may manifest itself in the individual straightening up, becoming more excited or showing increased muscle tone when the sign is presented. Gradually, the person may perhaps start to look in the direction of or move towards the place where the activity takes place, or where specific things are kept. Such reactions are not only visible when, for example, signs in the form of

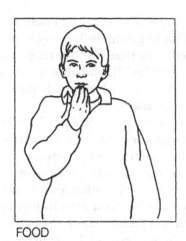
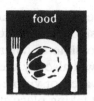

FOOD

objects have been included intentionally, but may also be indicators of the individual's comprehension of natural markers in daily routines.

When teaching signal signs, it is of vital importance that they are presented immediately before the activities. If too much time passes between presentation of the signal and the activity taking place, distracting events may interfere and make it difficult for the individual to understand the relationship between the signs and the activities that they signal.

> Hannah is a learning-disabled girl aged 7 years. She is led by the hand to feel her bathing costume as a signal that she is going swimming. She is then dressed, led to the bus stop, waits 15 minutes for the bus, sits on the bus for 20 minutes, walks for 5 minutes, goes to the changing room, undresses, puts on her bathing costume and finally goes swimming.

Using signs in the manner indicated above is unsuitable in the early stages of intervention. It may be difficult to understand that the bathing costume signals a visit to the swimming pool and not one of the activities that always occurs beforehand.

When teaching the significance of signal signs, it is also important that they are not presented at too late a stage. For example, it is not very useful to use the sign FOOD to inform individuals that they are going to eat when they are already seated at the table. The sign is redundant, and thus meaningless, because it does not signal a change in the situation. The fact that they are going to eat has already been conveyed through a large number of natural markers: the food is on the table, there is a smell of food, they are wearing bibs, etc. The sign should be performed before they enter the room or, at the very least, before they are seated at the table.

Once the signal sign has been learned, the interval between presentation of the sign and the situation should gradually be lengthened, so that it becomes possible to talk about activities that will not take place immediately. This will also lay the foundation for the individual either to ask for things that are not visible or to express a wish to participate in activities that are not taking place at the time of asking.

Signal-controlled frame structuring may be combined with the use of a timetable with pictures or graphic signs or a *day box* with rows containing objects, as is common in structured total communication. However, the signal signs and the fixed order of the various activities are the crucial elements in the intervention. These must be understood in the context of the particular situation before they can be presented independently of it. Reviewing signs for the day's activities before the individuals can clearly demonstrate an understanding of what they signal may make it more difficult for them to learn the signal function of these signs.

Structuring is a means to the learning of communication, but communication and structure should not be confounded. The use of signal signs in order to provide the individuals with a better understanding of their own environment is not dependent on frame structuring. Manual, graphic and tangible signs may be used to signal activities and events, even though the events do not occur daily or at the same time on every occasion. They may be used with all activities and events that are repeated often enough, so that it may be a reasonable assumption that the individuals will be able to understand the signs. Using signal signs in daily routines or in other situations in which the same activities or events occur in the same order is especially useful, because the fixed order and use of signal signs have a mutually enhancing effect. The signal signs facilitate the individual's understanding of the situation, and an understanding of the situation facilitates understanding of the signs.

In environments where use and comprehension of manual signs are taught, it is usual to use signal signs also outside the planned situations. This is more unusual when graphic and tangible signs are used. These signs should also be used so that the individuals have the possibility to learn from non-planned comprehension experiences, if they are able to do so. In cases where the individuals need to learn that a sign corresponds to a specific spoken word, the graphic signs should be used in conjunction with speech whenever this is practical. In this way, the individual's comprehension (and possibly use) of the sign and the word may be associated with several situations. For people with a poor understanding of spoken language, the simultaneous use of signs and speech may also make it easier for them to understand the words that are being spoken.

Special training

Comprehension training in special teaching situations can be classified according to the person performing the sign – the individual or the teacher. When teaching manual sign comprehension, the teacher generally displays a picture or points at an object, and the person has to perform the manual sign that corresponds to that picture or object. When teaching tangible or graphic sign comprehension the individual has to point at the sign. This is the equivalent of naming. However, the most common form of comprehension training is where the teacher performs a manual sign or points at a tangible or graphic sign. The learner has to point to the corresponding object or picture, pick it up or perform an activity. The teacher points at or performs the sign, and simultaneously says the word that corresponds to it. In this type of comprehension training, the individual generally has to choose among several objects or pictures. The positioning of the pictures or objects should vary, so that the individual does not merely learn to pick up the object or point at the picture that occupies one particular position.

> Dan is a 15-year-old learning-disabled boy. A ball and a spoon are placed in front of him on a table. The teacher says *ball* while performing the sign BALL. Dan gives the ball to the teacher (Booth, 1978).

Comprehension training in which the teacher uses the signs and the individual points at an object is less common in tangible and graphic sign teaching than it is in manual sign teaching. This is partly because manual signs must be performed each time they are used whereas the other signs are present the whole time. The teacher becomes used to performing

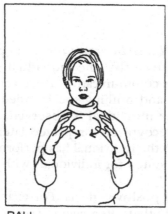

BALL

manual signs, but not to pointing at tangible and graphic signs. The main reason, however, is probably that many tangible signs are object models and graphic signs are stylized drawings, and the teacher seems to assume that the individuals understand them immediately.

There appears – with the exception of signal signs – to be no tradition of teaching comprehension of graphic and tangible signs. This is probably related to the fact that Blissymbolics was the first graphic system to be adopted. Many of the individuals who were first taught to use Blissymbols had a good understanding of spoken language (compare Vanderheiden et al., 1975). They needed to be taught which spoken word a specific sign corresponded to. The most simple and efficient way of teaching sign comprehension to such a group is for the teacher to say the words that the graphic signs correspond to without having to find objects or pictures that they may be used to referring to or describing. Comprehension training in which the learner has to touch or in some other way indicate objects or pictures is best suited for individuals belonging to the alternative language group and the supportive language group. For those who belong to the expressive language group and who have a good understanding of spoken language, a more appropriate approach is first to explain in speech the signs that are to be learned, and then perhaps check how well the signs are remembered by asking the individual to translate the words that the teacher has said into graphic or manual signs.

Teaching sign use

There are many ways of training the use of signs, and they may be classified in different ways. Most of them may be used in both special training and natural environments.

Watch, wait and react

This strategy is part of *structured overinterpretation*. Its purpose is to transform to signs the casual activity that the individual produced by reacting as though that activity was communicative. The teaching may take place in unstructured situations, and nothing special needs be done to encourage specific activities. The individual is observed. As soon as a movement is made that may be recognized if repeated later, the teacher reacts to this movement as though the individual has performed a specific manual sign. This method is best suited for individuals with a low degree of self-initiated activity.

The strategy may have several positive effects. For example, there is reason to believe that the passivity that often characterizes children with poor language and communication skills is related to the fact that they display behaviour that causes reaction from others less than other children (Ryan, 1977). The watch, wait and react strategy increases the chances of an individual's activities causing a reaction, which will probably stimulate the level of activity and initiative to communicate. The objective of this strategy is that the teacher's reactions to the individual's casual activity should have a spiralling effect, with the reactions causing new activities on the part of the individual. This will improve the learning opportunities for individuals with severely impaired communication skills. The new activities may then in turn be ascribed a similar sign function. In this way, a positive spiral of development is started. For this to happen, it is best that the activities that the teacher reacts to are, to start with, expressions indicating that the individual is attentive and motivated. This also increases the likelihood of the individual becoming aware of the interrelationship of what is happening in the situation, his or her own activities, and the reactions of people in the surroundings.

> Harold is a 4-year-old learning-disabled boy. He is passive and shows very little self-initiated activity. He likes to be lifted up and played with roughly. Sometimes he beats his breast. It is decided that this should be 'interpreted' by his parents and the nursery school staff as 'I want to play'. Each time he beats his breast, he is lifted up and played with.

The watch, wait and react strategy has clear limitations. The person who administers the intervention has little control over when a selected casual activity will occur, and can run the risk of having to wait for a long time before it is repeated. It is crucial that the individual is attentive and that the reactions manage to catch the individual's interest. One may secure these conditions to a certain extent by beginning with an activity that occurs relatively often and basing the sign's 'content' on information about the learner's interests.

Reacting to habitual behaviour

This strategy is most suitable for individuals who have some degree of self-initiated activity, but where that activity is not functional. For example, reacting to habitual behaviour is a strategy that suits children and adults who, when left to their own devices, wander aimlessly around a room, kick walls and furniture, hit a table if they pass one by, or pull objects down from shelves. The strategy is based on knowing what the individual is interested in and what he or she will do in a given situation. The objective is to make a non-functional activity communicative and socially acceptable. To achieve this, one must produce an intervention situation in which it is possible to trigger off the activity and utilize it for sign teaching.

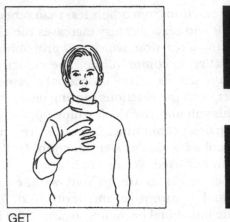
GET

Andrew is an 8-year-old boy with autism. He has a tendency to empty any handbags he can get his hands on. He is placed in a room in which a person is sitting with a handbag, and where nothing special is happening. The teacher follows him as he walks around the room. As soon as he reaches for the bag, he is held back by his teacher who forms the manual sign HANDBAG with his hands. He is then given the bag by the person who is sitting there.

Alternatively, Andrew could have been taught to use a general sign such as GET or GIVE, depending on what the teacher thought was most useful at the present stage of the intervention.

The purpose of this strategy is to give habitual behaviour that has previously been non-functional a sign function by systematically reacting to the behaviour as though it was communicative. This strategy is based on the learners relating their own activity to the reactions of the communication partner. For the strategy to succeed, it is therefore essential that the individuals pay attention to both their own behaviour and the reaction of the teacher, so that they will want the reaction to be repeated.

Many individuals with autism and learning disability show behaviour problems. When using the strategy of reacting to habitual behaviour, what is generally regarded as problem behaviour may be taken as a starting point and exploited to the individual's advantage. As the behaviour is replaced by a sign and given a positive function, the sign teaching may lead to a reduction in the problematic behaviour. An advantage with this strategy is that the teacher will be able to decide the time of the teaching by planning a situation in which the behaviour occurs habitually. This provides the teacher with control over the sign teaching which, among other things, will ensure a sufficient number of repetitions.

Build-and-break chains

This strategy is based on constructing a chain of activities that the individual is motivated to carry out, and then obstructing the chain so that it is impossible to complete it without help. When the individual shows confusion or frustration, he or she is guided to produce a manual sign or to point at a tangible or graphic sign. The teacher then provides the individual with a possibility to continue the behaviour chain. This strategy can be utilized among individuals with varying levels of activity, and is especially suitable for people who need to learn to do things on their own initiative.

Both learned activity chains and naturally occurring chains (routines) may be used as a basis for the build-and-break chain strategy, providing that the individual is sufficiently well motivated in the situation. The chains need not be long.

> Carl is a 10-year-old boy with autism. He has learned to complete a simple jigsaw puzzle when the pieces are placed from left to right. Carl has learned to take the correct piece of puzzle. The chain is broken by placing the pieces out of his reach, so that Carl needs help to get hold of them. There are two teachers. One is behind Carl and helps, while the other sits in front of him and tends to the pieces. As soon as Carl discovers he is missing one of the pieces of the jigsaw puzzle (preferably not the first piece), he reaches for it without getting hold of it and looks at the teacher sitting in front of him. The helper guides his hands to perform the sign PIECE. Then the other teacher gives him the piece of jigsaw puzzle that he needs.

It is essential that the individual is motivated to carry out the chain before it is broken for the purpose of sign teaching. This is not always an easy task. One way of ensuring the individual's motivation is to begin by

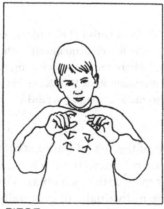

PIECE

breaking the chain when the last link in the chain precedes something that the individual wishes to do. For example, for someone who is fond of going for a drive, the fixed routine of getting dressed before going for a drive can be interrupted. Sometimes humour and surprise can be used to break the chain.

The build-and-break chain strategy involves frustrating the learner. Frustration works because a need for communication arises and may make it clear to the individual that using signs can be useful. It is vital that the frustration that the individual is subjected to – in the eyes of the learner – appears to be the result of situational circumstances; it should not appear to be produced by the conversational partner, who should act as a helper. Otherwise, the individual may be confused about the role of the partner, and may react as if teased or punished without a reason.

Reacting to signal-triggered anticipatory behaviour

The strategy of reacting to signal-triggered anticipatory behaviour assumes that the teacher has constructed a frame structure in which known activities or events occur in a specific order, and where the activities or events have a precursory sign. When the individuals begin to demonstrate that they understand what is going to happen, the anticipatory reaction that they show may be used in the teaching of new signs. If the anticipatory reaction is appropriate, it may be used as a sign, or the individual's hands can be guided to form a manual sign or to point to a tangible or graphic sign immediately after the anticipatory reaction.

The strategy assumes that the activity or event that the individual has anticipated will follow naturally once the individual has reacted. In practical terms, this means that a chain is produced by placing a sign between the links. The chain will end with the activity indicated by the sign.

> Elaine is a 19-year-old girl with autism. She enjoys basket-weaving. This activity is signalled with WORK. She is well acquainted with this situation and looks in the direction of the shelf where the basket-weaving materials are kept when the teacher says *work* and manually signs WORK. As Elaine looks towards the shelf, her hands are formed to make the sign MATERIAL and the materials she needs are then fetched.

This is one example of the use of frame structure, where a manual sign is used to signal a group of activities. These may be various activities pertaining to 'work' or gymnastics, which are often suitable for producing a situation in which the individual will gradually learn to choose between different activities with the help of signs.

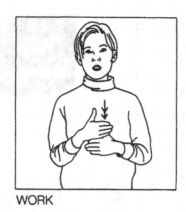

WORK

If the individuals display signal-triggered anticipatory behaviour, several of the basic conditions that are essential to the success of the teaching are already present. They are attentive, motivated and have an understanding of what the situation entails. This makes it easier for them to learn to understand and begin using the sign. In addition, the teacher has control in advance over what is going to happen, and is able to use the structuring as a tool with which to encourage activity in the individuals if their behavioural repertoire is limited.

Fulfilling wants

This is the most commonly used strategy. It may be used in both natural and special training situations, and is a strategy that may be used with all the three main groups. For the supportive language group and the alternative language groups, it is an instrument with which to teach the individuals that they can achieve something by using language. For the expressive language group, the strategy is expedient for unlearning learned helplessness, and showing individuals that they can achieve a particular goal by using signs. The same strategy can thus have different objectives.

When fulfilling the desire of individuals to carry out a particular activity, their likes and interests should be borne in mind and used as a starting point. The teacher should create a situation that makes the individuals want to carry out the activity, and mould their hands to make the manual sign or point at the graphic or tangible sign, and then let them perform the activity that they want. Similarly, the teacher fulfils an individual's wish for a particular thing by using an object that he or she knows the person wants. This may be an object that the individual likes to do something with or play with, an item of food or drink, etc. The teacher waits until the individual shows, in one way or another, that the particular object is wanted, guides his or her hands to form the sign or point at a tangible or graphic sign, and then provides the object.

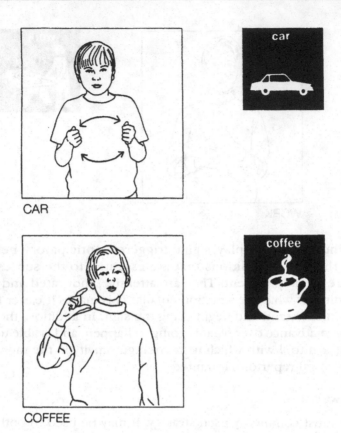

CAR

car

COFFEE

coffee

Henry is a 7-year-old autistic boy. He likes to crank the ladder on his toy fire-engine up and down. The teacher walks together with Henry and makes sure that they pass the fire-engine. When Henry clearly looks at the fire-engine, stops or reaches for it, the teacher moulds his hands to perform the sign CAR, where-upon Henry is given the fire-engine.

Elaine is a 43-year-old multiply impaired woman, who is dependent on a wheel-chair. She is fond of coffee, which she drinks with a straw, but she never herself takes the initiative to get coffee. She can press the keys on a communication aid with digitized speech output. The teacher has recorded the word coffee on her talking aid and placed the PIC sign *COFFEE* on a key that she can press. The teacher sits close by Elaine with two cups and a coffee pot. When Elaine looks at the teacher, she approaches her and helps Elaine to press the key with *COFFEE*. The machine says '*coffee*' and the teacher pours Elaine a cup.

Although many individuals with limited comprehension of spoken language who are taught manual, graphic or tangible signs generally perform few activities and appear to like few things, this is not the only reason why these same things and activities are repeated. Those who plan the teaching often show little imagination and creativity. There are, after all, many areas from which to chose. There are toys and games, household objects, food, sweets, fruit, clothes and shoes, cassette players, television and radio, cuddling, gymnastics, outdoor activities, etc. Physical activity may be DANCE. Looking at a MAGAZINE is enjoyable. In northern Norway, for example, REINDEER may be a useful animal sign. It is also easy to overlook the fact that preferences and interests change as the individual becomes older and learns new skills. It is not only the overall activity that needs a sign. A craft session may include DRAW, PAPER, CUT and GLUE.

Sometimes the objects indicated by the signs being taught are too easily available in the environment. An open shelf located high up on the wall may be practical. As the shelf is open, any objects placed there are visible, which may help the individual to remember them and have a wish to get hold of them. As a result of the fact that the shelf is placed high up on the wall, the individuals are unable to reach the object on their own, and this provides them with the opportunity of approaching another person for help. The aim of this strategy is not to make it difficult to get something,

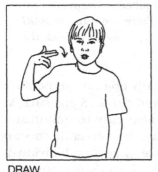

DRAW

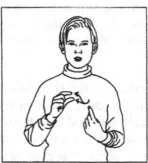

PAPER

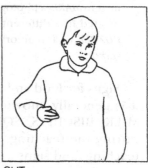

CUT

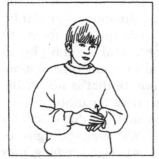

GLUE

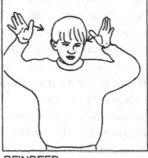

REINDEER

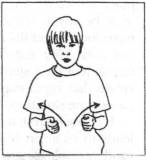

MAGAZINE

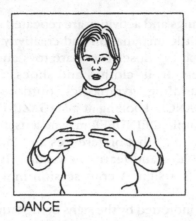

DANCE

but to help the person understand that an object out of reach, even out of sight, may be obtainable with signs.

> Mari is a 6-year-old girl with autism and profound learning disability. Her communication aid is a miniature doll's suitcase that contains about 20 strips with four photographs and PIC signs each. She is doing various activities together with a teacher in the main room of the pre-school. She puts *PUZZLE* next to *MARI* (a photograph of herself) in the lid of the suitcase. The puzzles are located in a different room. Mari and the teacher therefore transfer *MARI PUZZLE* to a 'memory strip' and bring this along when they go to fetch the puzzle.

Signs for food and drink are often chosen as early object signs because it is generally known what people like to eat and drink. Signs such as MILK, BISCUITS, SQUASH and SAUSAGE are also easy to administer during the teaching. However, it may not always be advisable to start teaching food signs at meal times. It is easy to take away from individuals communication skills that they already possess and ruin a pleasant situation at the same time. Instead, the sign teaching can be carried out in the place where the meals are usually served, but a short while before the meal begins. Once the signs are mastered in this situation, they can be introduced carefully during real meals. One way to do this is to 'forget' to put something that the individual likes on the table, and use this ploy to implement food signs in natural situations, and at the same time demonstrate that signs may be used for getting something that is not in the immediate situation, i.e. they may be tools to improve a situation.

It is essential that sign use does not become a ritual, but that it actually leads to an improved situation for the individual. Although the signs for food or drink are often well suited to the first stages of sign teaching, they are occasionally unsuitable because they do not lead to increased

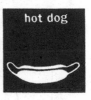

draw | dance | milk | squash | hot dog

functional communication. If a boy already has a means of expressing clearly to the people around him that he wants orange juice – by smacking his lips, for example – and expects to be given orange juice when he does so, the purpose of using a conventional sign to achieve the same thing may be unclear to him. He would have to be taught not to smack his lips before he could be taught to use the sign JUICE. In such instances, learning signs to express things that the individual is already capable of communicating in other ways may lead to a confusion about their purpose, and it will be more expedient to begin with teaching other signs.

Some motor-impaired children have difficulty chewing and swallowing, and eating is therefore an activity that they do reluctantly. In such cases, choosing between different types of food is not a suitable teaching strategy. On the other hand, it can be advantageous for children to achieve improved control over meals in terms of when the next bite of food will be consumed and when they want to drink (Morris, 1981).

Focusing on expression and comprehension

The objective of teaching alternative communication is to provide individuals with better means to express themselves and to understand what other people are communicating. In expressive training, the individuals are taught to express themselves to others. In comprehension training, they are taught to understand what other people are communicating to them.

In reality, most language and communication intervention consists of both comprehension teaching and expressive teaching. However, there are both theoretical and practical arguments for giving priority to either comprehension or expressive use in the first stages of teaching. Among other things, the theoretical arguments stem from different views on the relationship between language and cognition in human development. Those who give priority to comprehension training base their arguments on the theory that children must first acquire concepts before they can learn words or signs. From this point of view, it is natural to begin with concept training and assume that the signs will be used once the concepts have been understood. It has generally been assumed that comprehension always precedes use in language development, but nowadays it has become more common to hold that expressive use and comprehension

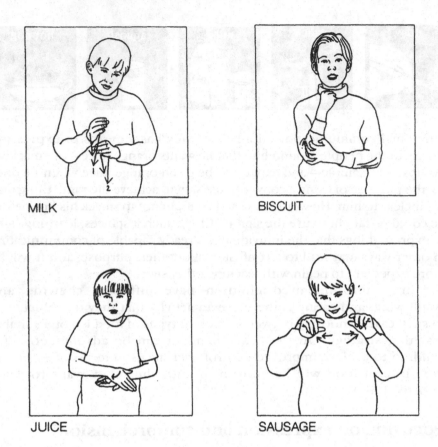

MILK   BISCUIT

JUICE   SAUSAGE

developed simultaneously complement one another. Sometimes individuals' use of a sign or word will be more advanced than their comprehension of that same sign or word; at other times comprehension is acquired first (Clark, 1982; Bates, Bretherton and Snyder, 1988). A developmental order of concepts and words may vary, and children can learn concepts by using words or signs.

In instances where it is necessary to give priority to one or other form of teaching, it is, in our opinion, most productive to give emphasis to expressive teaching. There are several reasons for this. There is no clear relationship between individuals' understanding of how other people use a sign and their beginning to use that sign for themselves in the same way, whereas teaching use of signs also implies training in what the sign means. When others react to the signs used by individuals, these reactions will, over time, make it possible for the individuals to understand how the signs are used. It is therefore more likely that expressive teaching will lead to comprehension than that comprehension teaching will lead to expressive use.

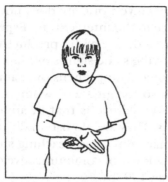

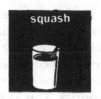

JUICE/SQUASH

In traditional intervention with children who have delayed language development, comprehension training does not lead to improved use (Leonard, 1981). Autistic children who had been taught expressive use both understood and used manual signs better than autistic children who had been taught comprehension (Watters, Wheeler and Watters, 1981).

In a study of children with Down's syndrome, Romski and Ruder (1984) found that simultaneous use of manual signs and speech did not produce better results than teaching in which only speech was used. This finding is rather unusual because the use of supportive signs among this group has generally produced very good results (compare, for example, Kotkin, Simpson and Desanto, 1978; le Prevost, 1983; Johansson, 1987; Launonen, 1996, 1998). What distinguishes this study from others in terms of method is that *the children themselves did not use signs*. It was the teacher who used simultaneous signs and speech, or speech alone. This study gives support to the assumption that motor performance plays a role in the acquisition of manual signs, and it emphasizes how important it is that the individuals produce the signs themselves.

Another significant reason for giving priority to expression instead of comprehension in intervention is that expressive training directly teaches individuals to influence their surroundings. In comprehension training, it is the teacher who takes the initiative, whereas the language-impaired individual provides the teacher with answers or carries out instructions. Expressive training shifts the communicative initiative to the individual. A lack of communicative initiative is one of the most fundamental problems among individuals with extensive language disorders. By teaching these individuals expressive use, there is greater reason to hope that communicative initiative on their part will be encouraged. A focus on expressive teaching is also supported by the emphasis that developmental psychology puts on the active role of learners in knowledge acquisition (e.g. Nelson, 1996).

The fact that expressive teaching is given priority does not mean that comprehension teaching has no place in the intervention. Especially once a good deal of signs have been learned, it may be productive to teach expressive use and comprehension of the same signs simultaneously.

For some groups of disabled people, comprehension training should be given priority. This is especially so for girls and women with Rett's syndrome, whose most characteristic feature is that of apraxia, i.e. an inability to perform voluntary actions. They are almost totally incapable of expressing themselves, and the primary aim of the teaching should therefore be to increase the girls' understanding of communicative expressions and everyday activities (von Tetzchner, 1997b).

Nor does an emphasis on expressive training imply that comprehension is of no significance when choosing signs. It is quicker for individuals to learn to use signs that correspond to known spoken words than it is to learn signs corresponding to unknown words (Clarke, Remington and Light, 1986). An understanding of some of the relevant aspects of the situation – a shared context – will also facilitate sign acquisition. There are examples showing that, in the early stages of normal language development, children use words in familiar situations. For example, Bloom's daughter used *car* only about the cars she saw from the window (Bloom, 1973). In terms of sign or speech teaching, it is similarly easiest to start learning signs or words in known situations, where the individuals have some cues to the possible function of the signs or words.

Incidental teaching

'Incidental teaching' is the term used to describe a situation in which the teaching or subject matter has not been decided on in advance. However, this does not mean that the situation is not planned. The teacher may know that the individual is interested in a specific activity and has planned that he or she should learn the sign for this activity, without setting the time for when the teaching should take place. Sometimes incidental teaching can take place without the teacher knowing what the individual is interested in. If a situation is created in which it is likely that the individual will want something, and the teacher then waits for the expression of interest in an unstructured situation, the incidental teaching will correspond to the *watch, wait and react* strategy.

Eric is a 6-year-old autistic boy. He stands in front of a cupboard and performs all the manual signs he knows. When the cupboard is opened he reaches out for a model air plane in the cupboard. His hand is quickly guided to make the manual sign AEROPLANE, and Eric is given the aeroplane.

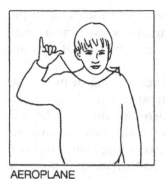
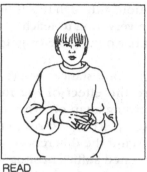
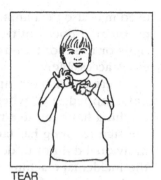

AEROPLANE   READ   TEAR

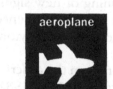

Claire is a 12-year-old learning-disabled girl. She holds a book in her hand and stands looking at her teacher. Her hand is guided to make the manual sign READ. Claire is then allowed to sit on the teacher's lap while the teacher reads for her.

Betty is an 8-year-old multiply impaired girl. She sits in a wheelchair. During morning assembly at nursery school she looks intently at the pages of the large calendar that one of the children is allowed to tear off. The assistant fetches the PIC sign *TEAR*, puts it together with the other PIC signs on the tray attached to the wheelchair and guides Betty to point to it. The calendar is taken to Betty and, with help from the assistant, she tears off the page.

The advantages of incidental teaching are that it provides more teaching situations, and that the teaching takes place in situations in which the individual is motivated and has a use for the sign. Incidental teaching may be used with both new signs and signs that are being practised, depending on the situation. However, this is conditional on signs being easily accessible, i.e. that the person in charge of the incidental teaching knows the manual signs that are needed, and that both trained and untrained tangible or graphic signs are available in all situations.

Professionals often have reservations about teaching signs that are not a part of the planned programme. They are afraid that the situation will be too difficult for the individuals to grasp and that they may find it confusing. The teacher's own knowledge of the communication system used may also be a limitation, although this is not usually the cause of the problem. It does not take very long to teach someone a few new manual signs or to set out a number of tangible or graphic signs so that they are easily accessible.

There are also examples of instances where the learning of new signs has stopped, and where the effect of the introduction of incidental teaching has been like turning a tap on. The reason for this *may* be that the sign teaching has taken place in too restricted a situation, so that the individual did not understand the difference between the signs, and that the incidental teaching created sufficient situational variation. It may also be the case that the teaching situation itself had become monotonous and ritualistic, and thus no longer contributed to the learning of new signs. Unexpected events have been demonstrated to have a positive influence on children's attempts to communicate (McClenny, Roberts and Layton, 1992).

This presentation of incidental teaching differs in part from the descriptions that are given in a number of other contexts (Oliver and Halle, 1982; Carr, 1985). The main difference is that, for us, incidental teaching has as its aim that *the communication should be successful.* In much of the literature, incidental teaching is regarded as *an opportunity to establish a teaching situation.* Despite the fact that the teaching begins on a communicative initiative from the individual, the language goals are decided on in advance (Warren and Kaiser, 1986; Hamilton and Snell, 1993). The teacher also uses methods employed in special training, such as prompting, imitation, etc., and thus interrupts the communication. The approach seems to be founded mainly on the environment's function in terms of people being available to provide reward and feedback to children imitating and performing other forms of structured training, and to interpret and formulate in spoken language the non-vocal messages produced by the children. Although basic mechanisms of learning, such as classic and operant conditioning, may be important constituents when designing language intervention for people with profound learning disability and language impairment, restricting the theoretical basis of intervention only to this technology may hinder professionals in taking advantage of contributions of other elements of the language learning context. For people who are less cognitively and linguistically impaired, this conditioning is not likely to be the central intervention strategy.

Structured waiting

As a way of making life easier for disabled people, many parents and professionals anticipate their needs and give them what they require.

However, by doing this they may also remove one aspect of the situation that makes communication useful. The result may be that the individuals are not given the opportunity of taking the initiative in situations where this would otherwise have been natural. This may create a form of learned passivity. To increase the probability that the individuals themselves will initiate communication, structured waiting can be introduced in natural teaching situations and in incidental teaching when one believes that the individual will use a *known* sign. This implies that the teacher or communication partner waits a little while before taking the turn, making prompts or giving the individual help to perform or indicate a sign. It is usual to begin with a very short interval and gradually increase the time to about 10 seconds. It is possible to wait even longer, but longer periods of waiting seldom seem to lead to self-initiation among people without motor impairments (Oliver and Halle, 1982; Foxx et al., 1988). Among motor-impaired individuals who have difficulty in pointing or performing manual signs, it may be necessary to wait longer (compare Light, 1985).

> Jay is a 7-year-old boy with learning disability. He was taken to the changing room to change clothes before exercising. He needed help with the button on his trousers. The teacher held her finger on the button but waited 10 seconds before Jay, on the occasions he needed it, was given help in performing the manual sign HELP.
> Jay used to push a scooter together with his physiotherapist as a means of training his arm muscles. The physiotherapist would stop and wait 10 seconds for Jay to perform the manual sign PUSH before she helps him to perform the sign (Oliver and Halle, 1982).

By waiting, the chances that the individuals will take the initiative in a communicative situation are increased. This may make them more active and decrease their learned passivity. It has also been shown that the time it takes to learn new signs is reduced if structured waiting is included as part of the teaching strategy (Bennet et al., 1986).

Structured waiting can also be very important for people with motor impairments who belong to the expressive language group, but for a different reason. The motor impairment means that they spend longer both answering and taking the initiative. For their communication not only to be responsive but also to have initiative, the communication partner must give them sufficient time. Learning-disabled people who belong to one of the other main groups can also be slow and take time responding and showing initiative. Thus, structured waiting has a double function: it creates a need for communication and places restrictions on the communication partners, so that they become more aware that they

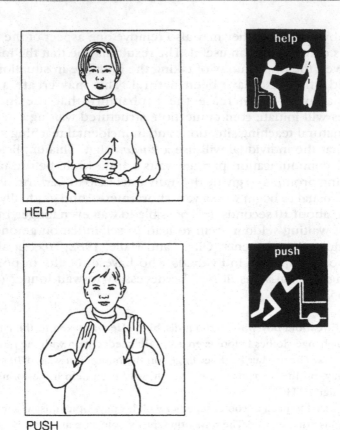

HELP

PUSH

should not give help unless it is absolutely necessary. Intentional postponement of help may be used even with small children (compare Light, 1985).

Naming

Naming contains elements of both comprehension and use. Giving names to objects and events is a normal linguistic activity, which is found in the very early stages of language acquisition, often in situations where children and parents look at a book or toys together. In intervention involving alternative communication systems, naming is typically used to teach the individual the name of objects and pictures, not to use them. The teaching usually takes place in special teaching situations. It is the learners who point at the graphic sign or perform the manual sign, and they do not learn to use the manual or graphic sign in new ways, only to answer questions when the object is present or they are shown a picture of an object or an event (compare Fischer, 1994).

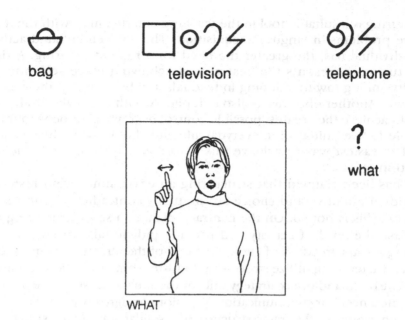

bag   television   telephone

?

what

WHAT

Peter is 4 years old. He has motor impairment, but shows good language comprehension, and uses Blissymbols. He sits with his teacher at the nursery school. She has different objects around her and points at an object or a picture of a particular object while simultaneously pronouncing the word that corresponds to the Blissymbol. Peter points at the Blissymbols on his board as the teacher says the words.

Kate is an autistic girl of 14 years. She uses a number of signs and a few spoken words. She sits with her teacher, who points at various objects and says *What is that?* while performing the sign WHAT. Kate then performs the appropriate manual sign, and is given help where necessary.

Naming can be an appropriate way of learning new names but requires that the individual has learned to use a number of signs in order to obtain objects and participate in activities. It is useful to be able to answer questions, but this is not a goal of the initial intervention. For children and adults with good language skills whom it is thought will be able to translate their comprehension into functional use, naming is a good method of acquiring new signs.

Structured and unstructured situations

Structuring of the teaching situation is one of the best tools available in language and communication intervention. In particular, conscious structuring is a suitable tool in the teaching of individuals with the most severe problems in language acquisition. The less self-initiated activity an individual has, the greater the need for a rigid structuring. A rigid structuring represents the best way of achieving more self-initiated activity among low-functioning individuals and breaking up their life of passivity. Another objective is also that people with extensive disabilities should achieve the greatest possible control over what happens to them, be able to take initiative in everyday life and choose what they want to do. The easiest way to achieve this is to create a structured teaching situation.

It has been claimed that structuring an environment and fostering individual initiative and choice are mutually contradictory but, in our opinion, this is not so. On the contrary, planned use of structuring can increase the level of activity and provide individuals with a basis for gaining greater freedom of choice. Several of the strategies employed in expressive teaching utilize structuring to foster communication and initiative. The build-and-break strategy utilizes the situational structure in order to create a need for communication. Reactions to signal-triggered anticipatory behaviour use the frame structure in a similar way. Frame structuring is also suited to the task of establishing choice between activities.

Although structuring is one of the most useful tools available for developing situational understanding and communication, it is also important to be aware that structure is a *help condition* and not a goal in itself. Most people have a relatively structured existence. They get up in the morning, eat breakfast, go to school or work, eat dinner, watch television, etc. However, the structure is fairly flexible; watching television may be replaced by a trip to the cinema, an evening playing bridge, a social gathering with friends, etc. A correspondingly flexible structure is the ideal objective for people who receive structured intervention. Thus, the aim of structuring is to form the basis of the development of flexible behavioural patterns and the ability to make decisions. This means that the structure is changed as soon as there is a basis for doing so.

Once a successful frame structure has been established, i.e. when the day's activities seem to be understood and are carried out well enough, it is probably time to begin dismantling the structure. In many cases, the situations for the individuals concerned may be so structured, have taken place with virtually no complications and have remained unchanged for such a long period of time that there is no natural need for communication in their daily routines. The signal signs have become rituals, and no longer help to build up new understanding about the environment. The individual may be so tied to the frame structure and the signals that these now preclude the development of new skills and choices, instead of strengthening this development. This may be called *learned dependence*.

After an over-routinized structure has been dismantled, the individual may still have a need for a *time aid*. Such an aid may be a calendar that helps the individual to understand the differences between the days: weekdays and public holidays, vacations and working days.

Edward is an 18-year-old boy with autism who understands a little speech. When his daily routine was broken up by holidays he had violent temper tantrums. It was difficult to quieten him down and he had to be held so that he did not hurt himself or others. Edward's mother drew a calendar for him on which were included things that she knew he liked (Figure 28). To represent the days he spent at school, she drew a picture of a bus because he always looked forward to taking the bus. On some of his days off from school, he is allowed to drive his uncle's tractor. On Saturdays they always mop the floor. On Sundays he has egg for breakfast. Christmas shopping, the Christmas holidays and New Year's Eve are all represented with drawings that are easy for him to understand. The calendar hangs in one place in the kitchen. Every morning Edward looks at it to find out what that particular day will bring. Each evening he crosses off the day that has passed. Since Edward was given the calendar, his holidays have been much more peaceful. It appears as though it was important for him to know that he was going back to school, and that this part of his life was not over even though the holidays were long (Steindal K, personal communication, 1990).

Also other case studies suggest that a calendar should become an integrated part of the alternative communication means as soon as the individual starts to have expectations about events outside the immediate time frame (e.g. Møller and von Tetzchner, 1996).

Many individuals with limited communication abilities react negatively when a routine activity is omitted or changed. The behaviour problems may be prevented or considerably reduced if the activity is always replaced with another, and the disabled individuals are informed about the change in a manner that they understand. This may be done by indicating the changes that will happen on a calendar containing the activities of the day or the week. Both activities are represented on the calendar. The graphic sign of the activity that is stopped is marked with *NO*, e.g. in the form of a red X, whereas a green arrow points from this activity to the sign of the activity that is replacing it (Hawkes, 1998).

Preparatory training

Language and communication teaching often begins with the learning of skills, knowledge or activities that are regarded as preconditions for language acquisition. It is often a stated requirement that these conditions

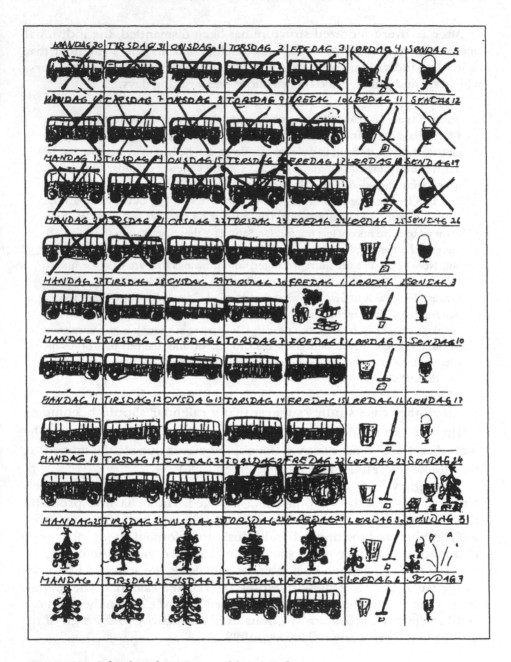

Figure 28. *Calendar of an 18-year-old autistic boy.*

must be present before the language teaching can commence. One example of this is the requirement that the child 'be in possession of' concepts that correspond to the words before these can be learned, which is based on the theory that concepts must exist before language. Other examples are the requirements that the child has concepts of amount or object constancy (Chapman and Miller, 1980; Shane and Bashir, 1981). The ability to imitate has also been regarded as a necessary precursor to language acquisition (Skinner, 1957; Piaget and Inhelder, 1969). The assumption that such fundamental preconditions must exist in order for the child to acquire language has little empirical basis, however, and has often led to inefficient teaching and hindered the acquisition of communication. There are many examples of individuals who have not reached Piaget's sensorimotor stage V or VI, but who have nevertheless been able to use language (Bonvillian, Orlansky and Novack, 1981; Reichle and Karlan, 1985). Matching has been regarded as an important skill for graphic communication, but seems to be useful rather than necessary (Franklin, Mirenda and Phillips, 1996; Stephenson and Linfoot, 1996).

Another type of condition that is stressed concerns the practical implementation of language teaching. Some skills or activities are regarded as necessary, or extremely advantageous, if language teaching is to be effective. One example of such a skill is being able to sit still on a chair in front of a table for a certain period of time. Other examples are the ability to be attentive and look at the teacher. Motivation to communicate has also been emphasized as a practical condition (compare Vanderheiden et al., 1975; Bryen and Joyce, 1985).

Teaching the individual skills and activities that may contribute to a more effective language teaching at a later stage is positive, and in line with the necessity of regarding different intervention measures in the perspective of gradually emerging abilities. This teaching should not, however, be at the expense of communication teaching. Such skills and activities are a part of the total intervention and not a necessary requirement for starting communication teaching. Teaching of such skills should take place together with the language teaching and will thus not lead to a loss of time.

There are a number of theoretical and practical conditions that have been given special attention, including eye contact, direction of gaze, attentiveness, sitting still, behaviour chains, imitation and motor skills.

Eye contact

In intervention involving people with autism, the establishment of eye contact is often considered of major importance and as a primary aim before the implementation of language teaching. This is because the lack of eye contact has been regarded as a sign of contact disorder. However, there is no support for the theory that the establishment of eye contact is a necessary precondition for language acquisition. In addition, it is difficult to look another person in the eyes and simultaneously look at one's own or others' manual signs, or attend to the graphic signs on a communication aid.

Gaze direction and attentiveness

In particular, individuals with autism and learning disability have been given training in gaze direction and attentiveness, but individuals in the expressive language group have also often been taught to look at objects to relay messages before they are taught to use graphic sign systems.

There are two different types of arguments that are used to justify the special emphasis on training gaze direction. The first justification is that intended communication skills are essential to the learning of language, because it precedes words in normal development. A change in gaze direction, i.e. the child looking alternately at an object and the adult, has been used as a measure of intended communication (Bates, 1979). Training gaze direction has thus been regarded as training in intended communication.

The second justification is more practical. Gaze direction is regarded as an expression of attentiveness, and training the child to direct his or her gaze at a person or object is a form of attentiveness training.

Joint attention is a fundamental prerequisite for the success of language teaching, and initiating contact with another person may be a prerequisite for the use of a manual, graphic or tangible sign to be perceived as communication. For example, autistic individuals often look away from the direction in which they are pointing and the pointing is therefore not considered communicative (Sarriá, Gómez and Tamarit, 1996). Many people with extensive motor impairments are not perceived as communicating because the listener does not notice that they are attentive. They may not have the ability to hold their head up, change the direction of gaze, etc. However, practising these skills in advance is not particularly productive. An understanding of how to initiate contact and get the attention of another person can be expected to be understood only in a functional context. Similarly, it can be futile to teach an individual to direct the gaze at another person unless it is clear why this has a purpose. Reinforcing such behaviour, e.g. by giving sweets, may only cause greater confusion. Both attentiveness and the initiation of contact are easier to bring out in an actual communicative situation than by special training. Moreover, in typical language development, talking about something to which the child is already attentive seems to promote word learning better than when the adult first tries to direct the child's attention to something before it is named (Masur, 1997).

Looking at the object that the communication is about is often a part of the actual sign teaching, e.g. by the teacher using this as a first indicator of the individual's choice or attentiveness. In turn, this is a basis for helping the individual form the manual sign. In graphic sign teaching, the teacher may point first at the object to direct the individual's gaze and then move

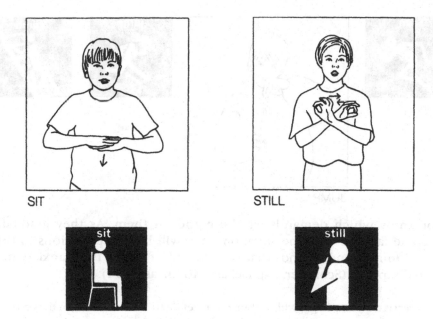

SIT STILL

the gaze onwards to the graphic sign (Berg, 1998). If the individual is learning eye-pointing, the gaze direction is the actual communicative expression and should be taught in a functional communicative setting.

Sitting still

The requirement that an individual sits still by a table for a certain length of time is very commonplace in the teaching of alternative communication. It is usually learning-disabled and autistic individuals who are taught to sit still, but also some restless children with less extensive disorders belonging to the supportive language group.

It can be expedient to teach the individuals to sit still by a table because it facilitates the performance of a large number of activities that are generally performed at a table: painting, building with Lego bricks, doing jigsaw puzzles, etc. Such activities have their own value and may also be utilized in communication intervention. Training in sitting still is thus not justified on the grounds of communication teaching, but rather because of the objective that the individuals take part in activities that are performed at a table. If one teaches the individuals to sit still, by using, for example, the command signs SIT and STILL, and then make them unlearn this so that they can carry out an activity (point at or perform a sign), this necessitates a good deal of extra work and loss of time. At the beginning of the communication teaching, the individuals may be anxious and unsettled because the situation is new, they have very little grasp of what is going on and do

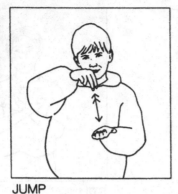

JUMP

not know which demands will be made on them. As they gradually become familiar with the situation, they will have expectations to that situation and understand what is expected of them. Their anxiety may then disappear (Schaeffer, Raphael and Kollinzas, 1994).

> Tracy is a 6-year-old girl with autism. Her chief interest was running in the corridors at school. The first thing she learned was therefore the manual sign RUN. When she ran towards the door in order to run out into the corridor, she was stopped and guided to make the manual sign before she left the room. There were many opportunities to repeat this, and the sign was used spontaneously from the very first day. The teaching continued in the gymnasium with the signs JUMP and CLIMB (Steindal K, personal communication, 1990).

This example shows that restlessness can also be the expression of an interest that may be utilized in the intervention.

Behaviour chains

Skills and activities that give one something to communicate about are fundamental to all language teaching. When starting language intervention for autistic and learning-disabled people, the teacher often finds that they possess few such skills and activities. This may mean that they need to be taught behaviour chains, i.e. several activities that must be performed consecutively. A simple behaviour chain might consist of fetching building bricks and building a small tower. Learning to ride a bicycle involves a chain of advanced motor skills.

The teaching of behaviour chains usually takes place at the same time as language intervention, often with the use of signal signs. The primary purpose of building behaviour chains is to improve the individuals' independence and understanding of their own environment, but the behaviour chains may also be used in language teaching. In the case of profoundly disabled individuals, not all behaviour chains will be identified with tangible, graphic or manual signs, and behaviour chains that have been established without signs can be practical to use when the sign teaching is expanded.

Imitation

There have been arguments for imitation training both as a prerequisite for other learning and as a skill that is functional in itself. Imitation as a necessary prerequisite for learning has led to an emphasis on training of imitation as a 'metaskill', i.e. as a general ability to follow the instruction: *Do as I do.* This type of metaskill usually appears late in development, however, and the first actions children imitate are *actions that they already master.* One-year-old children can imitate someone combing the hair with a comb, but will refuse to comb with a toy car. Even children who are a good deal older can appear fairly frustrated if they are asked to do the same as, for example, someone who places her hand on her head (Guillaume, 1971). This implies that imitation is an unsuitable strategy for teaching new skills in early development.

In the preliminary stages of imitation training, children are often given help in performing the action that they have to imitate. When later they are able to imitate the action, this may be taken as an indicator that the *action* has been learned, rather than that imitation has been learned as a general principle. So, although the imitation training appears to have been successful, in the sense that the individual imitates specific actions or sounds, this does not necessarily mean that the skill will be generalized, i.e. that the individual will more easily begin to imitate signs or words that other people are using.

The fact that imitation is not a prerequisite for language acquisition has been fully demonstrated by children and adults with extensive motor impairments. Many individuals who are barely able to imitate any action nevertheless develop the ability to solve problems, good language comprehension and use of language through writing or graphic signs. Also, severely learning-disabled people who failed to learn to imitate have learned to use graphic and manual signs.

Several studies show limited effectiveness of imitation compared with other strategies in speech training (Gibbon and Grunwell, 1990; Nelson et al., 1996). There are few studies that have compared imitation and hand guidance in manual sign teaching. Iacono and Parsons (1986) used these two strategies in intervention with three severely learning-disabled youths between the ages of 11 and 15 years. Two of them had never been taught manual signs. The third adolescent had been taught to use the sign DRINK several years earlier, but had never used the sign spontaneously. In an

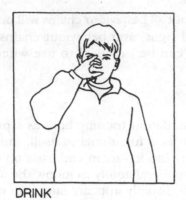

DRINK

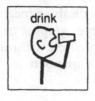

evaluation of their imitation skills, one of the youths (F.L.) managed to imitate six of ten gestures, whereas the other two did not manage to imitate any of them.

The teaching was designed so that the manual signs BISCUIT and DRINK or BISCUIT and LOLLIPOP were first attempted to be taught with the aid of imitation. Then one sign was attempted to be taught using imitation and the other with hand guidance. Finally, both the signs were trained with hand guidance. The results demonstrate clearly that imitation was not a good strategy for teaching these individuals (Figure 29). Even F.L., who had managed to imitate gestures, did not benefit from the imitation training.

These results gained support from a study in which seven pre-school children were taught to imitate speech and manual signs, and were hand guided to give graphic signs in communication training. After 20 sessions, six of the seven children did not imitate speech or manual signs, but rapidly learned to hand over graphic signs. Moreover, during vocal and manual imitation, the children showed frequent problem behaviours, whereas few such behaviours were observed during the graphic sign training with hand guidance. The seventh child learned to imitate spoken words and manual signs, and to give graphic signs at similar rates (Bondy and Frost, 1998).

The necessity of being able to imitate on practical grounds is to a large extent a legacy from traditional speech training, where imitating sounds is a major element. It is difficult to carry out speech training without the imitation of sounds, because it is not easy to form the lips, tongue and other parts of the individual's articulatory organ in order to get him or her to pronounce a specific word. One of the great advantages of alternative communication systems is that imitation is not necessary, because help and guidance in pointing at tangible or graphic signs, or performing manual signs, can be given in other ways. Imitation *can* be a useful strategy, provided that the individual is aware of what imitation is about, i.e. has acquired imitation as a metaskill.

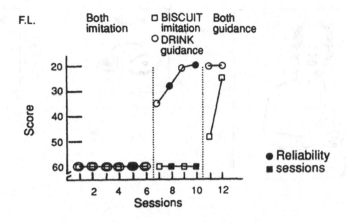

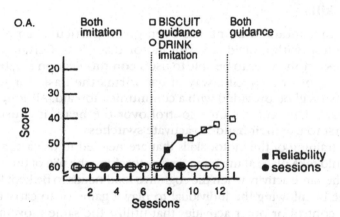

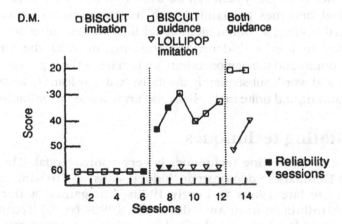

Figure 29. *Learning curves of imitation and hand guidance (Iacono and Parsons, 1986). The lowest possible score is 60, the highest 20.*

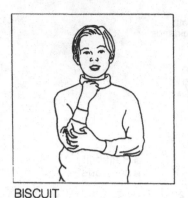

BISCUIT

Motor skills

Preparatory motor training has been given particular emphasis in the intervention with individuals with motor disorders. Certain motor skills are necessary in order to be able to use a communication aid, but often the mastering of one specific way of use forms the basis for whether the individual will be provided with a communication aid. Although, as a rule, individuals have most motor control over the head, it is usual to teach them first to use their hands to activate switches.

The training of the motor skills that are needed to use a communication aid should take place at the same time as teaching the use of the aid, although not in the same activity when the cognitive load needs to be kept low. This can be done by allowing the individual to play a game or to carry out environmental control or other activities that utilize the same movements. At the same time, the sign system can be used in a dependent way so that the individual becomes acquainted with its function. For example, if the individual is given a communication aid that utilizes automatic scanning, it can at first be used with dependent scanning, in which the conversational partner points and the person indicates when he or she is pointing at the right column and word. Subsequently, the individual may learn to master independent scanning and unite motor skills and knowledge of communication.

Facilitating techniques

The use of facilitating techniques is very controversial. They were first used in Denmark to demonstrate 'hidden skills' and to some extent in the USA in the late 1960s and early 1970s, but gained wider popularity through influence from Australia in the 1990s (von Tetzchner, 1997c). They consist in somehow physically assisting a communication-impaired person in pointing at a traditional communication board with letters, pictures or graphic signs, or in writing on an electronic communication aid or a computer. The *facilitator*, i.e. the person assisting the disabled person, may provide hand-over-hand assistance, holding the hand of the communication-impaired person, and typically isolating the index finger for pointing; many of the communication-impaired individuals seem, however, to have the mechanical motor skills necessary for pointing independently, and may do so on other occasions. The facilitator may also hold the arm or sleeve, or place a hand on the shoulder, leg or somewhere else on the disabled person. He or she may slow down the disabled person's movements, make the person withdraw the hand from the board and avoid obvious mistakes. In addition, the facilitator may provide verbal prompts and encouragement (Crossley, 1994).

In a revival of 'hidden skills' in Denmark, a group of severely disabled youths at a home for learning-disabled people were, in 1986, said to be able to use letter boards when they were given help with the pointing. They were unable to speak or use sign language, nor were they able to point at the letters on the board on their own. The claim was that, when helped, they were not only able to give voice to their needs, but also to advanced thoughts and feelings towards other residents, their family and staff (Bo-enheden M-huset, 1986; Johnson, 1989).

GOOD PEOPLE ARE
ALWAYS HAPPY
KARINA

JESPER THE COWARD
SHUTS HIS BODY AND
CAN'T OPEN THEM
NOT EVEN WITH
HELP AND ONE DAY I
WILL CHOOSE MY
OWN LIFE
JESPER

I SLEEP ON A SOFA ALL
DAY WITH BEANS IN MY
BELLY
KARL

NOW YOU HAVE
YOUR DOUBTS
KARSTEN

I DON'T WANT TO BE
STERILIZED BECAUSE
THAT MEANS AN
OPERATION. I'VE
USED THE PILL
BEFORE SO I'D LIKE
TO USE IT AGAIN
MAJA

OUR FRIENDSHIP IS
GOOD
KARIN IS ALSO MY
FRIEND
LEO

LOVE BETWEEN
FRIENDS IS
DIFFERENT
I CAN'T EXPLAIN IT
LOVE BETWEEN
ADULTS IS GREATER
THAN INFATUATION
PERNILLE

The overriding issue in discussions of facilitating techniques is how the messages are generated. Von Tetzchner (1996a) distinguishes among facilitated, false and automatic communication. In *facilitated communication*, the messages produced originate in the mind of the communication-impaired person. They may or may not indicate an understanding of language and communication that is apparent only when the person is given sensitive hand guidance by a facilitator. In *automatic communication*, messages are produced by facilitators without their being aware of this. In *false communication*, messages are consciously produced by facilitators in order somehow to meet their own ends.

The fact that some communication-impaired people may be able to express themselves with the help of facilitating techniques is not disputed. However, even if it is genuine, facilitated communication is of little interest if the disabled person communicates as well or better via other means. The real issue is whether the person communicates better when facilitating techniques are applied than when he or she is communicating independently. Many communication-impaired individuals are claimed to demonstrate undiscovered communication and spelling skills with no or minimal instruction (e.g. Johnson, 1989; Biklen, 1990; Crossley and Remington-Gurney, 1992; Sellin, 1992). It is this claim that is the core matter and focus of empirical studies.

A number of studies have been designed to 'validate' the use of facilitating techniques, i.e. to demonstrate whether the messages produced, which indicate an unexpected level of linguistic competence on behalf of the communication-impaired person, are genuine facilitated communication. The aim of validation studies makes the basic design quite simple, and it is agreed that some kind of true communicative situation is needed, meaning a situation where the disabled person provides information to a communication partner that the facilitator cannot know or guess. There is, however, considerable disagreement with regard to the type of situations that may be used and how the results of facilitating techniques should be assessed. Most proponents of facilitating techniques, i.e. those who claim that unexpected skills are really revealed, seem to favour 'qualitative evidence'. Others maintain that controlled studies are needed, with designs similar to laboratory or field experiments, or consisting of written dialogues where the communication partner's utterances are not seen by the facilitator. The methods used are basically similar, but differ somewhat in control conditions applied. In some studies, ear phones have been used to provide auditory screening so that only the disabled person hears the spoken question or instruction. Other studies have applied visual screening in order to hide cards with words or sentences, pictures or objects from the view of the facilitator, or the facilitator has simply been asked to look away. In some studies, the disabled person has done or been told something or been shown an object or a video without the facilitator present, and then asked to relay information about this with the aid of facilitating techniques.

The experimental approach is based on a need to ensure that the facilitator does not know or can guess the information provided with facilitating techniques and thus cannot be its source. The existing evidence clearly demonstrates that facilitating techniques usually lead to automatic writing, displaying the thoughts and attitudes of the facilitators. The controlled studies show that the facilitators tend to attribute skills to the person that he or she does not possess. With regard to the communication-impaired person, facilitating techniques tend to be directive rather than supportive, and it seems considerably easier to demonstrate 'unexpected' influence from facilitators than from the people who are exposed to facilitating techniques. (For reviews from different perspectives, see Crossley and Remington-Gurney, 1992; Haskew and Donnellan, 1992; Biklen, 1993; Green, 1994; Klewe et al., 1994; von Tetzchner, 1996a).

Chapter 8
Choosing the first signs

The first signs an individual learns are special because they form the basis of an understanding of how signs may be used. They are also the most difficult and time-consuming signs to teach: learning later signs generally takes less time. The choice of the first signs is therefore especially important. Making a 'correct' choice may facilitate the teaching process. This chapter covers the first 10–20 signs. Its aim is *not* to provide a recommended list of signs, but rather to discuss the principles that should be applied when choosing signs.

Signs should be chosen on the basis of their general usefulness. The most important criteria to be taken into account are the needs, interests and desires of the individual who will be using them. It is therefore a good rule to ensure that the first signs are signs that the teacher knows – or has good reason to believe – that the individual will wish to use. This will ensure motivation and attentiveness, and make it easier to understand the purpose of signing. The significance of these advantages cannot be valued too highly. Motivation, attentiveness and an understanding of the usefulness of communication are conditions that are often lacking in the education of individuals with extensive language and communication disorders.

There is general agreement that signs should be selected on the basis of their usefulness, but there is less agreement about what is useful. Usefulness for the individuals' environment may often be placed before that of usefulness for the individuals. Usefulness implies that the individuals are able to make themselves understood in such a way that they can initiate participation in activities and obtain the objects that they want. This type of usefulness is especially important for individuals who belong to the alternative language group, but it is also the basis for choosing signs for individuals who belong to the other two groups.

For individuals who belong to the supportive language group, there may be specific objects or activities that are difficult to ask for or situations in which they find it difficult to make themselves understood. If arguments over toys frequently occur, MINE, YOURS and HIS/HERS may be useful.

$$\underset{\text{mine}}{\bot 1_+} \qquad \underset{\text{yours}}{\bot 2_+} \qquad \underset{\text{his}}{\wedge 3_+} \qquad \underset{\text{hers}}{\triangle 3_+}$$

FIRST may be used in the sense 'I had it first'. There are also examples where signs for emotions such as ANGRY and CRY ('sad') have proved useful among children with a difficult temper. However, it must be stressed that such words can be very difficult to teach and, if they are to be used as first signs, they should be taught to children with a good understanding of spoken language.

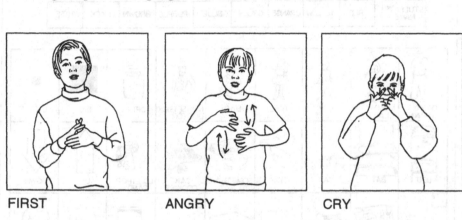

FIRST   ANGRY   CRY

Many individuals who belong to the expressive language group have a fairly good understanding of spoken language. The main purpose of the first signs is therefore not to teach them how the signs are used, but to instil in them a sense that signs are useful. Communication boards are often not used in spontaneous communication (Harris, 1982; Glennen and Calculator, 1985), and many of the graphic signs and words typically placed on communication boards may not encourage their use (Figure 30). The first signs should give the individuals better access to the activities and objects they want, as well as improved possibilities for directing the attention of communication partners towards matters in which they are interested and towards initiating conversations.

Other people also have a need for one or more specific signs. The family and others in close contact with the individual need to be able to make themselves understood, and the usefulness of the signs should also be seen in terms of their needs. For the purposes of upbringing, the parents and significant others in the children's environment need to be

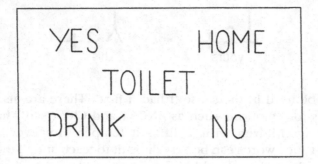

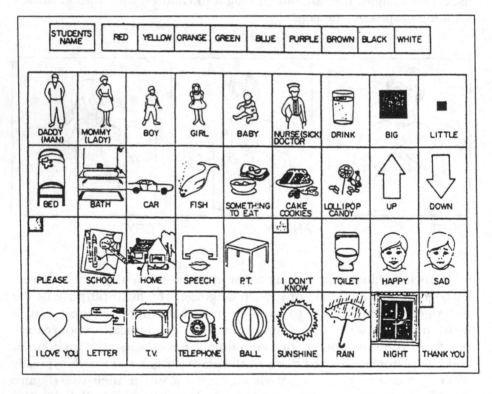

Figure 30. *Examples of communication boards that do not encourage use. (Source: Feallock, 1958; McDonald and Schultz, 1973.)*

able to explain what the child is allowed to do, what is dangerous and how best to behave. They also need to be able to communicate what is going to happen, because the behavioural problems and anxiety experienced by linguistically impaired people are often related to their lack of understanding of what other people want them to do (Frith, 1989). This means that the individuals in the alternative language group should be taught to

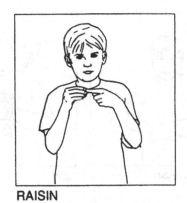

RAISIN

understand signal and command signs, which may make their life easier and reduce misunderstandings and conflicts.

Existing communication

Only seldom will an individual totally lack communication skills when communication intervention begins. Existing communication skills should be taken into account when selecting signs. This communication has generally developed through interaction between the individuals and their families, and it may have taken many years to establish sounds, gestures, facial expressions, etc., that the family and others who know them well are able to understand. It is also essential that this 'private' communication is not used as a starting point by trying to make the individuals express things that they are already capable of communicating in new ways. For example, if a boy smacks his lips to express the fact that he would like some raisins, RAISIN should not be one of the first signs that he learns. If the teacher had chosen to teach the boy the manual or graphic sign RAISIN, this would mean that he would have to unlearn what he already knew, i.e. he would be robbed of some of the communication skills that he already possessed. The aim of the intervention is to provide more communication skills, not to change the form of those that already exist. An important part of the preliminary intervention therefore consists of making professionals aware of, and understand, the communicative expressions that the individual already possesses. It is only at a later stage, when a vocabulary of conventional forms has been acquired, that the original communication can be replaced with other, more commonly used manual, graphic or tangible signs. Individuals who receive communication aids will generally continue to use vocalization, gestures, their eyes, etc., even though graphic signs or script forms their conventional communication (Light, 1985; Heim and Baker-Mills, 1996).

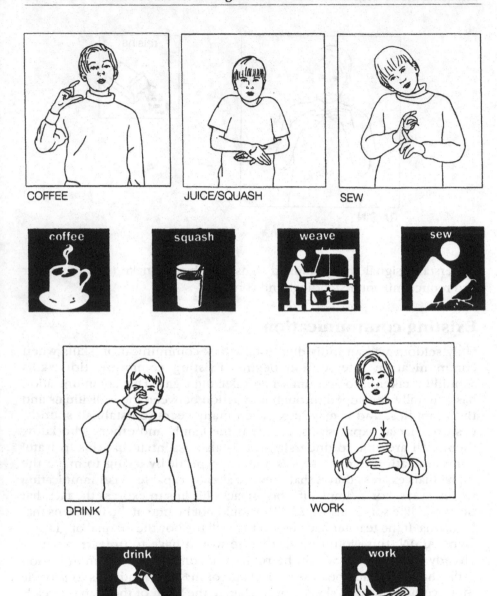

General and specific signs

In our opinion, the first expressive signs should be *specific*, i.e. related to narrow or basic categories of objects and actions. The alternative is to link the signs to more general or broader *classes* of objects, activities or events. COFFEE, SQUASH, WEAVE and SEW may be regarded as specific signs,

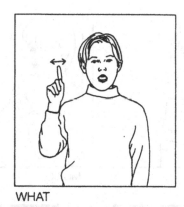

WHAT

whereas DRINK and WORK are *general*. For example, WORK may be used to indicate sewing, weaving and cutting grass.

The reason for choosing specific rather than general signs, whenever this is practically feasible, is to avoid problems that may arise when the individuals learn new signs. If, for example, the individuals have learned to use the manual sign DRINK in a situation where they are given squash each time they use the sign, it may subsequently be difficult to teach them to use the sign SQUASH. To teach SQUASH, the teacher must either combine DRINK and SQUASH to form a sign sentence, or perhaps introduce a practice where the individual begins by using DRINK, the teacher then asks WHAT and the individual answers SQUASH. The teaching process becomes laborious and provides plenty of opportunities for misunderstanding. Learning a specific sign may also involve the unlearning of the general sign. This may be the case if the individual interprets the general sign as more specific than the teacher had intended, i.e. in a way that either partially or totally corresponded to the use of the specific sign. For example, someone might take DRINK to mean 'squash'. The risk that individuals will misunderstand is great, because it may be easy for them to interpret a general sign as a specific sign when the sign is used to denote an interesting object or activity.

Signal signs can be both specific and general, but in contrast to expressive signs the first signal signs are often signs that signalize a general situation, such as *FOOD* before a meal, *SPORT* before physical activity and *MUSIC* before music therapy and other musical activities.

The aim of expressive teaching in the use of tangible, graphic and manual signs is that the individuals should be able to give expression to wants and thoughts, and influence their environment in a way that is socially acceptable. They have to learn the consequences that use of the sign may have. Each sign should have a different consequence, so that not all signs are interpreted as variations of one general sign. An individual

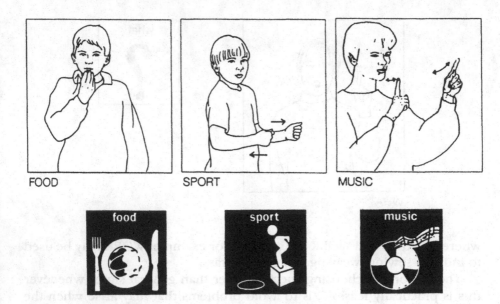

FOOD   SPORT   MUSIC

who is given a piece of chocolate as a reward for performing the signs BALL, BOAT and SCISSORS, when these objects are present, will learn that BALL means 'chocolate' when there is a ball on the table, BOAT means 'chocolate' when there is a boat on the table, and SCISSORS means 'chocolate' when there is a pair of scissors on the table. Thus, the chocolate makes it difficult for the learner to understand the connection between BALL and the act of rolling or throwing a ball, between BOAT and playing with the boat in the bathtub, and between SCISSORS and the act of cutting paper.

A primary objective for individuals who belong to the expressive language group is that they should be able to initiate conversation and other forms of interaction. In addition, the signs that they learn should be useful in a variety of situations and discussions of many subjects. Useful general first signs may, for example, be *COME*, *LOOK*, *PLAY* and *TALK*. With

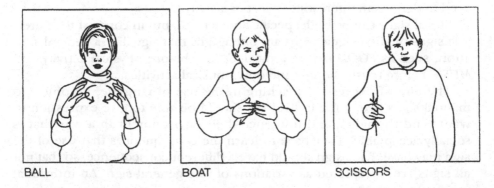

BALL   BOAT   SCISSORS

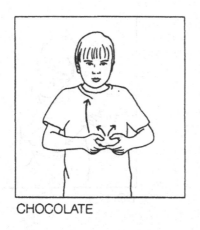

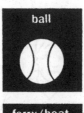

CHOCOLATE

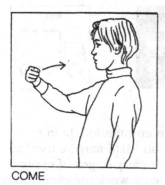

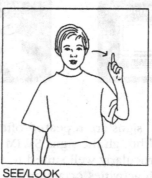

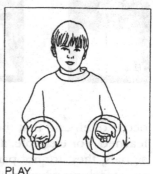

COME   SEE/LOOK   PLAY

such general expressions, there is still a risk that individuals remain passive and that the activities in which they take part are chiefly decided by others. To foster independence, they must be able to take the initiative in deciding activities, so specific signs such as *BOOK*, *COMPUTER*, *DOLL* and *LORRY* may also be useful early signs for this group.

Repetitions

For all three groups, it is essential that the signs chosen are possible to use fairly frequently. For the alternative language and supportive language group, it is important that the potential communicative settings selected

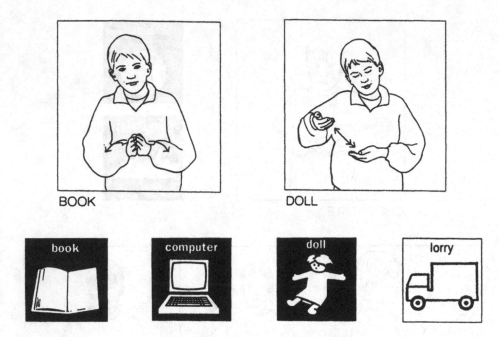

occur often and that the signs are repeated often enough for them to be learned. For example, although the signs SWIM and RIDE may be used as signals, they are not particularly well suited to the early stages of expressive teaching when such activities occur only once a week, or even less. When the teaching takes place in the individual's natural environment, the best strategy is to use signs that can be used in connection with routines and other frequently repeated activities. Usual first signs are the names of food, and other objects and activities that are not usually mentioned very often. In special training and planned teaching situations, the teacher has greater control over how often the signs will be used, and it may be advantageous to design a situation that gives individuals the chance to learn such signs through intensive or mass practice – on the condition that they do not become bored. Activities enjoyed by the individuals are easier to repeat in the natural environment.

Studies have demonstrated the importance of frequent adult use for the acquisition of the very first lexical forms (Harris, 1992). Tangible, graphic and manual signs should also be used frequently enough by people in the environment to support the structured teaching.

Motor skills

The learners must be able to perform the sign so that it is easily understood. Manual signs place the greatest demands on motor skills, and they should not be used if motor disorders prevent their performance. The

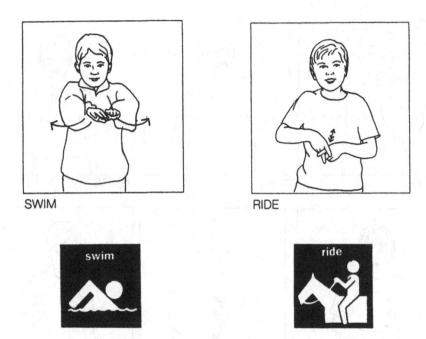

SWIM   RIDE

individuals should not have so much difficulty in performing the signs that
their attention becomes focused on the articulation and they lose track of
their function.

Many people in need of augmentative communication are clumsy, and
it may be difficult to recognize the manual signs that they are performing.
If an individual performs manual signs childishly or clumsily, the conversational partner may, for example, confuse such signs as FOOD and DRINK.
A problem that is often encountered is that the individual is unable to
make the distinction in hand shape, with the result that both FOOD and
DRINK are performed by leading the hand to the mouth without forming
the hands to produce the specific hand shape required. It is therefore
more practical to use THIRSTY rather than DRINK, because THIRSTY is
performed with the hands in a different position relative to the
individual's body. In this way, both signs may be used without placing too
much emphasis on their articulation. It is the function not the articulation
of the signs that should be emphasized, especially when teaching the first
signs. CAR and MILK are two other manual signs that are frequently used,
but are difficult to distinguish from one another. DRIVE may be a better
sign to use than CAR because its articulation is easier to distinguish from
that of MILK.

On occasions when it is not possible to find manual signs that are easy
to perform, another strategy is to simplify the signs. However, it is important to be aware that simplifying the way in which the signs are articulated

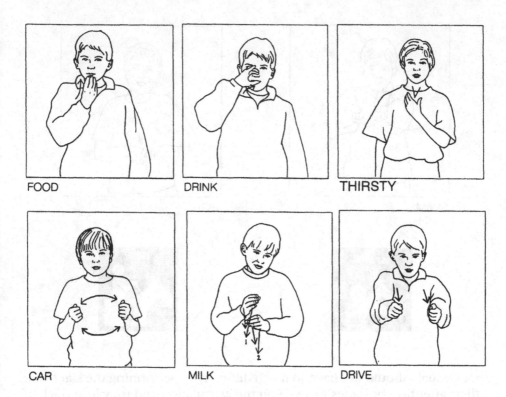

FOOD   DRINK   THIRSTY

CAR   MILK   DRIVE

does not *always* make them easier to learn. Many individuals with extensive communication disorders find it easier to learn manual signs than graphic signs, even though graphic signs are always easier to produce. It appears as though the actual motor production of manual signs – which differs for each sign – is an aid to distinguishing one sign from another. This also requires the signs to be different in terms of motor articulation.

There are no fixed rules about what distinguishes manual signs that are easy to learn from those that are difficult, but there are studies that give some cues about the type of simplifications that should be made. The hand shapes should be simple and the fingers should not need to be placed in unusual positions. Two-handed signs are easier to learn than one-handed signs. Symmetrical signs, i.e. signs where both hands perform the same movement, are easier to learn than asymmetrical signs, where the hands have different functions. It appears that touch is a good aid to learning and performing signs. Manual signs where the hands touch the body are easier to learn than signs where the hands are not in contact with the body. As might be expected, complex signs are more difficult to learn than signs with only one movement (Dennis et al., 1982; Grove, 1990). More information is needed before it is known how signs should best be simplified, and individual differences should be taken into consideration. It makes good sense to take these circumstances into account, however, when both selecting and simplifying manual signs.

The primary motor skill required when using graphic signs is the ability to indicate in such a manner that it is clear to the communication partner which sign is indicated. Indication may be done with the hands, eyes, feet, etc. (see p. 46). If pointing is performed with the hands, accuracy of hand and arm movements determines the size of the graphic signs, the distance between them, and how many signs there will be room for on the communication board. The location on the communication board is also important, and it may be necessary to use only some areas of the board (Figure 31). When the individuals begin graphic sign training, it is essential that they have as few problems indicating them as possible, so that they experience positive results immediately. The individual's environment is not accustomed to using graphic signs either. The fact that the individual is able to indicate reasonably quickly may help conversational partners to break former communication patterns in which they wholly dominated the communicative situation.

Perception

The individual's ability to perceive sensory impressions is of crucial importance for the choice of both sign system and individual signs. A visually impaired individual may have difficulty in distinguishing between and identifying manual signs used by others, unless they are used in a deaf–blind mode in which the hands are moved through the sign by the communication partner. Sight is also an aid when learning expressive

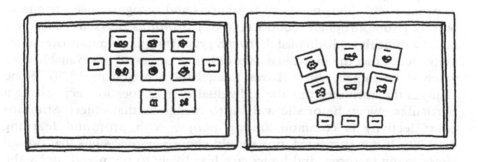

Figure 31. *Boards may have an unusual design owing to perceptual or motor limitations on the part of the user.*

signs. Manual signs that can be seen by the individuals themselves while they perform them may be easier to learn than others (Luftig, 1984). Visual acuity will determine the size of graphic signs and their choice. Reduced visual acuity may make it difficult for the individual to distinguish between graphic signs that resemble one another. In cases where individuals have lost part of their field of vision or are blind in one eye, it may be necessary to use only part of the communication board. With individuals who have severe visual impairments, communication aids with artificial speech output may be used. Such communication aids may utilize several switches or a concept keyboard with a different texture in each square (Mathy-Laikko et al., 1989). A visually impaired user may utilize the location of the area to press to say certain words and phrases. The communication aid should then be fitted with tactile guidelines and other cues to orienting. It is also important that the words and phrases remain in stable positions.

Graphic systems have to some extent been made perceivable or tangible for people with visual impairments. For example, sculptured three-dimensional PIC signs have been produced that enable individuals to perceive the signs by feeling them with their fingers. These may be of use to people with partially impaired vision, who use the sense of touch as a supplement to sight. For individuals who are totally dependent on perceiving the differences between signs by touch, however, PIC signs of this sort are not particularly suitable. Perceiving forms with one's fingers is difficult. Many of the differences that are easy to perceive using sight are not so easy to perceive by touch. It is better to use a tangible sign system, which takes into account the possibilities and limitations offered by tactile perception. For example, Premack's word bricks consist of forms that can be recognized fairly easily and manipulated for further investigation.

Not only visual disorders in the usual sense are of significance for the visual perception of visual impressions. Brain damage may make it difficult to process and interpret visual sensations and recognize even common objects (Humphreys and Riddoch, 1987). *Stimulus overselectivity* may make it difficult to distinguish between graphic signs. Stimulus overselectivity means that the individual uses only one or few of the available cues when identifying an object (Lovas, Koegel and Schreibman, 1979). If one changes the attributes that the individual uses as cues for recognizing a particular object, he or she will fail to recognize that object. Stimulus overselectivity is common among people with profound learning disability. If it is suspected, one should choose graphic signs that do not share many features, and hence are less likely to be mixed up by the individual.

If the individual has problems seeing the differences between the PIC signs or between signs in other graphic sign systems, it may be necessary to simplify or change the form of the signs. This can be done with a black felt-tip pen.

If the individual has some understanding of spoken language, it is important to utilize this understanding. For example, people with developmental dysphasia often have difficulty in distinguishing between words that sound alike (homonyms). Care should therefore be taken not to chose signs that correspond to similar sounding words.

Iconicity

It is a general assumption that iconicity may facilitate the acquisition of both manual and graphic signs.

- *Iconicity* means that there is a similarity between the performance or appearance of a sign and obvious features of the object or action for which the sign is used. Iconicity is measured in terms of transparency and translucency.
- *Transparency* indicates the ease with which people who are unfamiliar with the sign are able to guess the meaning of the sign. Transparency is sometimes called 'guessability' and is the feature usually associated with iconicity.
- *Translucency* indicates the ease with which one can perceive a relationship between a sign's meaning and its appearance or performance when the gloss of the sign is provided.
- *Opaqueness* means that no relationship between the sign's meaning and its appearance or performance is perceived even when the gloss is known.

A sign can be translucent even though the relationship perceived is not the true connection between the sign's meaning and its form. For example, GIRL in American sign language is highly translucent because

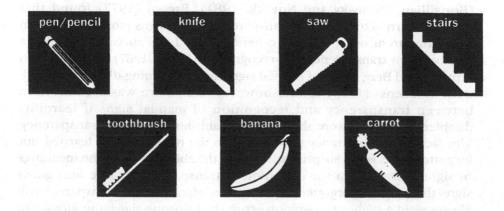

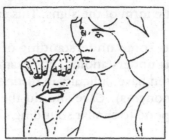

GIRL (American Sign
Language)

many people perceive a connection between the way the sign is
performed – the thumb is stroked across the cheek – and the fact that girls
have soft cheeks. The sign actually originates from the fact that girls in the
USA in the last century wore bonnets, which were held in place by a band
attached under their chin. The stroking movement indicates the bonnet
band (Klima and Bellugi, 1979).

Manual signs

The relationship between iconicity and the acquisition of manual signs
depends on the diagnostic group being studied, and whether transparency or translucency is used as a measure of iconicity (Doherty, 1985).

There is no clear connection between how easy it is for adults to
guess the meaning of manual signs and how easy it is to learn them. The
transparency of manual signs, measured by the adults guessing at the
signs' glosses, is not always significant with regard to the ease with which
those signs may be acquired. Deaf children do not learn more iconic
manual signs in their early development than one would expect on the
basis of the share of iconic signs found in American sign language
(Bonvillian, Orlansky and Novack, 1981). Brown (1977) found that
children learned to recognize transparent manual signs more quickly than
non-transparent ones, whereas others have had less success in finding a
link between transparency and recognition (Miller, 1987) or production
(Trasher and Bray, 1984) of manual signs among learning-disabled individuals. Goosens' (1983) found, however, that there was a connection
between transparency and recognition of manual signs if learning-
disabled individuals were also used to establishing the signs' transparency.
The fact that transparency plays a role in the recognition of learned but
forgotten signs is not surprising, because the ability to guess the meanings
of signs follows from the definition of transparency. As one may guess
signs that one has forgotten, the forgotten signs that are transparent will
always yield a higher recognition score than opaque signs, the glosses of

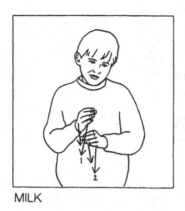

MILK

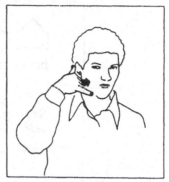

TELEPHONE (American Sign Language)

which are less easy to guess. However, signs that are transparent for some people, e.g. university students, are not necessarily so for others, such as language-impaired nursery school children. MILK was perhaps fairly transparent for children during the last century because many of them had seen a cow being milked by hand. Today, there are few children who would associate the sign with milking.

The differences that exist in the perception of translucency manifest themselves clearly in a study of 100 American manual signs for object words, which are often used in the teaching of learning-disabled individuals. A group of normally developed 6-year-old children rated only one sign (TELEPHONE) as being highly translucent. Hearing and deaf students rated 26 signs as being highly translucent. For the children and the hearing students, 55 and 48 signs, respectively, were given a low translucency rating, whereas the deaf students rated only 16 signs as being of low translucency (Griffith and Robinson, 1981).

With regard to the use of manual signs, research has not found that a high or low degree of translucency plays a role for the ease with which severely learning-disabled individuals learn signs (Kohl, 1981). In terms of recognition of manual signs, it has been found that signs that were rated high in translucency are remembered better than signs rated low in translucency (Griffith and Robinson, 1980). This is to be expected because many highly translucent signs are also highly transparent.

It is not surprising that university students benefit from translucency when remembering signs. Perceiving a relationship makes it easier for them to recall a particular sign, and the establishment of such connections is a memory technique that is commonly used (compare Luria, 1969; Klima and Bellugi, 1979). For normally developed 3-year-old children, however, it seems that iconicity is of no help when recognizing manual signs (Miller, 1987). When learning-disabled people do not learn translu-

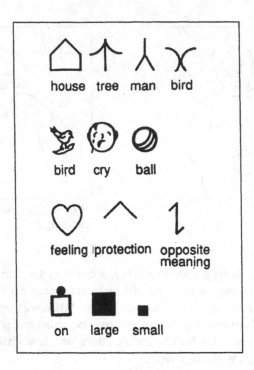

cent manual signs any quicker than non-translucent signs, this may be the result of their lack of the skills needed for them to be able to utilize such similarities, i.e. they are unable to see the connection between the sign they are making and a specific aspect of the object or action represented in its performance.

There is thus little to support the theory that iconicity facilitates the acquisition of the first manual signs by small children and learning-disabled people. However, iconicity does facilitate recognition and production among other adults. Choosing iconic manual signs may therefore help the adult to remember what the sign is supposed to express, and thereby create a more responsive language environment by increasing the chances that the sign will be recognized. For this reason, iconic signs should be chosen where there is a choice of signs that otherwise seem equally functional and easy to learn.

Graphic signs

When assessing iconicity in graphic sign systems, pictorial similarity is clearer. Many of the sign systems consist of more or less stylized drawings, and even drawings that are not part of a graphic sign system have been called iconic (compare Hurlbut, Iwata and Green 1982). Signs of this type are said to be *pictographic*. A number of graphic signs are not pictographic in the strictest sense of the word, but portray an object or action that is usually associated with what the sign is used to refer to. Such signs are often said to be *ideographic*. Many ideographic signs are a natural result of the fact that not all words are easy to illustrate. There are also graphic systems with little or no iconicity, such as Lexigrams.

Roughly speaking, the Blissymbols and Rebus signs that are described as pictographic are transparent, whereas the signs that are characterized as ideographic are translucent. The Blissymbols *HOUSE*, *TREE*, *MAN* and *BIRD* are regarded as pictographic and so are the Rebus signs *BIRD*, *CRY* and *BALL*. The Blissymbols *FEELING*, *PROTECTION* and *OPPOSITE* are ideographic, however, as are the Rebus signs *ON*, *LARGE* and *SMALL*. *HELP* is a typically ideographic PCS sign. Most PIC signs are pictographic, but signs such as *HELP*, *HOME* and *FRIENDS* are ideographic. Although this has not been studied, there is reason to believe that iconic graphic signs that correspond to object words are transparent, whereas iconic graphic signs that correspond to verbs and other classes of words are more translucent. In probability, there are also relatively more iconic signs among object groups than other groups (Figure 32).

There are few comparisons of graphic signs within a single system. Using a simple association task, Fuller (1997) found that the glosses of translucent Blissymbols were easier to remember than less translucent ones. Attempts to ascertain the significance of iconicity have been concentrated on comparing different systems. The results from such studies show, for the most part, that systems with a greater degree of iconic signs are easier to learn than those with many non-iconic signs. Blissymbols are generally easier to learn than Premack's word bricks (as visual forms), and Rebus signs are easier to learn than Blissymbols. The differences reported come from studies of associative learning and recognition of the signs, where the subjects have to remember which signs correspond to particular words. Hurlbut and his colleagues (1982) found, however, that learning-disabled individuals also used drawings more spontaneously than Blissymbols.

Based on comparisons of the systems, it appears that iconic graphic signs should be chosen as a starting point. However, the basis for such a conclusion is uncertain. Severely learning-disabled individuals are not always able to perceive what a picture is supposed to represent. This may mean that figurative differences that seem great to most people because they convey meaning are not so clear for individuals who are unable to

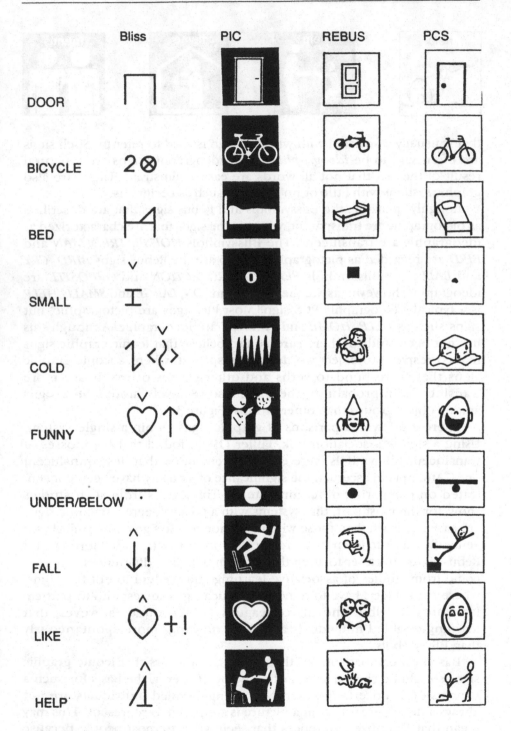

Figure 32. *Graphic signs that correspond to different word classes.*

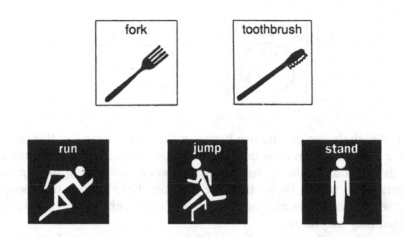

perceive the content of the picture. For example, some individuals may see little difference between the PCS signs *FORK* and *TOOTHBRUSH* if they are unaware of the objects' functions and do not notice the prongs on the fork and the bristles on the toothbrush. There is reason to believe that many profoundly learning-disabled individuals have difficulty in perceiving this type of difference, perhaps because of stimulus overselectivity or poor visual scanning strategies (compare Lyon and Ross, 1984).

Recognizing objects in pictures is only a small step in the development of pictorial perception. Perceiving action in pictures is learned at a later stage than the perception of objects (Kose, Beilin and O'Connor 1983; DeLoache and Burns, 1994). In view of the fact that many learning-disabled individuals have difficulty in recognizing objects in pictures (Dixon, 1981), one should be even more cautious about taking their perception of other sorts of picture content for granted. It is not easy to express actions, prepositions, etc. pictorially and unambiguously. If sign learners do not understand that the sign represents an action, or is supposed to signalize one, they may perhaps perceive it as depicting an object. The PIC signs *RUN*, *JUMP* and *STAND* may just as easily be perceived as 'man' or 'human'. Pictorial similarity may make the signs only appear more similar, which is more likely to confuse the learners than to help them (Oxley and von Tetzchner, 1999).

This discussion is not intended to be an argument against the use of iconic graphic signs in early teaching. There is reason to believe that such signs will facilitate the learning process for individuals who have developed the necessary pictorial comprehension. However, for many learning-disabled individuals this is not the case. If individuals appear unable to perceive the figurative pictorial content that has been stressed in the choice of signs, then the signs are not iconic for them and iconicity cannot make the learning process easier. It becomes more important to ensure that individuals can distinguish between the forms found in the signs that will be used, which may be done by traditional teaching of discrimination. If individuals are able to distinguish between iconic graphic signs, it is advantageous to use them, because this may help ensure that people in the environment react appropriately to the comprehension and expressive use that they may show.

The wish to illustrate and make clear the significance of the signs can sometimes produce very unfortunate results. For example, *YES* and *NO* are usually illustrated with a smiling face and a sad face. This does not correspond at all well to the use of these two words. The emotional expressions of these faces are clearly misleading when used in reply to such questions as *Are you sad? Are you angry? Did he go? Is it raining?* or *Is it broken?* The consequence may be that the individuals will generally regard the *NO* sign as negative and the *YES* sign as positive. There is also reason to believe that the conversational partners of the individuals will take notice of, and even mirror, the emotional content of the face drawings themselves and use them as cues to whether the individuals are happy or sad.

Tangible signs

There is no research into the role of transparency and translucency of tangible signs. Within the literature on iconicity, Premack's word bricks have been treated as visual forms. For individuals who can see, or who have been able so see and thus have the ability to make mental images based on visual features, transparency and translucency may be somewhat similar to graphic signs. However, for blind individuals who must rely on tactile identification, the features that are used in recognition, and which would make some tangible signs transparent or translucent, may be different from those used in visual recognition (see von Tetzchner and Martinsen, 1980; Warren, 1994). Often models of real objects are used as tangible signs. However, such models may not be immediately recognizable for a visually impaired individual, but depend on learning what they are, and they are thus translucent rather than transparent.

Simple and complex concepts

When one starts to teach language to individuals with extensive communication disorders, it is necessary to take into account what the learners can

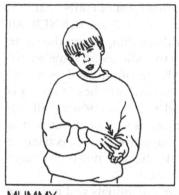

MUMMY

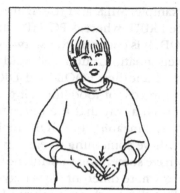

DADDY

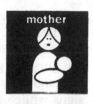

understand of the signs. In such circumstances, however, it is not always clear which concepts are difficult and which are easy. For example, 'mummy' and 'daddy' can hardly be regarded as particularly difficult concepts, but it may nevertheless be difficult to teach comprehension and expressive use of the signs MUMMY and DADDY.

Instead of speaking in terms of simple and difficult concepts, it may be better to speak of circumstances that make such concepts either difficult or easy to teach. Lahey and Bloom (1977) place great emphasis on 'ease of demonstration' when choosing first words, and cite, for example, the difficulties of demonstrating an individual's inner state as an argument for excluding words that express feelings when choosing a first vocabulary for language-impaired children.

When Lahey and Bloom prepared their guidelines, they probably had in mind children with delayed language development and less extensive disorders. They appear to assume that children with communication disorders are able to learn by observing other people, and ease of demonstration may thus be interpreted in a fairly literal sense. This is the case for many individuals who belong to the expressive language group, but, for people with more extensive language disorders, the 'ease of demonstration' for the first signs is a question of designing implicit teaching situations, i.e. situations that make the relationship between the sign and changes in the situation as clear as possible. When teaching signal signs, this means that the situation in which the sign is taught must be clear and defined. When teaching expressive signs, the objects and activities should be reasonably similar in function or design from time to time so that they are recognizable each time they are used.

It is also essential that the first signs are not too similar in terms of content, so that they do not cause confusion. However, determining whether signs are similar in terms of content is no easy task. Similarity may imply that both signs belong to the same category or that one is a subset of the other. For example, MILK and JUICE are both a form of DRINK. APPLE and BANANA are FRUIT, whereas POTATO and SAUSAGE are DINNER. All of these are FOOD. It is common to use two or three things from the same category in a given situation, but one should try to avoid using signs where one sign is part of another. FOOD and DRINK are often used as signal signs while other words for food are being practised, but these two signs are not used in such a way that the other food signs function as subcategories of them. The meaning of FOOD might just as well be described as 'eat' or 'You may have something to eat now'. Similarly, DRINK is used to signal 'You may have something to drink now'. In this way this type of sign denotes *domains* where different signs may be used.

When the first sign teaching is initiated, the individuals will not learn a general use of the words as found among competent language users. Competent users apply words such as *sausage* in a variety of combinations: *smoked sausage*, *sausage roll*, *liver sausage*, etc. Individuals with communication disorders first learn a *limited use* of the signs. SAUSAGE, for example, may best be translated with the phrase 'I want a hot dog'. Using SAUSAGE to say 'There is a sausage' or SAUSAGE RED to say 'I want a red sausage' or 'the sausage is Danish' is a skill that may be learned at a later stage. This depends on whether the sign SAUSAGE has been used in

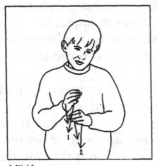

MILK

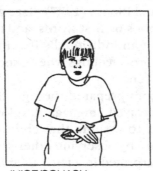

JUICE/SQUASH

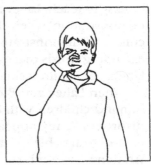

DRINK

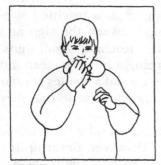

APPLE

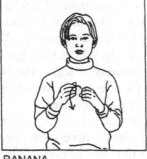

BANANA

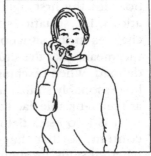

FRUIT

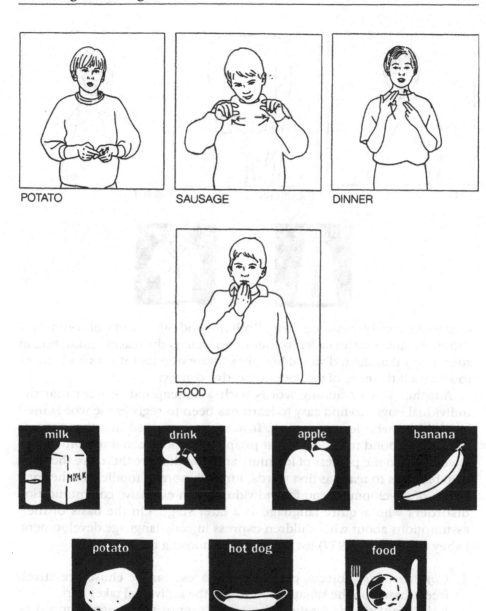

POTATO   SAUSAGE   DINNER

FOOD

milk   drink   apple   banana

potato   hot dog   food

situations that are functionally different. If an individual mixes up the signs TROUSERS and SHIRT after practising these signs in a single situation (Doherty, 1985), there is reason to believe that he or she has not systematically identified each of these garments with the particular routine of putting on either trousers or a shirt. The setting in which the dressing has taken place has not contained sufficient cues for the individual to be

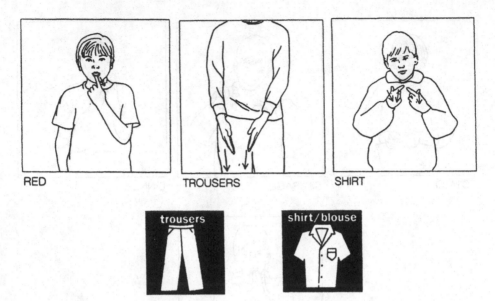

RED   TROUSERS   SHIRT

able to distinguish between them. Both this and other forms of confusions should be analysed, in order to attempt to change the teaching situation in such a way that the individual becomes aware of relevant cues and comes to share a little more of the communicative context.

Another way of finding words with a conceptual content that the individual ought to find easy to learn has been to register the words used by children who learn to speak. It has been assumed that these words must correspond to concepts that people with poor communicative skills have or are in the process of learning, and that they are therefore the most suitable ones to teach as first words, for both normal toddlers in the early stages of development and for individuals with extensive communication disorders who acquire language at a later stage. On the basis of their assumptions about what children express in early language development, Lahey and Bloom (1977) list six rules for choosing first words:

1. *Object words* (objects, people and places) can be chosen relatively freely, based on the situations in which the individual takes part.
2. *Relational words* (verbs, adjectives, prepositions, etc.) should be chosen so that they can be used with all or a large number of objects.
3. Avoid *words for inner feelings* because these are difficult to demonstrate, and thus to teach.
4. Avoid *Yes* and *No* as expressions of affirmation and denial. *No* can be used to express other important conditions.
5. Avoid pronouns because they are usually acquired at a later stage. Use *mummy* and *daddy* and people's names instead.
6. Avoid colours and opposites *(big–small)*. Use only one element of such

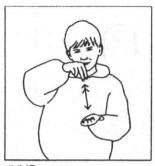
JUMP

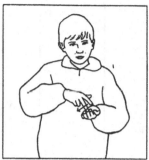
WALK

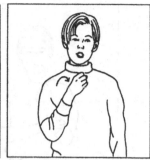
ICE CREAM

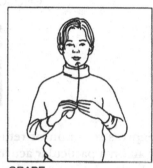
GRAPE

jump

walk

ice cream

grapes

pairs because opposites are acquired at a late stage and may confuse the child. It is better to use the word *not* instead, for example, *not-big* instead of *small*.

Most of these points make good sense. One should not, however, link the difference between object words and relational words with word classes. A word class may be defined only on the basis of the function of the words belonging to that class in the sentence. As long as an individual is not combining words to make sentences, there is little sense in saying that a sign belongs to a specific word class (see also Chapter 10). Thus, JUMP and WALK may not be regarded as belonging to a different word class from ICE-CREAM and GRAPE unless they are used to express different functions in multiple sign utterances.

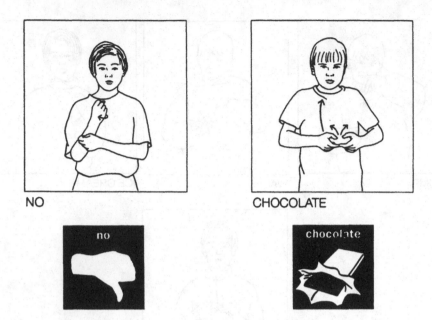

NO   CHOCOLATE

Emphazising NO to express rejection or refusal, non-existence, cessation of an activity and a ban on a particular activity, seems to be academically motivated. In the early stages of sign teaching, NO should be avoided as an expression of non-existence because adults should be able to use NO in order to deny the individual an activity or thing without being misunderstood. For example, if individuals say CHOCOLATE and the teacher says NO, they may interpret this as though there is no chocolate. If, at the same time, there is a bar of chocolate on the table, or the individuals have seen the teacher put a bar of chocolate in the cupboard, this may lead them to believe that they have not been understood and they will therefore continue to sign CHOCOLATE. As they are used to being misunderstood, this is a reasonable assumption on their part.

It is useful to be able to express the non-existence of an object, especially if the individual notices that a particular object is missing. However, GONE may be a better choice of sign than NO. It is questionable, however, whether GONE will be used any differently than the words GET, GIVE or HELP. These signs may also be used to obtain something that does not exist in a particular situation. It is a matter of finding out which sign is easiest to teach, and GONE may well prove to be the most appropriate sign.

What to expect

The teacher's expectations of the first stage of sign teaching will differ depending on which of the three groups is being taught, and on the stated

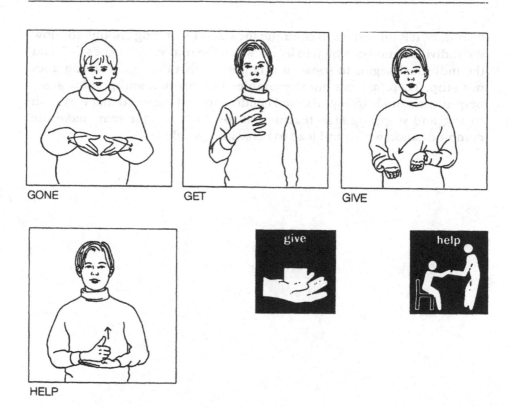

GONE GET GIVE

HELP give help

aims of the teaching. Many individuals who belong to the expressive language group have such a good understanding of spoken language at the start of the teaching that there is reason to expect them to learn quickly. However, it may take a long time before the signs are used spontaneously, which is the aim of the continued teaching. The supportive language group will also be expected to make rapid progress, because many in the group are able to use some spoken words and have a certain degree of language comprehension. The people with the greatest difficulties are found in the alternative language group, and it is here that one finds the greatest degree of uncertainty in terms of teaching progression. Even though it seems that most individuals acquire some communicative skills when they are taught to use graphic or manual signs, there are great variations. Wills (1981) summarizes 17 studies applying manual signs with 118 people. Nine individuals learned no signs, whereas the greatest number of signs acquired was 24 for each month of teaching. The average was three new signs for each month of teaching.

Even when the teaching is functional and takes place in the individual's natural environment, it may sometimes take several months before the signs are used spontaneously. For older people with communication disorders, a long history of learned dependence, helplessness and passivity may severely influence acquisition. For individuals with profound disorders, it is important to continue the training for long enough to allow the individual time in which to learn. When the intervention goes well and the individual begins to speak, it is important that the sign teaching does not stop. There are countless examples that manual and graphic signs help autistic and learning-disabled children to find the word that they wish to say, and stopping sign teaching at too early a stage may make the communication worse and lead to behaviour problems.

Chapter 9
Further vocabulary development

The construction of a functional vocabulary is the foundation of intervention with alternative communication systems. Once an individual can use 10–20 signs consistently, both spontaneously and in teaching situations, the character of the intervention changes. For many individuals who belong to the alternative language group, the preliminary teaching functions as a test period because the course of development is impossible to predict with any degree of certainty. Once the first signs have been learned, the teaching may become more flexible. An increased repertoire provides greater freedom of choice between the various teaching methods and enables greater versatility. This also places new demands on the teacher. It is particularly important to have long-term goals and intervention strategies that sustain the acquisition of future language skills.

The objectives of this continued development are the same for all three groups: to teach new signs, to lay the basis for the combination of signs to produce sentences, and to foster participation in conversations (see Chapters 10 and 11). However, these three aims will receive varying degrees of emphasis, depending on which group is being taught. The major difference is between the expressive language group and the other two groups.

Alternative and supportive language groups

When choosing new signs, a major goal is that individuals should be able to communicate in as many situations as possible. Signs should be integrated into new situations, in order for them to use signs throughout the day. This type of intervention approach may be called *surface oriented*. Another approach is to teach individuals new signs related to situations that are already used in the sign teaching. The individuals will learn to use more than one sign from within the same topic or domain. This approach may be called *domain oriented*. A domain-oriented expansion of sign vocabulary is semantically based and provides the basis for a more profound knowledge than that provided by surface-oriented vocabulary expansion. A domain-oriented intervention strategy may also enhance conversational skills because it gives the learners an opportunity to say more about the same subject.

> Jack is a 36-year-old learning-disabled man. He is interested in birds, especially those in the park, and has learned the manual sign BIRD. The domain 'birds' is expanded with DUCK, WING, BEAK and FLY.

One of the best ways to increase the sign vocabulary is to combine the teaching of new signs with the teaching of new skills and activities. Comprehension of new signs can be taught by introducing new signs in new activities, and by using signs to signal new activities.

> Paul is a 5-year-old boy with a developmental language disorder. He enjoys throwing a ball, playing snap and taking part in other games. He is keen on playing a variation on the game of quoits, but annoys the other children by trying to take the hoops when it is their turn. When it is his turn, he is guided to make the sign RING before he is given the quoits. This also helps him regulate his own behaviour.

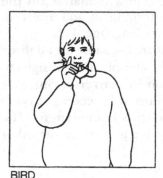

BIRD

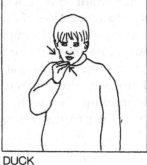

DUCK

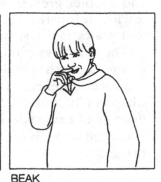

BEAK

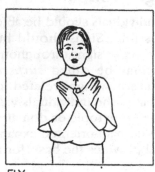

FLY

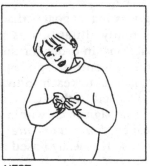

NEST

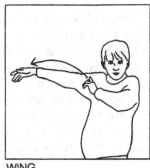

WING

The comprehension-based signs are naturally a mixture of signal signs and instructions. Some of the instructions are command signs, but *requests for action* will gradually become more commonplace because the main objective of giving instructions is no longer to control problematic behaviour. Also, naming and commenting on objects and activities gradually become more commonplace.

Teaching of signs in fixed routines both facilitates the introduction of these routines and makes it easier for individuals to understand the signs, because they know which activity is going to follow.

> Carol is a 20-year-old learning-disabled girl. She usually helps lay the table and this activity is signalled with the manual sign LAY-TABLE. Plates, glasses and cutlery are placed on the table. Carol places these on the table one piece at a time and always in the same order: plates, glasses, forks, knives and spoons. She is guided to perform the corresponding signs before she is given each of the objects.

It is also possible to use signal signs while carrying out an activity with the learner. If the activities are familiar and repeated frequently, they may provide good situations for sign teaching.

Among other strategies, the strategy of reacting to signal-controlled anticipatory behaviour is suitable as a means of increasing the number of expressive signs. The teacher can use a signal sign as a domain sign to give the individual the choice of at least two activities. The choice is made by training expressive signs. This form of domain-oriented intervention may be used not only in situations where the individual wants something or wishes to do something, but also in connection with naming.

> Irene is a 15-year-old girl with autism. She is fond of crafts and is being taught embroidery and knitting. Her craft lessons are signalled by the sign WORK. When her teacher brings out a basket of materials she is given the choice between SEW and KNIT.

One important aspect of domain-oriented teaching is that, as several signs are linked to the same general situation, it encourages the individual to narrow the use of each sign. This helps to increase the length of social interaction within a framework that is familiar for the individual.

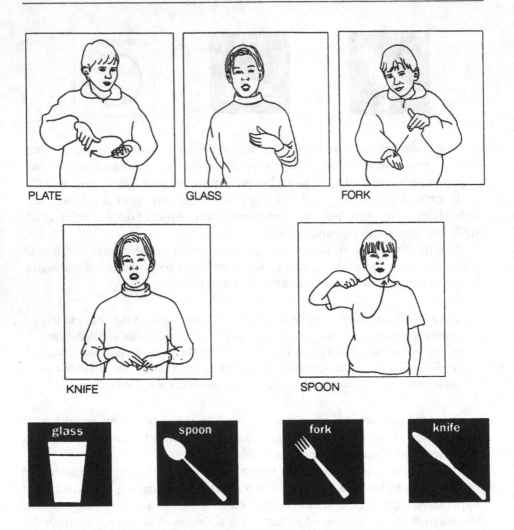

In both expressive training and comprehension training, a good way of beginning the process of sign expansion is to utilize signs that can be used to represent several activities that have one or more features in common. For example, OUT may be used to designate all sorts of outdoor activities. However, it is important that this sign does not interfere with the learning of other specific signs for outdoor activities that the individuals enjoy. SWING and SLIDE are examples of specific outdoor activities. Therefore, OUT should first be learned in situations where these other specific signs are not used. The best way to do this is to create a situation where OUT requires the individual to choose between two outdoor activities, so that OUT is not confused with signs used to represent specific activities. This implies that the teacher should begin by teaching the individuals to choose between two outdoor activities and then use OUT as a domain

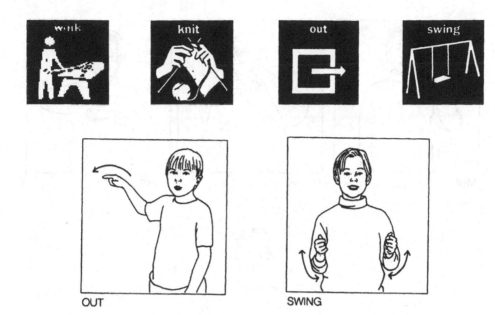

OUT   SWING

sign. Once OUT has been established, its use can be expanded to include more activities.

Contrasts between signs

When children learn to speak normally, it appears that they automatically assume that different words also have different uses (Clark, 1992). However, one should not immediately infer that individuals with severe communication disorders automatically assume that the signs they are being taught are used differently. This supposition has nevertheless given rise to an *exclusion strategy* as a means of introducing new signs when teaching comprehension to people with profound learning disability. The teaching consists of giving the individuals a particular type of food when a manual sign is presented. Once the individuals have learned to respond to the sign by taking the food, they are shown a new type of food together with the one they have already learned. The sign for the new type of food is then presented. The individuals respond to the new sign by taking the new food type because they exclude the food type for which they already know the sign. For example, *MEAT* is introduced together with *DRINK*, with which they are familiar, *POTATO-CHIPS* together with *CAKE* and *TOAST* together with *EGG* (McIlvane et al., 1984). This method seems best suited to comprehension training, but with some adaptations it could be used for expressive training as well. Exclusion may also be a useful strategy for teaching HELP or WHAT by presenting new, attractive objects together with objects with which the individuals are already familiar (in order to make it easier for them to understand that signs should be used).

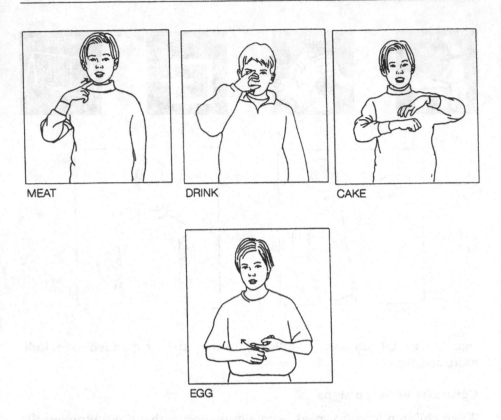

MEAT   DRINK   CAKE

EGG

If the tendency to perceive contrasts between signs is a robust phenomenon, this will be of great practical and theoretical significance. It implies, for example, that, when individuals appear unable to distinguish between the use of two signs, it does not result from the fact that they perceive them as being 'synonymous', i.e. as having the same meaning, but because they are unable to distinguish between their production or because the categories the signs referred to are not distinct enough. It is also conceivable that previous teaching, employing the use of praise and other general forms of reward with many different signs, has led to the unlearning of a 'natural' tendency to perceive and use signs differently, because they all result in the same consequence.

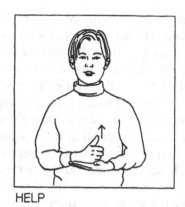

HELP

Signs for proper names

An environment consists not only of objects, activities and events, but also of people. Family and other people play a significant role in all aspects of the individual's life, and even profoundly learning-disabled and autistic people show person preferences. Name signs may be used to express the semantic role of Agent, and are therefore important for promoting the construction of sign sentences (see Chapter 10). However, it is often difficult to find good ways to teach people's names because the actual use of name signs has few immediate consequences. It may also be difficult for the individual to understand what these signs mean.

One solution to this may be to begin by using proper names as signal signs. In nursery schools, schools, institutions and sheltered houses, changes in staff members are often important events. The individuals generally have their favourites, people to whom they become particularly attached. Owing to the nature of shift work in such institutions, it can be difficult to get an overview of staff changes and it is often a problem for the individuals to know which staff members are present. Staff changes often take place without the knowledge of the disabled individuals, which makes it difficult for them to have a complete grasp of the situation and increases their feelings of uncertainty and confusion. The absence of a particular staff member whom the individual expects to be present may, for example, be perceived as punishment if the absence is felt to be caused by a previously occurring event. For many autistic individuals, the inability to anticipate events and to have an idea of what is going to happen often lead to panic reactions. Using people's names as signal signs may ensure that individuals with communication disorders are always informed about which members of staff are present. This may also increase the likelihood of communicative initiative on the part of the individual.

In practical terms, this may be done by each member of staff informing each individual that they have arrived. For an individual who uses manual signs, this is done by the member of staff guiding the individual's hands to sign the name. Each staff member should have his or her own sign. The name sign could be the first letter in the staff member's name using the hand alphabet, as is usual when presenting oneself to deaf people who use sign language, but it may be better to construct a manual sign because several staff members will have the same initial. If graphic signs are used, the name sign could be a drawing or a photograph of the person, at which the individual is guided to point. Tangible signs could, for example, be a distinctive form made in wood or a model of something that relates to the person. For individuals with somewhat more developed language skills, it may be sufficient to show them the picture or perform the manual sign. At a later stage, the manual, tangible or graphic signs may be used to talk about the staff and other people.

> Bodil is a 43-year-old woman with severe learning disability. One-third of her graphic vocabulary consists of 50 person names in the form of photographs. Her communication during intervention sessions has demonstrated that people are her major field of interest and that she has a genuine need for sharing experiences with others, and for putting into words and getting a hold on her own positive and negative emotional encounters with people (Møller and von Tetzchner, 1996).

Without regard to the type of signs an individual uses for general communication, in professional settings, it may be useful to have a wall board on which it is indicated who is and who is not present.

Expanding use

Expanding the use of signs is in many ways as important as expanding the sign vocabulary. Expanding use means applying one particular sign to communicate about several different exemplars of the same object, several performances of the same activity, in several different situations and in connection with various other signs. When teaching expanded use, the object or activity being taught is varied systematically. For example, PLATE can be used to refer to large and small plates, as well as different coloured plates. When practising the sign SQUASH, the situation may be varied by using different glasses and cups.

A significant feature of expanded use is that the signs are used in new ways. When the individual seems to have understood how to use a sign to obtain something, naming should be introduced. Practising naming is often linked to the act of responding to the sign WHAT, meaning 'What is

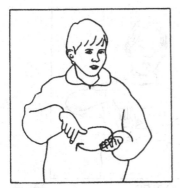 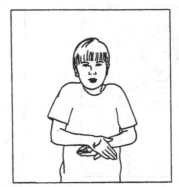 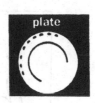

PLATE   JUICE/SQUASH

that?'. This skill is not particularly functional in itself, but the goal is that the naming will acquire a social function. Commenting about something without wanting it is a fairly advanced communicative skill, but the individuals and people in contact with them may enjoy sitting together naming objects, activities and pictures. It may be difficult to design situations that invite a commentary, but unusual and funny situations are often suitable.

> Billy is a severely disabled 3-year-old boy. It was attempted to teach him to name a ball but he showed no interest in the task. One day, a helper crept behind the teacher, who sat opposite Billy, held a large ball above the teacher's head and pretended that she was going to drop it. When Billy saw this, he pointed excitedly at the teacher and vocalized what sounded like ball (Halle, Alpert and Anderson, 1984).

One of the main aims of teaching naming is that the number of signs used by the individual to obtain something will increase without special training. Naming is therefore a more economical way of teaching new signs. Both this and the desire that naming be used to comment on events imply that naming should not unilaterally be linked to the conversational partner's WHAT. The signs should be useful for answering different communicative approaches. WHAT also allows the individual to direct the communication partner's attention to objects or activities of which they want to know the name, and to get comments about activities that are taking place. It is therefore essential that the teacher and the individual take turns at naming and asking questions in the teaching situations.

> Andrew is out for a walk with his teacher. A helicopter flies overhead. Andrew points at the helicopter and signs WHAT. The teacher shows him how to perform the manual sign HELICOPTER.

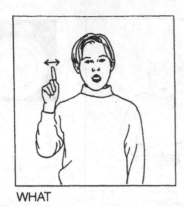

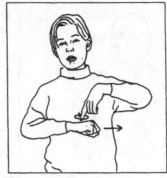

WHAT   HELICOPTER

Situations that begin with the individuals signing WHAT generally produce good conditions for teaching. The situation is initiated by the individuals themselves, based on their wish to gain information about a person, an object, event or activity. Both the individuals and their conversational partners focus on the same object or event, and the individuals are interested and motivated to learn new signs. By using the sign WHAT, the individuals will also be able to obtain information about *new* interests, thus gradually leading to a more user-controlled growth of sign vocabulary. In the case of individuals who, on occasion, ask the names of new objects or activities, it is a good idea to have a comprehensive dictionary of manual signs available whenever possible. Likewise, one should try to have as many graphic or tangible signs available at all times as is practically possible.

Individual sign dictionaries

An individual sign dictionary should be started as soon as the sign intervention is initiated. In the sign dictionary, the translation or gloss of each sign should be noted alphabetically, as well as which signs are being taught and which are being used or understood, or both. The book should also contain a description or drawing of how the manual signs are ordinarily performed, and how the individual performs them. In the case of graphic signs, in addition to the signs the dictionary should contain a description of how the individual points, and whether he or she uses combinations of signs to express special vocabulary items that are not on the board. There should be drawings of tangible signs, and how they are selected. The individual sign dictionary should follow the individuals at least in all their ordinary environments. With the help of the sign dictionary, anyone who is in contact with the individual can quickly get an idea of the signs that he or she uses and understands. If the sign vocabulary and number of sign combinations become large, the sign dictionary will also be an aid to keeping track of which signs have been learned.

The sign dictionary represents a way of discovering new ideas for expanding sign use. For example, one may look at the activity signs in the sign dictionary and try to find object signs that can be used in connection with these activities. Conversely, one may look at the object signs in order to find activities in which these signs can be used. Both of these approaches are examples of a domain-oriented strategy. The dictionary also makes it easier to ascertain whether there is anything that the individual may need but does not know the sign for.

The sign dictionary is not only useful for people in contact with the individual. The individuals themselves also benefit from it and, where possible, the dictionary should be made together with the individual. It may be divided into domains or something else that makes it easy for a non-reader to locate particular signs. The sign dictionary will become a type of reader of which the individual can be proud. As the written glosses are listed together with the signs, it is also practical when a manually signing individual is with people who do not know manual signs.

The expressive language group

The expressive language group is very heterogeneous. Also, in some cases where the major problem is a lack of expressive means, it may be necessary to employ some of the intervention methods discussed above. Other individuals who belong to this group have normal intellectual skills, or a mild or moderate degree of learning disability. However, by definition, in the expressive language group, learning difficulties are not decisive for the individual's need for expressive means. The criterion is a large gap between the comprehension and expression of the individual, and the limitations lie in the individual's lack of speech and, for many, the demands made on the individual's motor functions by the design of the aid.

Here, the focus is on individuals with good comprehension of spoken language and a substantial vocabulary. Exactly what is implied by 'substantial' is hard to say, but around 1000 signs or more is a reasonable estimate. However, it is rare to find such a large expressive vocabulary among users of communication aids who have not learned to write. The average graphic sign vocabulary of 5- to 10-year-old children with good comprehension of spoken language is around 300 signs (von Tetzchner, 1997a); 300 words are also the average expressive vocabulary for normally speaking 2-year-olds. Six-year-old children produce an average of 14 000 words (Carey, 1978; Bates, Dale and Thal, 1995).

User involvement

Even people with a good understanding of spoken language, who learn to express themselves with graphic signs, may have a limited vocabulary with one sign being chosen at the expense of another. This represents a consid-erable barrier to wider social participation. The sign vocabulary deter-mines which subjects can be discussed and which conversations are possible. Today, it is constantly repeated that the signs on a communica-tion board should be chosen on the basis of what is functional for the users in their particular environment. However, in many instances, too much emphasis is given to signs for care, nursing etc., despite the fact that the individual him- or herself seldom talks of care, nursing or similar situ-ations (Beukelman and Yorkston, 1984). The individuals need signs that can be used in a large variety of situations – signs that reflect their interests and make it possible for them to converse about a large number of subjects.

It is usually professionals who decide which graphic signs are on an individual's communication board. To make sure that the signs will be useful, it is essential that the users are involved as much as possible when selecting signs. User involvement in the sign selection process is especially important for older children, adolescents and adults, but attempts should be made to involve communication aid users at the earliest possible stage. This may be done by examining situations in which a child usually partici-pates or would like to participate: radio and television programmes, the dictionary of the graphic sign system used by the child, other lists of signs, ordinary dictionaries and books that have recently been read to the child. Thereafter, the child and his or her adult helpers can discuss words and their corresponding graphic signs and the situations in which the graphic signs can be used. Discussions of this type also give teachers considerable insight into the child's comprehension of spoken language and life situ-ation, as well as clues as to how conditions could be made more favourable for the child. As far as possible, children should be allowed to choose signs for themselves. If there are graphic signs that the adult believes are important for a child, these can be presented on another occasion, perhaps with the phrase: *I have a useful sign for you.*

Expanding the situations in which signs may be used

Many individuals who belong to the expressive language group are severely motor impaired. They have limited mobility and are likely to have a narrower range of experiences than their peers. To expand their sign use, the individuals must be given the opportunity to participate in a variety of situations. Nursery school and school form an important part of the environment of all children, but they are even more important for motor-impaired children and adolescents, who are less able to participate in leisure-time and outdoor activities outwith these environments. The teaching of communication use is often scholastic and planned with the requirements of nursery school and school in mind. Professionals should free themselves from these restrictions and expand the individual's situational repertoire. This is not an easy task and challenges the professionals' powers of innovation and imagination. Young helpers – brothers, sisters and peers – can play an important role in expanding participation in different situations, but they need guidance in how to adapt conditions so they become more favourable for participation of disabled children.

For an extended environment to lead to expanded understanding and use of signs, individuals must have access to their means of communication whenever it is needed. Any limitation in access means reduced communication. Access to communication aids is often poor outside school and special teaching situations. Many children and adolescents who sit in a pushchair or wheelchair have their communication board placed behind them in a carrier. This means that it is the adults who control when conversations may take place; the adults may take the communication board out only when they themselves wish to communicate, and when they believe the child or adolescent has something to say.

One of the difficulties with using communication aids is that it is not always easy to indicate graphic signs in situations where there would otherwise be a good deal of communication. This applies, for example, during washing, meal times, outings to the forest or country, in the car and in bed – situations that are often regarded as good for communication (von Tetzchner, 1996b). Eye-pointing may be an alternative, but there must be sufficient space between each of the graphic signs and they must be placed so that it is possible to follow the individual's direction of gaze without misunderstanding. One way of solving this may be for the conversational partner to wear a waistcoat with graphic signs on, so that the individual can eye-point or select signs by means of dependent scanning, i.e. the conversational partner points at the signs and the individual confirms when he or she is pointing at the correct sign (Figure 33). However, communication boards should, if possible, be fixed and not move with the conversational partner.

Meal times and care

Even people with situation-oriented communication boards will, as a rule, be unable to communicate in the bath, in the toilet, during mealtimes (with the exception of choosing between types of food), in bed, etc. It is important that the individuals are able to communicate in these situations, because individuals with motor impairment generally spend a long time over meals and care. Conversations during mealtimes also quickly become meaningless if they are only about food, i.e. what the individual wants to eat or drink. There is usually little to be said about this because there are

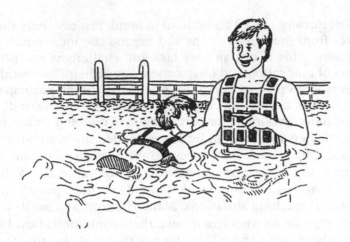

Figure 33. *A vest may be used as a communication board.*

few choices that need to be made during the course of a normal mealtime. The contrast to other people's conversations is considerable. Other children and adults talk mostly about what they have done or are thinking of doing, and a number of other topics. They spend very little time discussing the food that they are eating (Balandin and Iacono, 1998). To facilitate conversation during mealtimes, a set of signs that are useful for conversations may be placed where the child usually sits, fastened so that they do not end up under the plate or otherwise concealed. It is also a good idea to have some boards with domain signs easily available, for use when more specialized topics arise.

It is not easy to take a communication board into the bathroom, but PIC signs, Blissymbols or written words may be put on the bathroom wall. These should include signs that pertain to and are important in that particular situation. For very small children, this may be a picture of a bath-time toy of which they are fond; for somewhat older children and adults, the signs *HOT*, *COLD*, *STOP*, *MORE* and *SHOWER* are important so that they may say how they experience the situation, and whether it should be changed. In this situation, however, it is also a good idea to have something else to talk about, especially if the individual is fond of bathing and does so often. Care is time-consuming, and it is advantageous if the individual has the opportunity to communicate, even though this means that the care takes even longer.

Individuals with extensive motor impairments also benefit from access to signs that may be used to indicate the way in which other people handle them. Such signs enable them to instruct people who do not know them too well. When the individuals have access to signs that make it easier for other people to adjust, the adjustment will come naturally because the

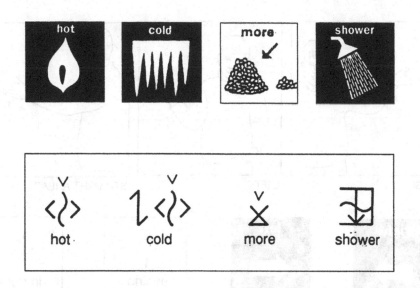

helpers become more sensitive and expect instruction. This helps improve the general situation (compare Hagen, Porter and Brink, 1973; Dalhoff, 1986). Similarly, a domain board for the dental setting may be important to give children and adults without intelligible speech better control and possibilities for expressing pain and discomfort, as well as when the dentist is doing the work in a good way from the patient's perspective (Sheehy, Moore and Tsamtsouris, 1993).

In the car

Communication in a car is often difficult because the driver has to keep his or her eyes on the road and because jolts and turns make pointing imprecise. At the same time, there is plenty to see and many situations that lend themselves to comment. Number plates, reckless drivers and road-hogs are often objects of attention for children. It is not so easy to give the individual access to a large vocabulary, but the situation can be made considerably more *active* and interesting if there are a few graphic signs available, in addition to manual signs if the individual has some motor skill. The communication aid user may be the 'navigator' and say *RIGHT*, *LEFT* and *STRAIGHT AHEAD* at junctions if the car journey follows a familiar route. *RIGHT*, *LEFT*, *BEHIND* and *AHEAD* may be used to indicate the location of points of interest. Synthetic or digitized speech may relieve some of the communication problems. (Technical aids can be attached to the lighter socket in the car.) If there are several people in the car, dependent scanning may be utilized, perhaps by reading aloud (auditory scanning) if the seating arrangements make it difficult to see the board. If

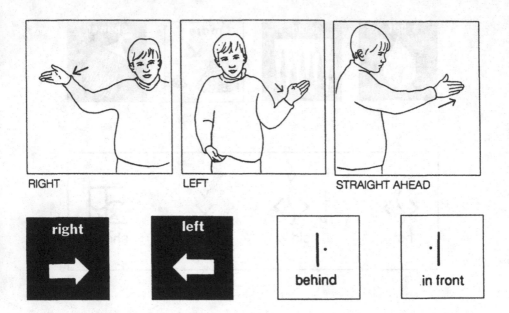

there is a specific destination, or the route passes particularly interesting places, it may provide a good opportunity to introduce new graphic signs, which the adult then uses to support his or her own comments. One may also stop from time to time if there is anything that should be looked at or talked about. If several children with communication aids are on a trip together, the adult can relay the conversations between them.

In bed and at night

Many disabled people need help both to get into and to get out of bed. Some are also frequently ill and spend a lot of time in bed, so it is important that they have the opportunity to communicate in the bedroom. The bedroom is often the place where children are cuddled and do small talk. Fairy-tales may be read aloud, and the child and the caregiver can talk about what is happening in them. This and other types of conversation help to provide disabled children with the same cultural base around which many child-like activities are built.

On occasion, it can be very important for children to be able to communicate at night. The reason why a child cries and is restless may simply be that he or she is thirsty and if the child is able to say so and is given something to drink everyone will get to sleep. But a child may also cry because of a nightmare or an ailment. It may take the parents a long time to find out what is wrong, which will result in a lack of sleep and perhaps grumpiness the next morning. A few graphic signs on the wall or a stand beside the bed may help to reduce the number of sleepless nights and make the child feel more secure.

Increased access to signs

The actual design of the communication board and the number of graphic signs that it can contain depend on the method of pointing or scanning and the user's motor skills. If direct selection is utilized, it is important that the signs are not so small that it is easy to misunderstand which sign the user is pointing at. As there is a limit to the number of signs that can be placed on a surface, the vocabulary should at all times be adapted to the user in the best possible manner. This implies, among other things, that the teacher or caregiver may have to swap signs instead of just adding new ones, and that it may be necessary to have more than one board.

There has been virtually no research into the consequences of different vocabularies. Carlson (1981) mentions that a child who did not use the communication board began to use it when the vocabulary was changed. However, except for the fact that vocabularies should be 'useful', little is known about the best way to construct a vocabulary in order to encourage the development of communication skills and competence. There is every reason to believe, however, that giving emphasis to a general vocabulary, i.e. a *surface-oriented* expansion of the vocabulary, may reinforce the lack of communicative initiative and limited conversational skills. The use of a *domain-oriented* strategy when developing vocabulary makes it easier for the individuals to say something new, and thus help them to make their own contributions to the conversation and continue it in such a way that the conversational partner does not lose interest.

In the discussion of communication boards, it is often emphasized that a small number of words constitute a large part of what is said. This fact has been used to argue that it is possible to communicate effectively with a small number of words, which is true as long as the conversation is kept at a very superficial level. At the same time, there has been a strong focus on signs that provide the individuals with the opportunity to express basic needs in everyday life. If the individuals are to have a chance of conversing at anything other than a superficial level and expressing anything more than basic needs, their vocabulary must be adapted to fit the situation at hand. Increasing the vocabulary alone is not a suitable method of developing conversational skills, because the user will almost immediately become dependent on the conversational partner to formulate questions and comments.

There are a number of reasons why reorganizing the individual's vocabulary requires swapping graphic signs. If new signs were added all the time, the vocabulary would become too large, even if some of the signs were transferred to other boards. It is necessary to give priority to some graphic signs over others. Moreover, the vocabulary that the conversational partner sees is important for how the individual is appraised, and determines which subjects he or she will discuss and how the conversation will start. Conversational partners tend to treat users of communication aids as though they are younger than they actually are (Shane and Cohen, 1981). If the signs on the communication board are childish, this tendency will be reinforced. Signs that are too childish should be replaced. For example, the picture of a teddy-bear on a child's board should be removed when the child becomes older.

Even when the user has several boards, there will be clear limits to how large the vocabulary can grow. One main communication board and its sub-boards, and any sub-sub-boards, in principle constitute a tree-like structure. Using several boards makes it difficult to keep tabs on the vocabulary, and in time it will become impractical. Communication aids based on computer technology with dynamic screens may relieve this problem, because the boards do not take up so much physical space. If an individual is able to choose between four graphic signs on three consecutive levels, this gives a vocabulary of 64 signs (Figure 34). Three levels with 16 signs on each page gives the individual access to 4096 signs (16 × 16 × 16). An individual with a reasonable degree of dexterity should be able to reach each sign quickly, but an individual with more extensive motor difficulties will take considerably longer to reach each one. However, the main

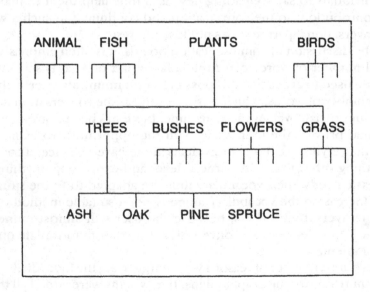

Figure 34. *Search structure when there are four signs on each screen.*

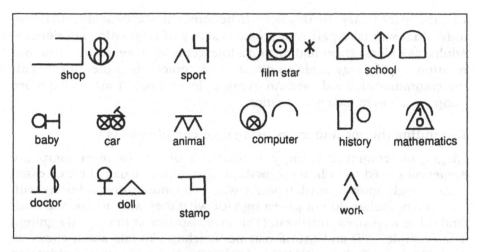

shop · sport · film star · school

baby · car · animal · computer · history · mathematics

doctor · doll · stamp · work

problem is to organize the signs so that the individual is able to remember the position at any given time without any other form of visual support than the view of the communication board displayed on the screen. There will be a total of 256 different screens (16×16) in a search structure with three levels of 16 signs each.

The development of the vocabularies in communication aids is still a field that needs further research. The sign structure in a technical aid should be designed so that the individual is able to grow with it. It should be able to retain those skills that are developed and build upon them. A tree structure is not the only conceivable form of search structure. One may also utilize technologies such as Minspeak (see p. 43). When describing the individual's everyday situation, the teacher should try to find central *domains* that may promote more profound conversation. For younger children, domain signs such as *SHOP, BABY, CAR, DOCTOR* and *DOLL* may be used in conjunction with role-playing, games and other activities. Older children and adolescents may use signs connected with special interests such as *SPORT, POP MUSIC, FILM STARS, ANIMALS, COMPUTERS, STAMPS* and *BOOKS*, or vocabulary associated with *SCHOOL* (*HISTORY, MATHEMATICS, GEOGRAPHY*, etc.) or *WORK*. More generally, single boards may also be adapted to specific environments. The vocabularies used may differ somewhat at home, school, in the youth club, on the street, etc. When producing such domain- and situation-dependent boards, both familiar and unfamiliar signs may be included, so that the board helps develop the individual's vocabulary. The boards should be reviewed systematically and revised regularly, e.g. four times a year, so that the individual is not unnecessarily restricted by the existing vocabulary.

The introduction of domain boards may have a positive effect on the environment and on professionals who are forced to design situations to suit the vocabulary. In this way, it becomes more probable that the individual will take part in a greater variety of linguistic experiences. Adults, as well as other children and adolescents who see the new communication boards, may begin to discuss new topics when they speak with the communication aid user. An exciting domain board may make more people want to initiate conversations.

Expanding the vocabulary by using sign combinations

In graphic communication, combinations of two or more signs are sometimes used to indicate something that would usually be expressed with a single spoken word, typically when communication aid users with limited vocabulary do not have a sign for what they want to say, and must find other ways of expressing it. (This may also appear in manual signing.) For example, *RED* and *SAUCE* may be 'ketchup'. To talk about chess, an individual may indicate *GAME* and *SQUARE*. However, this combination could just as well be interpreted as 'cards', 'Ludo' or 'Checkers' if none of these signs appeared on the communication board, and the individual might be obliged to give several more cues before the conversational partner understood what the user was trying to say. This kind of combination may be called *paraphrasing by analogy*.

The function of the most advanced graphic system today, Blissymbolics, is based on analogies. For example, *ANIMAL + LONG + NOSE* may mean 'elephant' or 'anteater'. In principle, the user may freely construct the equivalent of any spoken word from the basic Blissymbols, but a number of conventional meanings for Blissymbols have been established by the International Bliss Committee. The use of analogies as well as grammatical markers makes it somewhat difficult to estimate the real size of the expressive vocabulary based on Blissymbolics or other systems in which the signs may be combined. In the Blissymbolics system, combinations with *ACTION* change nouns into verbs. *ACTION + BICYCLE* becomes 'to cycle', *ACTION + SAILBOAT* becomes 'to sail'. Combining a sign with *OPPOSITE-MEANING* produces an antonym. Thus, *OPPOSITE-MEANING + LARGE* means 'small', *OPPOSITE-MEANING + HEAVY* means 'light'. However, such expressions also exist in the language of normally speaking children without such combinations being regarded as a word. When testing young children with the Illinois Test of Psycholinguistic Abilities (ITPA: Kirk, McCarthy and Kirk, 1968), it is not uncommon to receive the answer *Not heavy* to the question *Lead is heavy, feathers are . . .?*

Within augmentative and alternative communication, analogies are primarily associated with Blissymbolics because this system is explicitly based on analogy. However, analogies are also common in Rebus (Figure 35) and, in principle, the signs in all graphic systems may be combined to form new meanings. This applies also to script when the user has limited spelling skills, or when it is quicker to use a combination of words by

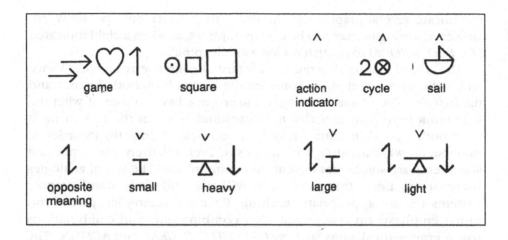

analogy rather than spelling out a long word. The PIC signs *HOUSE + SPORT* may mean 'gymnasium', and the Rebus signs *MAN + LIGHT* may mean 'electrician' if otherwise there are no signs to express these concepts (Figure 35). Analogies are also used in communication aids based on information technology. For example, with the *Words Strategy* applied with Minspeak (Braun and Stuckenschneider-Braun, 1990), it is necessary

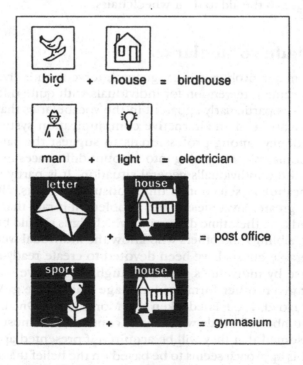

Figure 35. *Compounds of Rebus signs and PIC signs.*

to indicate several graphic signs in order to produce one spoken word. However, analogies may also be true metaphors, as when a child indicated *LEG BED + ROOM* to say that his leg was 'sleeping'.

The use of analogies requires substantial cognitive resources (Vance and Wells, 1994), and places considerable demands on both the user and the listener. The communication aid user must have an idea of what the communication partner is able to understand, whereas the partner must have both a good imagination and a good deal of empathy in order to understand what the user is trying to say. Even relatively uncomplicated statements are sometimes difficult to communicate. The use of analogies therefore assumes that those who will use and understand graphic systems receive appropriate teaching. Recent teaching has placed too much emphasis on ready-made sign combinations and combinations using grammatical signs such as *OPPOSITE*, *PLURAL* and *ACTION*. The users should learn to use the system in such a way that the conversational partners need not have prior knowledge of the construction to understand what is being said. The best way of doing this is probably to use technical communication aids with the maximum number of combinations, where the corresponding spoken word either appears on-screen or is articulated with artificial speech. Most graphic sign users who need an extensive vocabulary are severely motor impaired, and it may therefore be possible to attach the aid to their wheelchairs.

Ready-made vocabularies

One of the major problems in language intervention is the tendency to provide the same intervention for individuals with quite different characteristics. This is particularly apparent in the vocabularies that are selected for people who need an alternative communication system. There has been a tendency among professionals to suggest the same words for different people, without taking into account differences in terms of age, interests and the individual's general situation. It is partly related to the fact that vocabulary selection is time-consuming. Thus, although there seems to be greater awareness of this problem, it is rare that professionals sit down and take their time discussing which signs should be chosen with the parents, siblings and others who know the individual well.

Considerable efforts have been devoted to create ready-made vocabularies for use by individuals who are taught alternative communication systems or given other forms of language training (e.g. Walker, 1976; Fristoe and Lloyd, 1980; Fried-Oken and More, 1992). One tries to identify a limited number of words which have contents that most people need, and it is assumed that they will be acquired if presented appropriately to the user. This approach seems to be based on the belief that children learn approximately the same words, and in a more or less similar order.

These ready-made vocabularies vary in size. Some of them are intended to be used explicitly with a specific sign system, whereas others are intended as general guidelines, independent of whether the intervention involves speech, script, or manual, graphic or tangible sign systems. Two vocabularies that are supposedly suitable for use with children, and which have a central place in the literature, are shown in Table 5. There are approximately 80 words in each, and they are intended to be used as the individual's *first words*. Makaton (Walker and Ekeland, 1985) consists of nine stages. Only the first two stages are included here, because they contain approximately the same number of words as the vocabulary suggested by Fristoe and Lloyd (1980). Makaton is intended to be used by individuals with communication impairment and their teachers and caregivers. The second vocabulary is aimed especially at school-age children (Fristoe and Lloyd, 1980). In some instances the lists have also been used with children and adults with well-developed comprehension skills. In the sign vocabularies, no distinction is made between signs used in comprehension training and expressive training.

As the lists are general, it is impossible to take into account the special characteristics of each individual child. Fristoe and Lloyd take care in saying that the vocabulary is not suitable for everyone, but that many individuals will find it useful. Walker (1976) claims that the vocabulary in Makaton should be learned by everyone, although other signs may be included as well. Her choice of words to be signed, stages and the teaching procedures that make up the Makaton vocabulary has met with considerable criticism (Kiernan, Reid and Jones, 1982; Byler, 1985), but was later revised to be more flexible (Grove and Walker, 1990).

A review of the two vocabularies shows how difficult it is to design a first vocabulary that many individuals will find useful, and demonstrates at the same time which criteria have been used in the selection process. There are many missing words that children might well need. On the other hand, the lists have many words associated with cleanliness and self-help, which children may have limited interest in using. Nor do older children, adolescents and adults use such signs particularly often, most probably because care and washing usually take place at fixed times and without the individual having any particular influence over the situation.

The vocabularies are divided into *substantive words* and *relational words*, in accordance with the suggestions of Lahey and Bloom (1977). Substantive words include words that are used to indicate people, places or objects. Relational words are used to indicate relations between objects and include such word classes as verbs, adjectives and prepositions.

Despite the fact that the vocabularies are designed with children in mind, there are few words for toys. Signs for animals may be useful for children with a special interest in animals, or who have pets at home.

Table 5. *The words suggested by Fristoe and Lloyd (1980) (F&L) and the first two stages of Makaton (Walker and Ekeland, 1985) (W&E)*

Substantive words	W&E	F&L	Relational words	W&E	F&L
APPLE		X	AND	X	
BABY		X	BAD	X	X
BATHROOM		X	BATH	X	
BED	X		BIG/LARGE		X
BIRD	X	X	BROKEN		X
BOOK	X	X	CLEAN	X	
BOY	X		COLD	X	
BREAD	X		COME	X	
BRICKS	X		DIRTY	X	X
BROTHER	X		DOWN		X
BUTTER	X		DRINK	X	X
CAKE	X	X	EAT	X	X
CANDY		X	FALL		X
CAR	X	X	GET		X
CASSETTE PLAYER	X	X	GIVE	X	X
CAT	X	X	GONE		X
CHAIR	X	X	GOOD MORNING	X	
CHEESE	X		GOOD	X	X
COAT		X	GOODBYE	X	
COFFEE	X		HAPPY		X
COMB		X	HEAVY		X
COOKIE	X		HELP		X
CUP	X	X	HERE	X	
DADDY	X		HOT	X	X
DOG	X	X	KISS		X
DOLL	X		LEAVE	X	X
DOOR	X	X	LIE DOWN		X
DRINK		X	LOOK/WATCH	X	X
EGG	X		MAKE		X
FATHER		X	MORE		X
FIRE (HEATING)	X		NO	X	
FLOWER	X		NO	X	X
FOOD	X	X	OPEN		X
FORK	X		PLAY		X
GIRL	X	X	RUN		X
HAT		X	SHOWER	X	
HOME	X		SIT		X
HOUSE	X	X	SLEEP	X	
I	X		STAND		X
ICE CREAM	X		STAND-UP	X	
JAM	X		STOP		X
KNIFE	X		THANK YOU	X	
LADY	X		THERE	X	
LAMP	X		THIS/THAT/THOSE		X
LIGHT	X		THROW		X
MAN	X		UP		X

Table 5. *(Continued)*

Substantive words			Relational words		
	W&E	F&L		W&E	F&L
MILK	X	X	WALK		X
MUMMY/MOTHER	X	X	WASH	X	X
(Name signs)		X	WHAT	X	
PLATE	X		WHERE	X	
POTTY		X	YES	X	
SCHOOL		X			
SHIRT		X			
SHOES		X			
SISTER	X				
SPOON	X	X			
STAFF	X				
SUGAR	X				
TABLE	X	X			
TEDDY	X				
TELEVISION	X	X			
THERE	X				
TOILET	X	X			
TREE	X				
TROUSERS		X			
WATER		X			
WINDOW	X	X			
YOU	X	X			

HORSE may be used to signal riding, which is an activity enjoyed by many disabled individuals.

Signs for articles of clothing may be used as signal signs in a structured dressing setting. Surprisingly, Walker and Ekeland (1985) include no signs for clothes, but for some reason recommend pointing to clothes and body parts rather than using signs. Fristoe and Lloyd (1980) include the most common clothes. NAPPY is missing, as is DRESS. Signs for food types, fruit and sweets are among those signs that are taught first, because it is generally known what the individual likes to eat. Walker and Ekeland include no fruit but, somewhat surprisingly, have chosen to include BUTTER. Fristoe and Lloyd include APPLE, but have no signs for other types of fruit or food. Neither of the vocabularies includes ORANGE JUICE, which is a popular drink. CHOCOLATE is also missing.

There are many names for eating utensils and household goods. The names of eating utensils may be useful. Walker and Ekeland include KNIFE, FORK and SPOON; Fristoe and Lloyd include only SPOON, and omit CUP and GLASS. Some of the signs for household goods may be used for naming without any clear functional objective. TELEVISION is a good

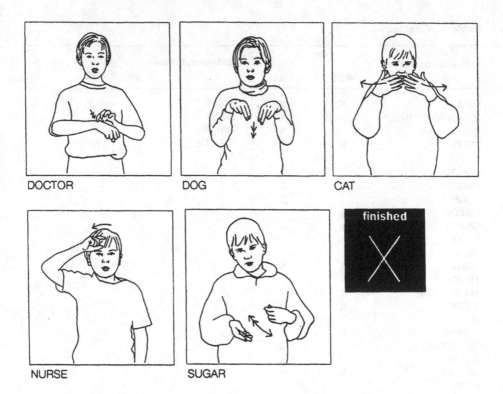

DOCTOR   DOG   CAT

NURSE   SUGAR

expressive sign. Signs such as BED and TOILET are best suited as signal signs.

It may be difficult to find good settings in which to teach signs for individuals (names), except as semantic Agents in sentences (see Chapter 10). One possibility is to use them as signal signs. I, ME and YOU seem rather inappropriate because they are often implicit in the utterance.

Relational words are selected in order to be used together with many objects, and are not as contingent on the individual's interests and environment as is the case with many other words. GET, SEE, PLAY and HELP may be used in connection with many objects and activities, and using them may facilitate the acquisition of new signs. Signs for specific activities are missing. Many of the signs may be of practical use when training self-help skills, and are thus suitable for use as signal signs. However, some of the signs seem to be rather unsuitable for an early functional vocabulary (e.g. CLEAN, DIRTY, HERE, HOT, COLD, EVIL, HEAVY, UP, DOWN, AND and WHERE).

Walker and Ekeland (1985) include YES and NO. Using these signs in answer to questions is only meaningful if the individual is able to understand yes–no questions. This is a condition that many of those who receive teaching in augmentative communication do not fulfil. Moreover, YES and

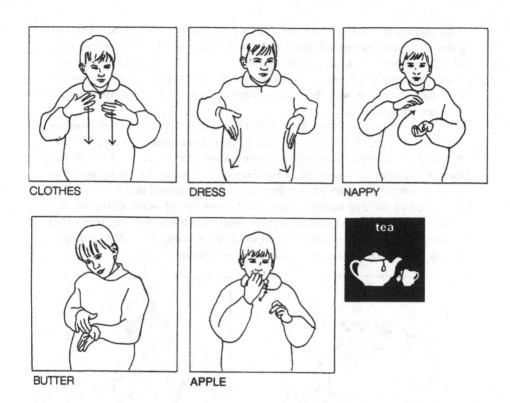

CLOTHES   DRESS   NAPPY

BUTTER   APPLE   tea

NO are dependent on the initiative of others. Fristoe and Lloyd (1980) do not use NO as an answer to a question but follow the arguments of Lahey and Bloom (1977) that NO may be used to express rejection, non-existence or the cessation of an action, and to deny another person an activity, i.e. as a signal sign (see Chapter 10). Rejection is something for which most individuals who start with alternative communication already have an expression, which means that it should be unnecessary to train them in this. As an indicator of non-existence, the word GONE may be more suitable, because the sign NO is used by others as a means of denying the individual an activity. STOP is better than NO when expressing the fact that an activity should cease. Nor is it easy to see how to design good teaching situations for rejection and non-existence. In general, YES and NO are unsuitable in the first stage of the intervention (see also Chapters 8 and 10).

How difficult it can be to find suitable signs in a ready-made vocabulary, rather than taking the individual's own situation as a starting point, is demonstrated in the following example (Yorkston et al., 1989).

G.T. was a 36-year-old woman with cerebral palsy who was unable to read and write. She had recently been given a board containing 24 Blissymbols. The board was in effect her first expressive vocabulary, but her comprehension skills suggested that she could use a far larger expressive vocabulary. She was given a communication aid with synthetic speech, and chose her vocabulary herself together with a team of professionals. Once she had begun to use some words, the team produced a description of her environment and a communication diary. Together with the team of professionals, G.T. also reviewed four standard vocabularies.

The total number of words on G.T.'s board was 240. Most of them were of a general nature, chosen on the basis of their presumed frequency of use. Words that occurred infrequently were avoided. The selection of words was thus in line with the needs that a standard or core vocabulary is supposed to meet. A comparison with 11 standard vocabularies showed that none of them contained all the 240 words on her board, even though some of the vocabularies were fairly extensive. Most of them covered well below 50 per cent of her words (Figure 36). Nor did the total of all the vocabularies' 2327 different words cover what was regarded as her core vocabulary needs.

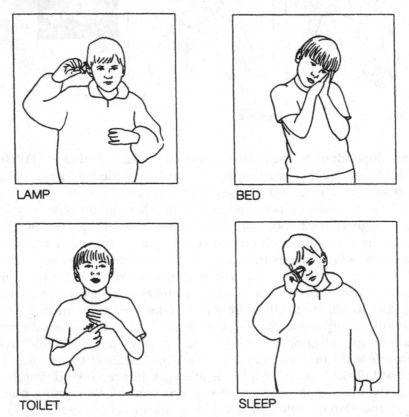

LAMP

BED

TOILET

SLEEP

There has been a lot of research time spent on trying to find general vocabularies that are suitable for teaching alternative communication. This is a seemingly impossible task. However, together with other word lists,

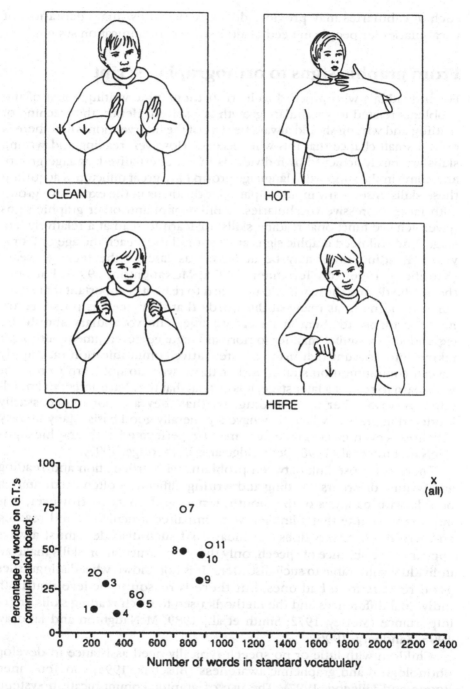

Figure 36. *Percentage of different vocabularies that a 36-year-old woman with cerebral palsy chose for her communication board. Her board contained 240 graphic signs (Yorkston et al., 1989).*

such vocabularies may provide ideas for the individual adaptation of vocabularies for people in need of alternative communication systems.

From graphic signs to orthographic script

For individuals who proceed to learn orthographic writing, most of the problems related to vocabulary growth are solved. Hence, the teaching of reading and writing should always be part of the intervention when there is even a small chance that this will succeed. However, reading and writing skills are rarely achieved by individuals in the alternative language group, and some in the supportive language group have great difficulties acquiring these skills. Also, many motor-impaired individuals in the expressive group with large expressive vocabularies of Blissymbol and other graphic signs never achieve functional reading skills, or learn to read at a relatively late stage, and will need graphic signs at least until they reach the age of 7 or 8 years. Reading skills may be achieved as late as the teenage years (Sandberg, 1996; von Tetzchner, 1997a; McNaughton, 1998). For both those who do and those who do not learn to read, it is important that signs, corresponding to as many of the words that they need as possible, are made available to them at an early stage. The vocabulary should be expanded in a similar manner to normal language development, although taking into account that users of alternative communication may apply special communication strategies. For those who do not learn to read or who learn to read at a later stage, it is crucial that they have access to knowledge in ways other than reading, so that they are not unnecessarily hindered in areas in which they have a generally good basis. Many literacy activities – even electronic mail – may be performed with graphic signs (McNaughton et al., 1996; Detheridge and Detheridge, 1997).

There is a close link between problems with articulation and reading and writing disorders. Reading and writing difficulties often occur among people with paralysis of the mouth, larynx and pharynx. However, it is important to note that a link between impaired articulation and reading and writing disorders does not mean that such disorders must always appear in the absence of speech, only that poor articulation skills make an individual vulnerable to such disorders. It is not known what distinguishes good readers from bad ones, but there is reason to believe that both individual differences and the methods used to teach reading skills are of importance (Morley, 1972; Smith et al., 1989; McNaughton and Lindsay, 1995; Sandberg, 1996).

Children with little or no speech typically need assistance to develop phonological and graphemic awareness (Blischak, 1994; von Tetzchner, Rogne and Lilleeng, 1997). The use of graphic communication systems may facilitate the understanding that print conveys meaning, but not awareness of the fact that they are built up of letters. This must be taught separately (Bishop, Rankin and Mirenda, 1994; Rankin, Harwood and Mirenda 1994). It should also be noted that the mere presence of the written word over or under the graphic sign is not sufficient for an individual to learn to read (Blischak and McDaniels, 1995). For example, unless taught explicitly, an individual may not be able to utilize cues from Blissymbols and letters at the same time.

> Rudi and the special teacher were gluing cards with Blissymbols and written words on the doors of the school. Rudi was shown the correct Blissymbol on a list and had to find the matching card. He did this correctly even with complex Blissymbols and Blissymbols he had not yet learned. Suddenly, he chose *SCHULHOF* (school yard) instead of *SCHAUKEL* (swing). He was prompted to change his choice but was very confident that he was right, pointing at the word printed on the card. Both words began with Sch and Rudi had paid attention only to their letters (Gangkofer and von Tetzchner, 1996, p. 300).

Thus, the transition from graphic signs to orthographic script do not usually happen automatically, but need to be promoted through explicit teaching.

To promote phonological awareness through sound play, children who are unable to talk but nevertheless are able to use a normal keyboard or concept keyboard, should have access to *synthetic* speech at an early stage and thereby be given the opportunity to learn to 'speak' before traditional teaching of reading is initiated. They can use the machine to 'babble' and to find words. The machine should be available at all times so that the children can practise using words and making narratives in a comparable way to children who learn to speak normally (compare Weir, 1966; Nelson, 1989).

A similar approach may be a good alternative to traditional teaching of reading. Instead of learning to read, the children learn to write. With the aid of synthetic speech, a computer pronounces what they have written. Children with reading and writing disorders do not usually have great problems recognising spoken words. Thus, the computer performs what the speech-impaired individuals find most difficult – articulating words or sequences of letters. The individuals can learn to write because the feedback from the computer's speech forms the basis of correcting spelling mistakes and ascertaining the correct spelling. This technology may be combined with programs that check spelling so that words such as *near* and *build* are not written n-e-r-e and b-i-l-d.

As yet, there has been little systematic research into the use of synthetic speech in teaching of reading. However, some studies indicate that such an approach may yield positive results (Koke and Neilson, 1987; Elbro, Rasmussen and Spelling, 1996; Schlosser et al., 1999). It may in fact be the

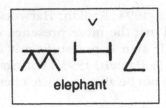

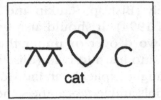

most efficient means to prevent reading disorders. According to E. Hjelmquist and A.D. Sandberg (personal communication, 1994), most of the severely motor-impaired children in Sweden who read and write well had access to computers with synthetic speech while learning to read. For children with difficulties learning to read, *predictive systems* (see p. ••), both alone and in combination with synthetic speech, may also be a useful tool (Newell, Booth and Beattie, 1991; von Tetzchner, Rogne and Lilleeng, 1997).

There are also examples where children who have been able to read have been given boards containing Blissymbols, and teaching in the use of Blissymbols has been favoured instead of reading instruction (Smith et al., 1989). This is probably the result of the fact that many professionals seem to believe that the graphic signs, e.g. in the Blissymbol system, express more than just their gloss. Thus, they feel that it is more meaningful to combine *ANIMAL* + *LONG* + *NOSE* to form ELEPHANT than animal + long + nose to mean 'elephant'. This is of course incorrect. One can just as well form analogies with script as with Blissymbols. The person who interprets an utterance in Blissymbols does in fact combine the glosses because they are written under the graphic signs. Although it is easier for children who are unable to speak to learn Blissymbols rather than normal script, once they have learned to spell they will find it easier to read script than Blissymbols.

Both Blissymbolics and Rebus use letters as an integrated part of the system. Single letters are used actively to give different meanings to signs as in the example of *CAT*. However, there are no ready-made procedures or teaching strategies that deal with the transition from Blissymbols to script. This is a serious flaw because many individuals use Blissymbols when they start to learn to read. It also means that the Blissymbols are not being used to develop language skills in the best way possible. The acquisition of reading skills may be delayed as a result of the lack of such strategies. The original Rebus system contains strategies that are particularly aimed at the promotion of reading skills. It may be useful to adopt some of these strategies and utilize them in conjunction with Blissymbols. The strategies traditionally used with Blissymbols may not be the most effective for individuals who are able to write.

Alan is a 20-year-old motor-impaired boy. He has a good understanding of spoken language and good writing skills. He uses a communication board with both Blissymbols and letters. When he wants to say 'cow', he points first at *ANIMAL* and then spells out the word c-o-w.

For people who are able to use orthographic script as their main form of communication, with the freedom of expression that it provides, it is necessary to acquire those strategies that are best suited to the communication form that they use, rather than continue to use strategies applied with Blissymbols. Many Blissymbols have short glosses. For an individual who is able to spell, it may be useful to have some ready-made words and phrases so that the communication process requires less time. It is not the short words that need to be replaced by analogies, but rather long words that are used relatively frequently. A decision should be made about which words these are, but it is clear that it will not apply to all the Blissymbols generally found on communication boards.

Finally, the teaching of reading and writing is often started too late and makes slow progress. Many children have limited independent access to books and magazines as a result of motor impairments. In spite of the educational problems that they have, many motor-impaired children spend less time than their peers with actual reading instruction in the classroom. They receive fewer literacy experiences, such as being read to and discussing the text with parents, and are given a less active role in such settings. Similar differences have not been found to distinguish good and bad readers within the group of children with limited speech. However, it is still suggested that an increase in number and quality of experiences with print and reading will support the development of literacy (Koppenhaver and Yoder, 1992; Light, Binger and Smith, 1994; Sandberg, 1996; McNaughton, 1998).

Chapter 10
Multi-sign utterances

The transition from single-word or single-sign utterances to utterances consisting of two or more words or manual, graphic or tangible signs is an important milestone in children's acquisition of language. Such utterances allow children to relay more complex meanings and thereby increase their expressive possibilities many times, both semantically and pragmatically. Language structure may especially help bootstrap (see later) or facilitate the acquisition of words or signs denoting categories other than physical objects. The present chapter discusses strategies that may promote the acquisition of language structure and use of utterances with two and more manual, graphic and tangible signs.

In normal development, the acquisition of the first 10–50 words takes several months (Bates, Bretherton and Snyder, 1988; Harris, 1992). In addition, the transition from one-word to two-word utterances happens gradually. The children must have sufficient vocabulary and good enough cognitive and productive control to plan and articulate two units within the same utterance (Peters, 1986). Some children use syntactic constructions at 15 months of age, whereas they may be totally lacking in some normally developing 2-year-olds. Ramer (1976) found that the time from the first two-word utterance until 20 per cent of the utterances had two words or more, varied between 6 weeks and 9 months. Deaf children using sign language start to use sentences at the same age as speaking children (Meier, 1991).

Early spoken utterances consist mainly of content words without inflections such as: *Doll sit*, *Sit chair*, *There Teddy*, *Teddy gone* and *Cat ear*. They comprise a small number of semantic relationships, typically Actions and Agents, reflecting different aspects of settings and events and thus the children's context, i.e. their focus and interpretation of the situation. Table 6 presents semantic relationships that are typical of young children's language. Table 7 gives examples of semantic roles in early two-word utterances.

Table 6. *Typical relationships in early utterances with one and two words (based on Bloom and Lahey, 1978)*

1. **Existence**: the utterance refers to an object in the situation and the child looks or points at it, touches it or picks it up, saying: *ball, there, there, ball, that there,* or something similar
2. **Non-existence**: some object does not exist in context or the child does not see, but there is some reason to expect it to be there or to look for it. The child may say *no* or *gone*, or say the name of the object with rising intonation (like a question) and look for it
3. **Recurrence**: an object – or a similar one – that has disappeared reappears, or an object similar to an existing one is brought into relation with the first object. The child may say *more*, *again* or *another*
4. **Disappearance**: some object has been in the context and then ceases to exist. It may suddenly be hidden from view, vanish or evaporate of its own accord. Children may say *all gone, away* or *bye-bye*. A girl pointed to the sun disappearing behind a cloud and said: *Gone.*
5. **Action**: the utterance refers to an action where the aim of the action is not to change the location of the objects or people. Marte looks at the sandwiches: *Taste! Eat!*
6. **Possession**: the utterance refers to a possessive relationship between a person and an object. John takes the ball: *Mine!!*
7. **Attribute**: the utterance refers to a quality or characteristic feature of an object. Marte points at the jam: *Strawberry. Red.*
8. **Negation**: the child denies the identity, condition or event that is expressed in another person's utterance, or in the child's own preceding utterance. Mamma offers a glass of milk to Anders asking: *Want milk?* Anders shakes the head and says: *No.*
9. **Rejection**: the utterance expresses that the child refuses an action or rejects an object. Mamma says: *Don't you want milk?* Anders pushes the glass away: *No.*
10. **Locative actions**: the utterance refers to an action that aims to change the location of people or objects. Anders places a doll in a chair: *Sit!*

Many individuals with autism and learning disability, who use an alternative language system, fail to make the transition to multi-sign utterances, and there may be several reasons why they seem to stop at the level of one-sign utterances. Neurological damage may to some extent hinder the acquisition of relevant cognitive and linguistic skills, but it may be noted that even severely and profoundly cognitively impaired people use spoken sentences (Rosenberg and Abbeduto, 1993). Moreover, children in the expressive language group with good comprehension of spoken language also tend to produce short graphic sentences, mainly one-sign utterances (Light, 1985; Udwin and Yule, 1990; von Tetzchner and Martinsen, 1996). For this group, and probably for most other language-

Table 7. *Typical semantic roles in early two-word utterances*

Agent	The one who performs the action
Action	The action
Patient	To whom or what something happens
Location	Where the action takes places or something is moved to or from
Possessor	The one who owns something
Possession	What is owned
Entity	Object or person with separate existence
Attribute	Characteristic of entity
Demonstrator	Indication of something
Agent + Action	*Baby cries*
Action + Patient	*Pulls wagon*
Agent + Patient	*Baby food*
Action + Location	*Sit chair*
Entity + Location	*Chair basement*
Possessor + Possession	*Mama glasses*
Entity + Attribute	*Big tree*
Demonstrator + Entity	*There apple*
Agent + Location + Time	*I school today*
Agent + Action + Patient	*Doggie eat food*
Agent + Action + Location	*Man sits car*
Action + Attribute + Entity	*Cut big flower*
Demonstrator + Possession + Possessor	*There scissors mama*

disordered children, it is not cognitive and linguistic impairments alone that hinder the development of multi-sign utterances. If they had not been motor impaired, they would probably have produced spoken sentences. Thus, factors related to other aspects of the communication, such as the language form itself and the interaction patterns in dialogues between natural and aided speakers, may to some degree determine the structure of utterances produced by communication aid users (Smith and Grove, 1999; Sutton, 1999).

One important contributing factor may be that many children who use an alternative language form have not been provided with the appropriate learning opportunities. The teaching and use of multi-sign utterances have received limited attention, and there is consequently a dearth of intervention strategies for syntactic development that take non-speaking children's possibilities and limitations into account. Language structure of graphic communication has mainly been discussed in relation to the expressive language of motor-impaired children with good comprehension of spoken language, and usually with reference to the syntax of ordinary written

Table 8. *Manual and graphic sign sentences reported to be used by children with autism and intellectual impairment*

Pete 20 years (age score comprehension 2;7)
CHILD EAT FORK (Premack's blocks)

Charlie 10 years (age score comprehension 3;9)
TEACHER PUT CANDY IN BOX (Premack's blocks)

Boy with autism
NO MOTHER CAR PLAY SCHOOL
Boy with autism (the only two-sign utterance in 9 months)
PAPER HEAD (request to play peekaboo)

Ted with autism 6.5 years
DADDY EAT
GO SCHOOL
MOTHER CAR
FATHER HAIRCUT
EAT CAKE
MORE CAKE
NO FOOD
NO GO

---

language. In fact, only a few studies have reported graphic or manual multi-sign utterances produced by autistic and learning disabled individuals (e.g. Fulwiler and Fouts, 1976; Bonvillian and Blackburn, 1991; Wilkinson, Romski and Sevcik, 1994; Grove, Dockrell and Woll, 1996; Grove and Dockrell, 2000). However, these studies indicate that the semantic relationships found in the expressive language of children in this group are comparable to those in the spoken language produced by young, normally developing children (Tables 7 and 8).

One result of this lack of appropriate strategies in the professional literature is that interventionists often do not know how to proceed when a child has successfully acquired an initial vocabulary of manual and/or graphic signs, and therefore continue to use the same intervention strategies directed at teaching single signs. Even if these strategies successfully contributed to promoting the child's acquisition of the first manual and graphic signs, they may not be optimal for teaching more complex utterances. Moreover, there is evidence that, even if non-speaking children have good comprehension of spoken language, the graphic expression is not a simple recording from 'inner speech' (Smith, 1996; Sutton and Morford, 1998). The consequences of this are cut off by the fact that these children receive hardly any support from adult language models. Normally speaking people in the environment seldom produce two (or more) syntactically connected signs when they use manual signs together with

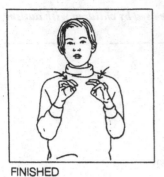
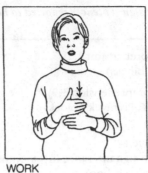

FINISHED   WORK

speech (Grove, Dockrell and Woll, 1996). Graphic signs are only rarely used together with speech by communication partners, and mainly during teaching sessions (Bruno and Bryen, 1986; Udwin and Yule, 1991; Romski and Sevcik, 1996).

Vocabulary

Choosing signs and encouraging individuals to use multiple sign utterances are closely linked. Sufficient and appropriate vocabulary is a prerequisite for making sentences. In normal development, children have typically learned 15–50 words when they start making sentences, and children using non-vocal language should be encouraged to use sentences at a similar stage. Many children with intellectual impairment remain for a longer time in the one-word phase than normally developing children, and have acquired bigger spoken vocabularies when they start to produce sentences. However, this development may not be directly applicable to communication aid users because they tend to have relatively smaller expressive vocabularies.

Signs that can be combined with more than one activity sign, as well as signs that can be combined with more than one object sign, are well suited to expanding an individual's sign vocabulary. For example, FINISHED and BALL can easily be combined with activity signs, e.g. FINISHED WORK, FINISHED JUMP, BALL KICK and BALL THROW. CARRY and SIT can be combined with many object signs, such as CARRY MILK, CARRY SACK, SIT CHAIR and SIT FLOOR. Command signs may also be used in sentences, e.g. FETCH CASSETTE, FETCH MINERAL WATER. With a little imagination, together with knowledge of the individual's interests and likes, this approach may be used in expressive training. The teacher and the individual can take turns at giving instructions, so that the teacher sometimes has to fetch the mineral water or cassette. Such utterances may also be used as a means of talking about events, often in combination with the name of one of the staff members or other residents: PETER GET TRAIN RAILS, MARY FINISHED MINERAL WATER.

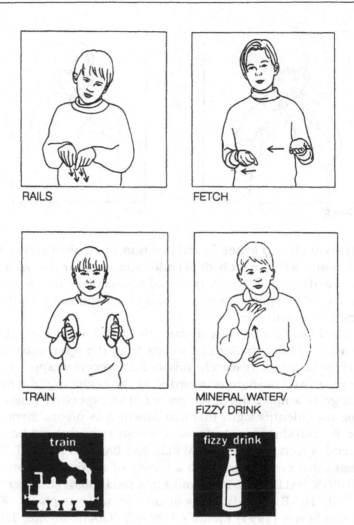

RAILS

FETCH

TRAIN

MINERAL WATER/
FIZZY DRINK

train

fizzy drink

Pivots

The vocabulary that has been chosen for a child by parents and professionals may or may not promote the use of utterances with multiple signs. Some signs are better suited to form multi-sign utterances than others, and these signs may help the user both acquire new signs and combine signs to form sentences. In the early stages of normal language development, certain words are used more frequently than others and these are often combined with other words. This class of words has been termed 'pivots' (Braine, 1963). The rest of the child's vocabulary, i.e. most of its words, belong to the open class.

In *Gone milk, Gone dog* and *Gone cake, gone* is pivot.
In *Me down, Doll down* and *Shoe down, down* is pivot.

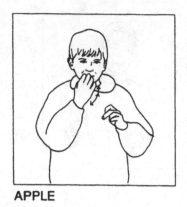

APPLE

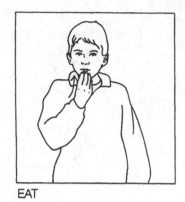

EAT

Pivots do not have a general fixed position, but a pivot is always used in the same position by the individual child. Some appear always at the front and others at the end of the utterances of a particular child. Some children may use a word as a pivot at the start and others the same word as a pivot at the end of the sentence.

There will not be a pivot in all early two-word utterances. Many utterances consist of combinations of words from the open class. However, within child language research, pivots have received special attention because their fixed position is regarded as the beginning of syntax. Thus, as a strategy to facilitate the development of an expressive language structure, one may identify signs that can function as pivots. Pivots may, for example, be introduced in the form of activity signs that can be combined with several objects, such as EAT APPLE, EAT BANANA and EAT BREAD, or object signs that can be used with a variety of activity signs, such as GET BALL, THROW BALL, ROLL BALL and KICK BALL. Signs such as FINISHED, GET, GONE, HAVE and GIVE may also be suitable as pivots. Wilkinson, Romski and Sevcik (1994) identified WANT, PLEASE, MORE, THROUGH, HELP, YES and NO as pivots, but these were not used in a fixed position by each child, and hence did not have the fixed distribution that gives a syntactic quality to pivots.

Pivot-oriented intervention has two aspects. First, it implies a selection priority for signs that may be easy to combine with other parts of the child's expressive vocabulary. Second, when selecting new signs from the open class, those that can be combined with the child's pivots may be given some priority. It should be noted, however, that the pivot-oriented vocabulary selection strategy implies only that awareness of the pivotal function guides the choice of signs, so that signs that may function as pivots are introduced to the child. Whether a particular sign will function as a pivot depends on the child's actual use of it. It is also possible to

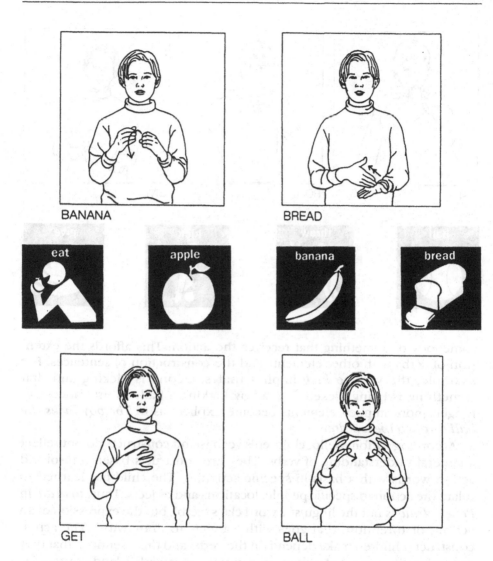

BANANA   BREAD

eat   apple   banana   bread

GET   BALL

combine signs from the open class, but, as pivots have a syntactic quality and are used often and in combination with different signs, they may afford the learning of new signs because they constitute a prototypical language structure (compare bootstrapping below).

Verb island constructs

Tomasello (1992) maintains that verbs play a central role in children's construction of grammar. Verbs are the organizing element for expressing intention, and represent an early conceptual frame for sentence construction because there is implicitly someone performing the verb action and

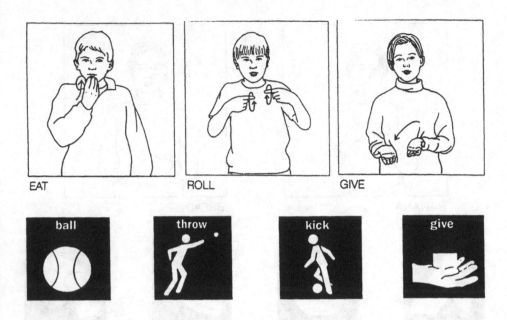

somebody or something that receives the action. This affords the extension of verbs with other elements and the construction of sentences. For example, the verb *to kick* implies that someone is kicking and that something is being kicked, e.g. a boy kicking a ball. As utterances get longer, more implicit elements become explicit, as in *The boy kicks the ball through the window.*

According to Tomasello, children's verb island constructs do not reflect a general understanding of verbs. They are constructs based on isolated action words with a basis in specific activities. The child has learned to relate the action to specific people, locations and objects. Thus, *to draw* in *Pencil draw* is not the linguistic word class 'verb', but the expression of an action, or intention, that goes with 'objects to draw with'. The actual constructs children make depend on the verbs and the intentions that they are trying to express. As children acquire more verb island constructs, these constructs become reorganized, or redescribed, into more abstract sentence constructions. Verb island constructs are thus both an experiential foundation and a model for later sentence construction.

One important implication of Tomasello's theory is that, in order to promote constructs with several signs, intervention should attempt to increase children's use of verbs in situations where the intentions expressed with the verbs may be combined with signs referring to elements that are contextually related to these verbs. This also means that the traditional tendency among professionals to focus on object words should be reduced.

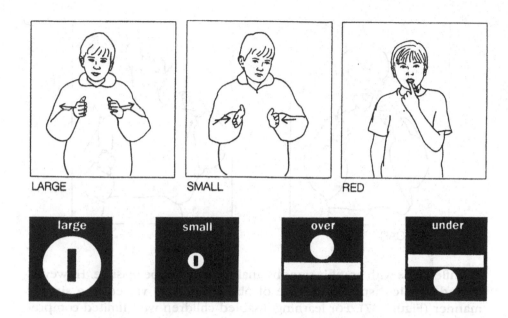

LARGE   SMALL   RED

large   small   over   under

New sign categories

As the sign vocabulary expands, it will be possible to combine more and
more signs. Although early vocabularies tend to comprise objects and
actions, children may have an increasing need for signs denoting qualities
such as LARGE, SMALL and RED, and spatial locatives such as ON, IN, ABOVE
and UNDER. People are usually central in children's environment and person
names may come to comprise an important part of the vocabulary. Signs
belonging to these categories may to some extent depend on language structure to be learned. However, even when children have reached a relatively
advanced linguistic competence, new signs should be selected on the basis of
assumptions about which signs may best contribute to improving their
communication opportunities, social function and overall situation.

Inflections

Although inflections are an integral part of sign languages, use of inflections is rarely reported for learning-disabled and language-impaired
individuals using alternative communication systems. However, investigations have demonstrated that some children with learning disability
modify their manual signs by analogy to express more precise meanings,
in spite of a lack of formal instruction and language models. Examples are
performing RUN fast to say 'run fast' and produce BOX with amplified
space to say 'large box' (Grove, Dockrell and Woll, 1996; Grove and
Dockrell, 2000). A similar inflection is used in many sign languages to
distinguish between, for example, SMALL-CAR and BIG-CAR.

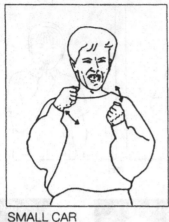
SMALL CAR

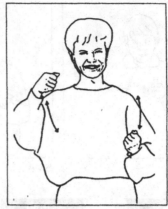
LARGE CAR

Inflections with graphic signs by analogy may not be feasible. However, with dynamic displays, the size of objects may be varied in a similar manner (Figure 37). For learning-disabled children with limited comprehension of spoken language, attributes expressed in this way may be easier to learn and use than graphic signs such as *SMALL* and *BIG*.

Sentences

The function of sentences is to express the interrelationships of two or more elements within a particular context. The message *Daddy car* is qualitatively very different from *Daddy* and *Car* produced separately. In the latter case, daddy and the car may or may not be related in some way. *Daddy car* expresses a definite relationship between Daddy and car, although the nature of the relationship may vary according to the context. It may mean that daddy owns a car, stands by a car, will be coming or going in a car, sits in a car, etc. Sentences thus usually comprise more precise statements than single words or signs, and thereby reflect more elements of the shared focus of the communication partners (von Tetzchner, 1996b).

Horizontal and vertical structures

Before children start using true two-word utterances, they produce one-word utterances that follow each other and are related to the same event, such as in this example from Bloom (1973), where Allison (aged 18 months or 1;6 years) hands the father a peach and a spoon:

Daddy.
Peach.
Cut.

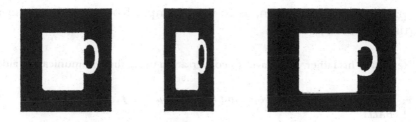

Figure 37. *Possible analogical inflections of PIC signs.*

Successive one-word utterances differ from 'true' multi-word utterances in that they are not expressed within the same sentence contour (Crystal, 1986). Scollon (1976) describes the relationship between such utterances as *vertical structures*. When making the utterances below, Brenda (aged 1;7 years) holds a shoe up to Scollon:

mama
mama
mam
s
sis
su?
sus

Brenda's vertically structured utterance may be interpreted as: '[This is] mama['s] shoe.' The many repetitions probably reflect the great effort Brenda put into the production of this meaning. A similar utterance with *horizontal structure* may have been *Mama shoe.* The elements of vertical structures are separated from each other in time, and sometimes also by utterances from the conversation partner that are unrelated in meaning.

The relational use of words interspersed with pauses, i.e. successive utterances in vertical structures, represents a transitional stage between one-word and two-word utterances. Utterances with a vertical structure are important developmentally because they demonstrate that children may relate words meaningfully to each other before they have learned to express them within the same sentence intonation. Such utterances are often found in the speech of children in the first half of the second year of life. When children are young, adults often say something in between the children's single-word utterances. Scollon demonstrates that a child's utterances may be related thematically even if the utterances inserted by the adult are not.

In addition, utterances produced by children using graphic language may be regarded as having a vertical structure, typically interspersed with the partners' interpretation, as in this example from von Tetzchner and Martinsen (1996, p. 78).

Henry and his father were having a conversation using the communication aid.

F: *Is there anything more you want to tell about this page?*
H: *BALL.*
F: *Yes, ball, yes. What do you do with the ball, Henry. Let's see if we can find something here that we use it for* [turns pages]. *Do we use the ball for anything here? What can we use the ball for?*
H: *FOOT.*

FOOT is related to BALL and Henry's statement may, for example, be interpreted as 'football' (one of Henry's great interests) or 'kick the ball'. From an alternative communication intervention perspective, utterances with vertical structure demonstrate the co-constructive nature of children's early multi-sign utterances, and how parents and other adults may facilitate relational structure by helping the child in the formation of such utterances. They imply a possibility of relating two and more signs to each other, even if they are not produced as one coherent utterance. Coherent utterances are often difficult to produce for children using communication aids. However, the single-sign utterances of children using communication aids tend to have a time-related narrative structure rather than a relational one, as in some of the dialogues discussed in the next chapter.

Topic-comment

Topic-comment is often considered a basic sentence construction where the topic is the theme, what one wants to communicate about, whereas the comment is what one wants to say about the topic. For example, in *Ball gone*, *ball* is topic and *gone* is comment. A related distinction is between 'given' and 'new'. The given is the topic, what is shared and may be considered as known, and the new is the comment, i.e. the particular aspect of what was known on which attention should be focused. In the next example, the child repeats the topic *look* (directing the mother's attention to an event that he or she wants her to see), until the mother acknowledges the shared attentional focus, and then presents the comment *Oy* (Martinsen and von Tetzchner, 1989, p. 62).

Child: *Look!*
        Look!
Mother: *Yes, look there.*
Child: *Oy* [expression of excitement].

Topic-comment, or given-new, may be used as a paradigm for creating utterances with more than one sign, in a vertical or horizontal structure. This strategy is also related to relevance, attention, shared focus and context (von Tetzchner, 1996b). It implies first directing the attention to the topic or domain of the conversation, and then making a statement about the situation, as in the example above. A child may indicate *BALL* to make the adult focus on it, and then *KICK* to make the parent kick it. This may be a more efficient communication structure even though *Kick ball* is the appropriate syntax of the spoken language in the child's environment (von Tetzchner, 1985).

One way to analyse a conversational or instructional situation in relation to relevance and attention is to attempt to identify the critical aspects of the communication situation. In a discussion about stuttering, Bjerkan (1975) defined *critical* in the following manner (pp. 108–109): 'In a situation with a given topic, the *critical* word is the word that is necessary for communicating about this topic.' Thus, the notion of the critical word or aspect of the message may serve to highlight what must be perceived and understood before a complex message can be understood, and which elements an utterance must contain in order to be comprehensible to others. Reaching an agreement about topic may involve negotiations or clarification about the critical information in the message. Learning language thus means learning to understand what another person considers to be critical and to relay one's own perspective.

Intervention strategies based on the notion of critical word or information may help the child and his or her caregivers to chose words that maximize the child's probability of being understood. They may also include situational adaptations, which makes it become evident to the child what the critical information is.

Semantic roles

The earliest semantic roles tend to be Agent and Action (see Table 7). However, interpretations of the utterances of young aided speakers often take it for granted that the child is the Agent. There is less talk about other people's actions. As the Agent is implicit, it is difficult to make the child aware of the possibility of changing it – to make somebody else the Agent. Many children have difficulties learning a fixed word order. One reason why sentence constructions based on semantic roles may be easier for language-disordered children is that they are not based on word order. The semantic role of each manual or graphic sign in a multi-sign utterance is based on the meaning that they have in the communicative setting.

If photographs are applied in the communication aid, the child is often present in the photograph, thereby making it difficult to distinguish Agent from Action, Location or any other semantic information that the photograph may be intended to relay. To avoid this problem and make children include and become aware of Agents in their utterances, one should introduce a separate photograph of the child, together with one or more photographs or signs from a graphic system that denotes other semantic roles. This is part of a semantic strategy to supply children with vocabulary items, which highlights the functions of different semantic roles.

A semantic strategy was applied when teaching graphic signs (photographs and PIC) to two preschool children with autism (von Tetzchner et al., 1998). One of the children, a boy called 'Robert', had a communication book with a small fold-out 'conversation' page in which he and his conversation partners could put the graphic signs selected. The other child, a girl named 'Mari', had a doll's suitcase containing strips of cardboard with four photographs and PIC signs. The lid of the suitcase functioned as the 'conversation location' where the selected signs were placed. The graphic signs of both children had Velcro on the back. Initially, a photograph of the child was always placed at the beginning of the graphic utterance, making the child the (implied) Agent. However, the photograph may not really function as a semantic Agent until different Agents are possible on the basis of the vocabulary and the communicative setting. The photographs of the children were, from time to time, replaced with another person, in order to signal a change of Agent and make them aware of the information intended to be relayed by their photographs.

Robert quickly understood the change in meaning related to the change of photograph, and started to use this productively. In the example below, the teacher (Kari) utilized the fact that Robert liked to play with Flip-flop, a 'pipe' for blowing a ping-pong ball into the air, although he was unable to blow the ball himself. This activity thus represented an opportunity for the teacher to introduce KARI (photograph of teacher) as Agent instead of ROBERT.

> Robert placed FLIP-FLOP after ROBERT which as usual was in the first position on the conversation page. The teacher placed the ping-pong ball on the pipe and put it into Robert's mouth. He tried to blow, not very successfully, and gave the pipe to the teacher. She replaced ROBERT with KARI saying Kari will blow, and started to blow into the pipe, making the ball dance in the air above it. She then changed the names again and gave the pipe to Robert.

One of the first clear indications that Robert had understood the semantic role of the Agent in the utterance on the conservation page appeared in the following situation:

> After a session involving taking turns with the pipe and changing names on the conversation page, Robert put FLIP-FLOP back into the communication book,

took out *ACTIVITY-BOARD* and placed it to the right of *KARI*, which happened to be on the conversation page when the play with the pipe ended. Kari started to play with the activity board and Robert watched for some time, looking puzzled but smiling. He then took away *KARI* and placed *ROBERT* on the conversation page, but Kari answered by putting *NO* (a red card with a black cross) on top of ROBERT. She then put *ROBERT* into the book again and *KARI* back on the conversation page, and continued playing with the activity board for a while. Robert then took *ACTIVITY-BOARD* away and replaced it with *BARREL* (a toy he liked very much). Kari showed great enthusiasm, made a lot of noise, and opened and closed the barrel. Robert watched, laughing and smiling.

The use of photographs of people to indicate Agent should be used as part of the intervention from the start, even when the individuals have not yet understood their function. The objective is to promote the use of expressive multi-sign utterances *before* the individual has learned it. It is a form of 'talking to learn' which is an integral part of typical language acquisition through co-construction with the teacher and other communication partners. Mari had not yet started to replace the photograph of herself to indicate another Agent or to show comprehension by reacting to such changes made by the teacher, but she did master communicative challenges that may guide her towards multi-sign expressions. In the situation described below, with the help of the teacher, she produced a two-sign utterance with vertical structure.

During lunch, Mari selected the photograph *CHEESE*. The teacher made a slice with a cheese knife and held it out to her without giving her any bread, saying: *Mari wants cheese*. Mari looked at it for more than a minute with a puzzled expression and then looked through her photographs and produced *BREAD*, thus linking two related objects, saying something like '[I want] bread with cheese'.

With graphic signs, the Agent is usually placed in the first position on the communication board, so that the individual can distinguish it from the semantic role of Patient. However, some individuals have problems following a fixed order, and this should not be taken as an indication that they cannot learn multi-sign utterances. Their placing of the graphic signs on the conversation location may, for example, be determined by the order in which they find the graphic signs that they intend to use. When constructing a message, Robert would sometimes take two person photographs from the same page of his communication book, place them next to each other, search for the action sign and place it next to them. Although a fixed word order may be practical, a failure to learn this should not be used as a hindrance to sentence development.

A variety of strategies may be used to help children produce manual and graphic sentences of varied complexity comprising different semantic roles. Interaction with several people one at a time may be a way of teaching Agent in a natural setting. This makes it necessary to communicate about actions that can be performed by several people, with several objects and in several ways, e.g. PER JUMPS, TEACHER JUMPS, PER SLIDES, OLA SLIDES, PULL CAR and PULL HORSE. HIDE and SEEK may be an amusing activity, in which an adult or child searches for the others. Such activities may also provide possibilities for training location and spatial terms, such as in JOHN UNDER TABLE and JOHN IN CLOSET. Such manual and graphic signs may be used both during an activity and when communicating about it and making narratives afterwards.

Negation

Children's early expressions are often modified by negation (Bloom, 1998). In intervention, it may be practical to introduce negations that do not reflect the child's wish because it usually has some non-verbal means to express 'don't want', and such negation forms are often difficult to teach because they, at least for a period of time, imply frequent introduction of something that the child does not like in order for him or her to reject it. If the use of negation is not linked only to the child's actions, it will be easier to promote the use of multiple Agents. Teachable negations may be 'not here' and 'do not'. As can be seen in the example with Robert above, Kari had introduced *NO* (a red card with a black cross) which meant something like 'no' or 'not'. Robert seemed to understand and accept NO much better than the spoken *no*, and he also quickly started to use it himself. This led to the creation of sentences with three items, as in *KARI NO DINNER*, where *NO* was put on top of *DINNER*. The way Robert used it, *NO* often had an inflectional quality because it was put on top of another graphic sign to modify it, but *NO* was also used alone.

The reaction to *NO* is not unique for Robert. It is our general experience that severely and profoundly learning-disabled children seem to understand and accept a graphic *NO* better than a spoken one.

Fill-in

In intervention based on semantic roles, the use of fill-in strategies may be a particularly useful strategy for making the semantic roles of graphic signs explicit. Robert and Mari used 'conversation locations' where the elements of each sentence were placed, in the form of a fold-out page and suitcase lid. This may be a prerequisite for applying the fill-in strategy in natural, non-instructional settings where communication is afforded (planned or non-planned), e.g. in the form of the presence of a popular toy or favourite food out of reach. Incomplete sentences may be laid out on the 'conversation' page or lid together with the child or while the child is watching, and the child is then encouraged to provide the rest of the information, for example:

OLA EAT ?
? EAT CARROT
? EAT CHOCOLATE
OLA PUZZLE ?
DOLL ? RED
? CAP

Preferably, the child selects a graphic sign from its total vocabulary (which should be present at all times). If the child does not respond, or seems at loss, the partner may help him or her by presenting two to three of his or her graphic signs from which to chose, or, if this fails, make a choice while demonstrating the function of the sign that is inserted as clearly as possible. For this kind of strategy to be used, the child must already have demonstrated relevant skills and the ability to make similar constructions in more structured settings. It is also important that the child experiences the provision of a 'missing' sign in the utterance as a communicative act that originates in the child's own needs, and not as some game performed only to please the teacher. Fill-in tasks may also be used in a reverse manner in comprehension (see Bootstrapping below).

Chaining

Behaviours, actions, and events and signs representing them may be linked to each other through chaining. Chains may have both a narrative-oriented (temporal) and a relationship-oriented (conceptual) foundation. For example, sentences may be produced by chaining specific expressive signs with more general ones. For instance, OUT may be taught as a signal sign (i.e. to indicate an activity that is going to happen), and SWING and WALK as expressive signs. These may then be combined as a means of informing a child that he or she is both going out and will either walk or swing, indicating OUT WALK or OUT SWING, and for the child to say that he or she wants to do such things. Later on, OUT may be used to construct OUT SHOP, OUT VISIT and other combinations. As a general sign will usually be produced before the specific one, chains may help create a topic-comment structure and approach a

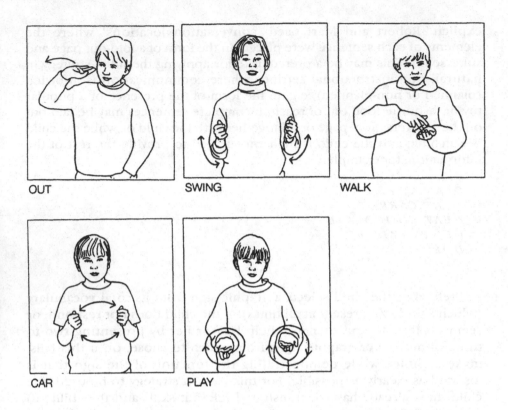

OUT   SWING   WALK

CAR   PLAY

pivot structure. Utterances may be expanded beyond two signs by adding more links, e.g. OUT CAR SHOP, OUT PLAY SWING and OUT VISIT GRANDMOTHER.

One objective of using sentences is that the individuals should also be able to communicate about sequences of activities – activities that are not taking place at the time of the conversation or objects that are not visible. This will enable them to obtain objects that are not present in the situation or suggest activities that are currently not taking place, specify to a greater extent what it is that they want, and give them a better grasp of what is going to happen. It may be difficult for individuals with intellectual impairment and autism to understand the order of events that will take place, or they may be too impatient to wait. In such instances, the sentence construction FIRST–THEN may be attempted to teach within a framework based on chaining. The individual may, for example, be told FIRST TIDY, THEN WALK or FIRST MUSIC, THEN SPORT. Even people with severe language and cognitive impairments may quickly demonstrate understanding of this and become more willing to wait when they know how to express it.

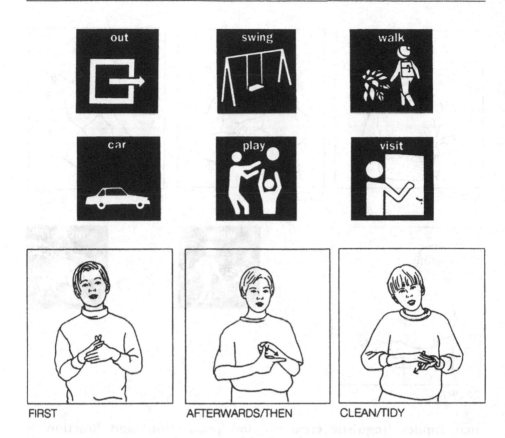

FIRST   AFTERWARDS/THEN   CLEAN/TIDY

Ready-made sentences

Modern communication aids based on computer technology enable users of graphic signs to produce 'holophrases', i.e. use one or several signs to say ready-made sentences. This might seem practical because the communication would then bear a closer resemblance to normal communication, and appear to overcome the problem created by lack of sentences. However, as long as a child is in an early stage of language development, the use of ready-made sentences may in fact make communication even more stereotypical because sentences are selected rather than constructed.

Single words may be interpreted in more ways than a sentence and will therefore provide more communicative flexibility. For example, *BOOK* may mean 'Give me the book', 'There is the book' or 'Take the book away'. '*Give me the book*' has only one meaning. Strategies for combining signs to form sentences are also based on single words, and the use of ready-made sentences may induce a gestalt strategy and possibly hinder the child's learning of the sentence-making process. Ready-made sentences

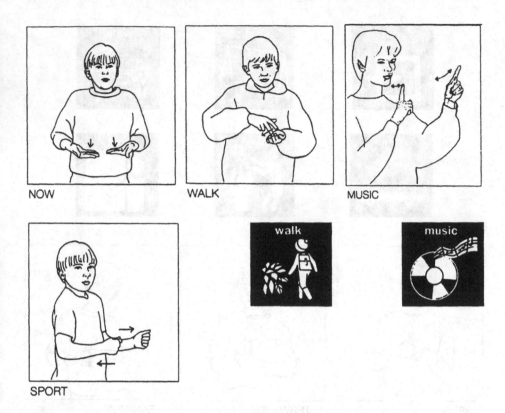

NOW   WALK   MUSIC

walk   music

SPORT

may hinder linguistic creativity and production, and function as 'formulas', i.e. they may always have the same fixed function, with limited adaptation to the situation. When children cannot produce sentences independently, such formulaic construction sentences do not function as models for later sentences, as may be the case in typical language development (compare Peters, 1983, 1995).

Cognitive effort

Several factors have been proposed which may contribute to the high proportion of single-sign utterances in the production of children with a good comprehension of spoken language (expressive group), as well as of children with limited speech comprehension (supportive language group and alternative language group). They include partner strategies, dialogue structure and intervention strategies. It is often assumed that children have fuller knowledge of semantic–syntactic relationships than is actually realized in their sentences, as a result of the cognitive demands on a young child's cognitive resources during production. Thus, one additional factor may be that graphic sign sentences are more difficult to produce because they require more conscious cognitive effort (von Tetzchner et al., 1998).

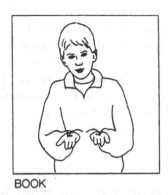

BOOK

In general, during development there seems to be some trade-off between different aspects of utterance production. It may take considerable resources to maintain an intended message in the mind and construct a longer utterance, and maybe at the same time remember a question or comment posed by the other person. Children working on their articulation may have fewer resources for content and vice versa. Normally speaking children tend to make longer sentences when using familiar words, which may be more automated, than with more recently acquired vocabulary. This may be caused by limited cognitive processing capacity, or interference between difference tasks, without implying that different aspects of language production are processed separately (Crystal, 1987; Masterson, 1997; Bloom, 1998). For people using graphic signs, however, the physical production process itself seems both more independent and to require more cognitive resources than for normally speaking individuals. It takes longer to select a graphic sign than to articulate the corresponding word. When the child has indicated one graphic sign, this must be kept in the working memory while searching for the next one. This search is not automated as in speech and may thus take a considerable share of the cognitive resources. Moreover, the search is likely to interfere with rehearsal, in addition to the fact that rehearsal strategies are not well developed in younger children (Guttentag, Ornstein and Siemens, 1987). As the adult has to follow the child's movements, this double-focused attention is required of both the child and the conversation partner.

The possibility of retaining the elements of a sentence while constructing the rest of the sentence, instead of pointing sequentially, may be an important strategy for facilitating the use of sentences. The temporary placement on a 'conversation location' may function as a 'rehearsal buffer'. It may also provide a means to 'bootstrap' new graphic signs. Although there is no way to know what, for example, Robert (see pages 254–256) would have achieved by pointing in a more traditional manner, his use of sentences surpassed both the limited use typically described for similar children and the lack of comprehension of spoken syntax indicated by his performance on the Reynell Developmental Language Scales. Moreover, his active use of variations around the existing structure of the graphic signs on the conversation page indicates that it helped him to keep the message structure in mind while sorting out how to solve communicative challenges. It seems unlikely that traditional pointing would have helped him in his endeavours in the same way (von Tetzchner et al., 1998).

Comprehension

Children in the three main groups differ in their ability to understand speech. Some have a good understanding of speech, whereas others understand speech only when it is augmented by alternative communication systems. Some understand graphic signs by themselves, whereas others understand the alternative communication form only when it is augmented by speech.

For children who understand some speech, one may ask to what extent the mapping of semantic–pragmatic content is similar in graphic signs and their corresponding words, typically written as glosses under the graphic representations. The underlying assumption seems to be that there is a close correspondence, but the diversity in mapping implied in any large difference in understood spoken vocabulary and expressed manual or graphic vocabulary would render this assumption invalid (Smith, 1996; Smith and Grove, 1999). One implication of this is that children who use manual and graphic signs need syntactic models from users of their own expressive language system so that they do not have to create their own structure. Thus, it would be an important aspect of the intervention that partners should not only augment their speech with separate key words as early as possible, but also apply at least two syntactically related graphic signs per spoken utterance when they augment speech.

In addition to their function as models, adults may expand children's utterances. Expansion is a characteristic of child-directed speech, and also a common technique for enhancing children's understanding and use of sentences on the basis of their own initiative and language production in traditional speech and language therapy (Snow and Ferguson, 1977; Nelson, 1996). However, because the aided vocabulary is usually very limited, it is important that adults expand the child's utterance in such a way that the child may be able to produce at least part of the expanded utterance.

C: BALL
A: {*THROW BALL I throw the ball to you*}

It is important to distinguish between the spoken interpretation of what the child is communicating and the expansion of his or her utter-

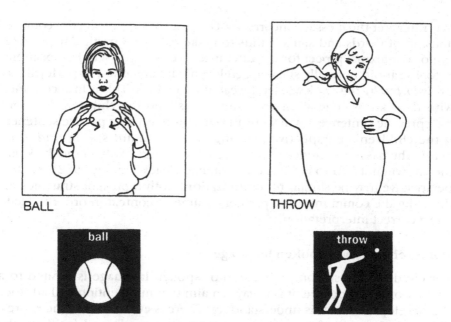

BALL   THROW

ball   throw

ance. The child is usually not able to produce the former, which is why the adult has to articulate it. In the example above, the adult expands the child's *BALL* to *THROW BALL* while saying *I throw the ball to you*. This acknowledges the child's request, but in the form of a reply, thus avoiding unnecessary and non-functional repetitions.

Bootstrapping

Fill-in tasks may be used to make children produce sentences. A related, but reverse strategy may be applied to facilitate comprehension of graphic communication by using a new sign in combination with known signs. *CHILD GIVE BALL TEACHER* and *CHILD ROLL BALL TEACHER* may be presented to teach the child *GIVE* and *ROLL* when *CHILD*, *BALL* and *TEACHER* are known. The question for the adult using fill-in strategies as an intervention to promote production is what the child must know in order to attribute the correct meaning to the sign. Incidentally, this is the same knowledge as the child needs to understand the sign. This strategy may utilize processes similar to the '*bootstrapping effect*' hypothesized for both normal and atypical language development (Pinker, 1984; Morgan and Demuth, 1996), where knowledge about the linguistic and/or situational frame is used by the child to derive the meaning of new words and signs.

Perspective

A shared focus will, to some extent, imply a shared perspective. If a child does not share the perspective of the communication partner, he or she may interpret the message incorrectly. One way of supporting the comprehension of words and signs is thus to make explicit a particular perspective or contextual aspect for the utterance that is expressed. For example, 3- to 4-year-old normally speaking children who are asked to perform *The cat is bitten by the duck* will let the cat bite the duck. This is in accordance with their knowledge about cats and ducks, and the children therefore interpret the sentence as if it were an active rather than a passive sentence. If the children's perspective is changed by the adult saying *Bad duck* before the passive sentence is presented, the children will let the duck bite the cat when asked to act out the sentence (MacWhinney, 1982). To give perspective may be similar to topicalization. Both represent strategies for directing the communication partners' frame or context in order to facilitate a correct interpretation.

Comprehension of spoken language

For children whose comprehension of spoken language is limited to a smaller or larger degree, it is always an aim that intervention will advance the development of this understanding. There is evidence that the expressive use of graphic language structure may precede and facilitate the comprehension of the syntax of spoken language. At the age of 6 years, Robert used graphic sentences, although he did not appear to understand spoken sentences when tested on the Reynell Developmental Language Scales (von Tetzchner et al., 1998). This development is in accordance with the assumptions underlying total communication – that all vocal and non-vocal language forms will support each other and that intervention aimed at supporting the development of an expressive graphic language structure may augment the comprehension of spoken language.

Variation

The ideas presented here represent a step towards the development of varied intervention strategies for promoting language structure in communication with alternative language systems. Such strategies have received relatively little attention and there is a great need for further elaboration and innovation in order to promote more versatile and flexible language use, and to prevent the boredom of monotone expression, i.e. the tendency always to let the individual communicate in the same small number of situations. This means that not only the disabled individuals but also their partners will have to vary their sentences. Language structure depends on distribution, and monotone language situations may reduce variation in expression, i.e. experiences that may enhance new aspects of language structure. For example, if an individual is always indicating wished for objects and activities or taking part in non-functional naming, motivation may run low. In assessments and evaluations of interventions, one may ask what the functions of the individual's utterances are in various settings, e.g. whether they always represent the topic. Semantic analysis may be a useful tool for describing an individual's communication – his or her use of Agent, Action, Object, Patient, etc.

For children in the expressive language group with sufficient comprehension of spoken language, explicit strategies may be applied when teaching structure. For this group, many sentence constructions may be possible for training in ordinary classrooms or in individual training sessions but, because all language use is embedded in context, whether this has an educational frame or not, it is essential that at least a substantial part of the teaching takes place in non-educational environments.

Chapter 11
Conversational skills

Individuals who belong to the alternative, supportive and expressive language groups are all characterized by poor conversational skills. However, the differences between these groups in terms of language comprehension, social skills and interests are so large that objectives and methods utilized to encourage conversational skills differ greatly. Despite these differences, an improvement in conversational skills will lead to increased independence and a sense of belonging and equality. Most users of alternative communication systems are dependent on others, both for performing daily tasks and in their leisure time. Conversation is a means of exchanging information and viewpoints, and influencing others. Improving individuals' mastery of conversation makes it easier for them to make known their own wishes and viewpoints, to influence others, to express interests and to make their own decisions.

In language development, conversations with adults imply training in language, concepts and values. Such conversations give the adults the opportunity to comment on what the children say and do, to tell them the names of objects and activities and how particular objects are used, and to explain to the children what they can and cannot do. For the children, conversations with adults form a significant part of the enculturalization process. Children with extensive language and communication disorders, and children who have difficulty in expressing themselves as a result of motor impairments, miss out on a great deal of this type of natural learning. A central objective of intervention is therefore that the alternative communication form should compensate for the lack of learning opportunities caused by the disability.

A lack of conversational skills also has the negative effect that children and adults who use alternative communication systems derive few benefits from interaction with other people. The problems that individuals in the expressive language group encounter in trying to express what they want to say are a daily source of frustration. Conversations become stereotypical and boring. For many of those who belong to the supportive language group, the experience of not being understood leads to shyness and embarrassment. For all three main groups with users of alternative communication modes, improvement in conversational skills may lead to increased and richer interaction with others.

The alternative language group

Traditionally, little attention has been paid to conversational skills when teaching language to people with language disorders. The main objective of alternative communication intervention has been to teach the individual to use single signs as a means of obtaining something or naming an object or activity. However, for some individuals in this group, communication may be a more fundamental problem than the acquisition of such language forms. The extent to which existing intervention programmes actually promote the skills that enable individuals to engage in dialogue is largely unknown. It is probable that new strategies and objectives are necessary to enhance conversational skills.

The basic conversational skills consist of starting a conversation and maintaining it, taking turns, changing topics, taking into account different conversational partners, and repairing any interruptions in the conversation caused by misunderstandings or other reasons. These skills are difficult for autistic people who belong to the alternative language group to acquire.

Keeping a long conversation going often proves to be a major problem, and it is extremely difficult to get autistic and severely learning-disabled people to make independent contributions to conversations. Typically, a dialogue will consist of only two utterances if it is the individual who starts the dialogue, or three if it is the conversational partner who begins. The most common types of conversations are those in which the conversational partner (C) asks about known things and gives the individual (I) assistance in answering by, for example, using WHAT or a prompt, i.e. help or encouragement.

I: COFFEE.
C: {YOU COFFEE *You can have coffee*}.
C: {WHAT *What do you want to do?*}
I: OUT WALK
C: {JACKET ON *Put on your jacket*}.

There is no simple answer about how this pattern should be broken, except in situations that are strictly structured or ritualized. However, it

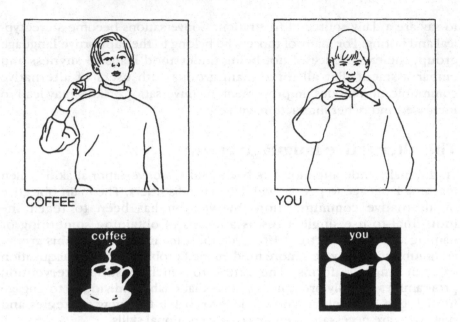

COFFEE   YOU

may be useful to try to find amusing and interesting topics. Children and adults who belong to the alternative language group may talk about experiences that they and conversational partners have had together, or perhaps common friends. Using a photograph album and pictures taken in familiar situations is often a good way to begin a longer conversation. However, it is important that the individuals use manual or graphic signs to communicate about the photographs, so that the interactions do not turn into a situation in which the individuals point at the picture and only the normally speaking people comment.

There is, as may be expected, a relationship between conversational skills and other linguistic skills. However, there are no fixed rules about how many signs or spoken words the individual must master before attempts are made at conversing. It is more a question of finding a suitable topic. Normally developing children in the early stages of language development, with very limited vocabularies, take part in simple dialogues with their parents and other adults. There has been success in teaching autistic and severely learning-disabled people, who had acquired 40–80 signs that they seldom used spontaneously, to participate in conversations.

Routines, plans and scripts

In sign intervention, structuring and fixed routines are used to teach the individual what is going to happen. The structure helps individuals to get an idea of what is happening, facilitates their understanding and use of the signs that they are going to learn, and builds up their expectations. In general, all people have a set of expectations about what different situations will contain and what will happen. Descriptions of these situations are called *plans* or *scripts* (Schank and Abelson, 1977), plans being more detailed than scripts. Plans contain a description of a specific course of events, whereas scripts describe a more general situation with possibilities for variation. In a communicative situation with strict structuring, the description will be a plan, whereas a more flexible structure may be called a script.

Scripts have been used to describe the development of early dialogue skills among children who develop language normally (Nelson, 1996), and strategies for developing conversational skills among individuals in the alternative language group may be based on scripts. The use of scripts is a continuation of intervention based on structuring and routines. Thus, it is an aim that interventions should advance from routines to scripts and dialogues. This means that the teacher should build up both plans or scripts and utilize them to make conversations.

The first conversations that children normally take part in come about because adults structure and design conversations by prompting and coaxing answers out of the child. It is the adult (A) who *links* the child's (C) utterances together and produces a meaningful entity.

A: *Yesterday you went to* . . . .
C:
A: *You went to Grand* . . . .
C: *To Grandmothers*
A: *And you travelled by* . . . .
C: *Train*.

Typical conversations concern things that one is in the process of doing or has done. They may be about the food being cooked by the adult, a visit, the children at nursery school, etc. Many conversations recur frequently, so that the child gradually learns what to say to the various cue words. Some conversations are repeated on a daily basis.

Attempts should be made to establish similar conversations with people who have communication disorders. The conversational partner controls the course of the conversation and prompts for the individual's conversational turns, i.e. gives encouragement and helps the individual to answer. Some individuals who belong to the alternative language group may require this procedure for the rest of their lives. For these individuals, the greatest gain is to learn the role of conversational partner, and that significant people can gradually weave new elements into the conversation, elements that may lead to new learning.

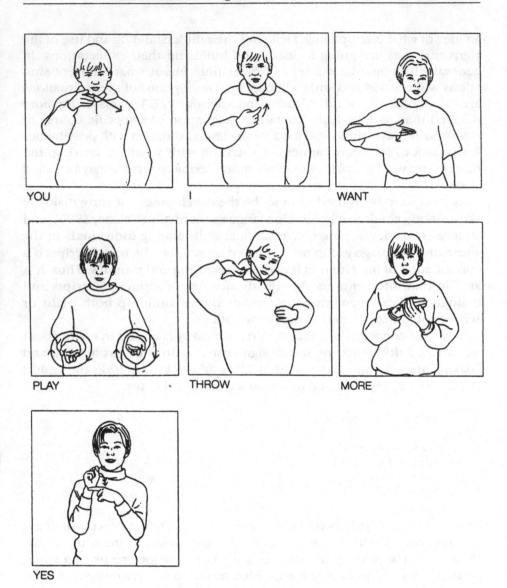

YOU

I

WANT

PLAY

THROW

MORE

YES

Sommer, Whitman and Keogh (1988) taught six learning-disabled and autistic adolescents to have a conversation about a game of quoits. The adolescents were between the ages of 8 and 25 years and had little or no speech. Their manual sign vocabulary varied between 40 and 80 signs, but these signs were rarely used spontaneously. Seven signs were used in the teaching situation: YOU, I, WANT, (TO) PLAY, (TO) THROW, MORE and YES. The dialogue itself was formulated as a plan.

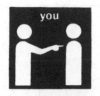

 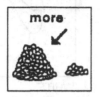

P1:   YOU WANT [TO] PLAY
P2:   I WANT [TO] PLAY
P1:   THROW
P2:   [Throws]
P2:   YOU THROW
P1:   [Throws]
P1:   YOU THROW
P2:   [Throws]
P2:   YOU THROW
P1:   [Throws]
P2:   PLAY MORE
P1:   YES

To begin with, the conversation was performed with each of the adolescents and a teacher. Then the teacher helped the adolescents to perform the conversation together in pairs. The help consisted of prompts if one of the participants stopped. Two of the adolescents learned to perform the whole sequence, whereas the remaining four learned to perform parts of it. The quoit dialogue was based on a situation in which the individuals generally interacted, and where the sign sentences fulfilled a functional role. The adolescents continued to use some of the signs when they played quoits, even after the training sessions ended.

The two most capable adolescents in this study had previously taken part in a study in which they had to learn to perform a conversation about orange juice and biscuits. They learned to use a number of the sign sentences together with the teacher, but not with one another (Keogh et al., 1987). In this study, they used 15 signs and three different plans, and there is reason to believe that this was too complex. At the same time, it is conceivable that the good results achieved by the two adolescents in the second study were a result of their previous experience.

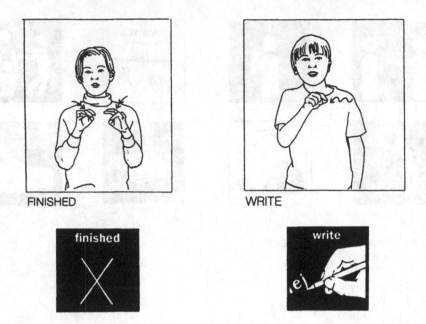

FINISHED

WRITE

finished

write

In both studies a plan was used, i.e. a dialogue written beforehand, rather than a script. The aim in such situations should be gradually to change the dialogues from plans to scripts with greater flexibility. It is believed that this will lead to increased generalization and more spontan-eous use than in these studies. The strategy of teaching conversational skills with the help of a plan still needs to be investigated in a variety of situations before we shall know how this method should be applied for developing conversational skills in everyday settings. In the study carried out by Sommer, Whitman and Keogh (1988), only parts of the conversation were used more generally. In particular, the comment YOU THROW was omitted, probably as a result of this remark being redundant because the turn of the next player was signalled by the fact that the first player had finished throwing. Perhaps it would have been better to have introduced FINISHED into the conversation. It is also conceivable that the participants would like to make a note of the number of quoits that had landed on the peg. Thus, WRITE and FINISHED could have been introduced at the appropriate stages of the game.

The communication skills of learning-disabled people are often too focused on just school and work-related activities. Script approaches are useful for developing broader situation-appropriate communication. Heller and her associates (1996) used a script-like approach to promote social interaction communication about things other than work tasks in a sheltered work setting for three individuals with learning disability, hearing loss and no severe motor impairment. They had vocabularies of about 200 manual signs; the signs were not used in communication with co-workers but they were provided with two communication boards with PCS and drawings of manual signs for this purpose: one with work task items and one with non-task vocabulary such as *HOW-ARE-YOU*, *FINE*, *TIRED*, *SHOPPING*, *FOOTBALL* and *TELEVISION*. The intervention consisted of teaching the three individuals scripts for greetings, being offered an object, conversations about a topic and closing conversations. After a training period in an educational setting, the three individuals were helped to use the new skills with co-workers in their sheltered work setting. The results included more communication about things other than work tasks and increased social participation at work. As a follow-up, the co-workers could be taught to understand and use relevant manual signs.

The little experience with regard to the usefulness of direct training of conversational skills for this group is mixed. However, it is a good idea to try this approach with individuals who have learned a number of signs. Also, for severely learning-disabled individuals, communication should not only be a means for expressing needs and gaining control of their environment, but also be used for other forms of talk. In particular, it is important to attribute normal feelings and relationships to them, and their need to communicate about such matters. For example, Bodil, a 43-year-old woman with no speech and limited comprehension of spoken language, acquired a graphic vocabulary of about 150 items, of which a third were person names in the forms of photographs. Her main interest was people and she demonstrated a genuine need to share experiences with others and to put into words her own positive and negative emotional encounters with other people, as well as for 'presenting' herself. The degree to which she began to manage this, in the course of a 1-year intervention phase, emphasizes the need for setting the language intervention within a conversational frame (Møller and von Tetzchner, 1996). Moreover, in both small and large institutions, learning-disabled people who use alternative communication communicate almost solely with staff members. Therefore, conversational training should aim at getting individuals with impaired communication skills to communicate more with one other.

The supportive language group

Conversational skills have not been a chief concern in the teaching of individuals who belong to the supportive language group either, although it is expected that they will begin to take part in conversations.

For children who belong to this group, the first conversations are often frustrating experiences. This applies particularly to children with develop-

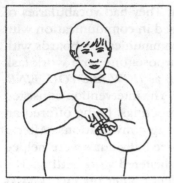

WALK

mental language disorders and other individuals who have such extensive articulatory problems that it is difficult for the listener to understand what they are saying. Conversations tend to come to a standstill. These individuals often develop the strategy of answering yes to all questions, whether or not they have understood them.

Even for adults in close contact with the children, their speech is inadequate for them to be understood. The adults depend on situational cues in order to understand what the children are trying to say. In situations where there are no such cues, very little will be understood. For example, parents relate that it is especially difficult to understand their children when they are out driving (Schjølberg, 1984). The problems encountered by adults when trying to understand the children often lead – in the same way as for the children – to them answering *yes* and *no* to questions in the hope that the reply given is the correct one. This way of answering does not encourage continued conversation, and the children often stop communicating when they receive incorrect and meaningless answers. The adults, in an effort to keep the conversation going after not having understood the children, take control of the conversation by asking them questions, or by deciding for themselves the course of events. This exerts pressure on the children's communicative ability, so that they are able to do what they want. If the adults always decide, the children may find the time spent with them uninteresting.

The objective of the intervention is to make it easier for the children to participate in conversations and experience being understood. The use of graphic or manual signs helps the conversational partner understand, with the result that the conversation does not come to a halt as easily or is not diverted from its objective through lack of understanding. This may provide the children with increased opportunities for indirect learning and give them greater benefit from contact with adults.

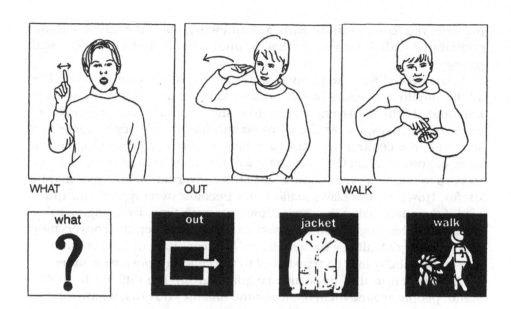

The intervention will not differ appreciably from that given to the alternative language group, although strategies employed with the expressive language group may also be utilized (see below). Emphasis should be given to dialogues in natural settings, in the form of structured conversations about a clearly defined topic. The conversations should begin by establishing a topic, e.g. by saying *Let's talk about your bicycle* or *You know that walk we're going on tomorrow.* To make sure that the topic has been understood, and that the children are attentive, one should make sure that they confirm the topic. This may be clear if the children sign BICYCLE or WALK. To make it easier for the adults to understand, scripts may be useful. This means that *new* situations are designed which are easy to grasp and understand, but in which the children are able to make a contribution, i.e. relay something that the person with whom they are communicating does not know.

In addition to using manual and graphic signs and establishing a topic of conversation, the intelligibility of the speech of children with articulatory disorders may be improved by designing situations in which the adults have several situational cues for what the child is interested in. Such situations may be arranged simply, e.g. a child and the adult play together with the same toys from day to day, but the game differs somewhat. The adult is encouraged to comment on what the child does with the toys. In such a situation, the child is likely to experience that more of what he or she says is understood without having to resort to boring repetition, and the adult will gradually learn more about how the child speaks and articulates sounds. Conversations may be centred around pictures or toys to provide the conversation with a framework, but the child should contribute with information that is unknown to the conversational partner.

It is essential that the partners in the conversation change roles. The adults should not always be the ones to ask questions while the speech-impaired children answer. The children should also ask for information, encourage activity, etc. As the conversation has a tendency to come to a standstill, the children typically have little experience of keeping to one topic of conversation. One important aim is therefore to help the children to keep to one topic and follow it up in the conversation. Role-play may be useful. However, the play situation may become stereotypical and ritual-ized if the adult makes the same comments each time. By changing roles, the adult's chaining, which is important initially to keep the conversation going, may gradually be broken down. A larger share of the communica-tive responsibility may be transferred to the child in a positive manner.

As children in the supportive language group are difficult to under-stand, people around them often assume that they do not have anything of significance to say. One aim of the intervention is therefore to demonstrate to people in the children's environment that they are able to participate in conversations and do have something to say. This helps lay the basis for a more natural form of language learning, which for this group will usually replace the formalized teaching over time.

For some individuals who belong to the supportive language group, e.g. children with Down's syndrome, the problem of establishing conver-sations in which the child takes an equal share of the communicative initia-tive is related to the fact that they need a long time to react to what the communication partner is doing and what is otherwise happening in the situation. It may be difficult for the conversation partner to wait long enough for the individuals to have a chance to take their turns. The best way of remedying this is to encourage the conversational partners to wait a little longer than usual, and to let them be convinced by personal experi-ence that this kind of waiting is not in vain. To ensure that the experiences will be positive, the waiting may take place in established situations in which it is highly likely that the individuals will take the initiative to communicate.

The expressive language group

There are often a number of factors that combine to produce problems for children and adults who belong to the expressive language group, when they participate in meaningful conversation, particularly those who have severe motor impairments. The type of aid that is used may have great significance for the course of conversation. However, poor conversational skills are also the result of an inadequate intervention and unfortunate experiences that the individual has had when communicating with others. Conversational partners often act in such a way that the conversations become more difficult and have little meaning: pretending to understand utterances that they have not understood, answering questions aimed at the individuals instead of allowing them to answer for themselves, and tending to raise their voice when speaking to these individuals (Shane and Cohen, 1981; Kraat, 1985; Collins, 1996). Similar strategies are found when speaking to people with a different native language (Ferguson and Debose, 1977).

Some of the most important problems that must be overcome are the individual's lack of communicative initiative, passive communicative style, slow communication and inadequate communicative strategies. In reality, these are intertwined. A good solution as a rule requires that both the individual and the conversational partner learn to act in new ways, that considerable thought is given when choosing a communication aid, and that circumstances are designed practically so that the aid can be used as effectively as possible.

For members of the expressive language group who have a good understanding of spoken language, the development of conversational skills is the most important aim of intervention. The lack of linguistic skills does not usually place restrictions on users of communication aids, but rather the lack of opportunities to use what they know. They do not need language intervention in the traditional sense; instead they need instruction in the technical and functional use of the aid. Traditional language intervention of the type that is not needed may lead to passivity and dependence. Their experience with communication has played a significant role in the development of a passive communicative style. The significance of learning good strategies in order to initiate and maintain conversations seems to have been underestimated. It was assumed that functional and varied use of communication aids would follow once the sign system and the aid had been mastered technically (Harris, 1982; Kraat, 1985; Basil, 1992). An emphasis on conversational strategies may help increase awareness of this problem, and thereby lead to less learned dependency and increased conversational responsibility.

Individuals who belong to the expressive language group are often motor impaired and have difficulty in performing a large number of commonplace activities that require motor skills. Above all, the different communication aids have practical consequences which, together with the user's motor impairment, produce physical restrictions in terms of how the conversations may be kept going. They often have best control over language, and linguistic comments replace a number of activities that occur naturally in ordinary interaction, e.g. pointing, and showing and

manipulating objects. The development of conversational skills is therefore of vital importance if this group is to be able to participate in a range
of social contexts.

The teaching employed to develop better conversational skills may be
divided into *environmental strategies, partner strategies* and *conversational strategies*. Environmental strategies and partner strategies aim at
increasing the individual's participation in conversational situations,
reducing routine situations and ensuring that the conversational partners
adapt to the language-impaired individuals. Conversational strategies are
strategies that the individuals themselves may use to make their communication more effective.

Environmental strategies

Many motor-impaired individuals have greater mastery of language skills
than motor skills. In fact, they may use communication skills to perform
actions through their helpers that other people can do independently.
They should therefore participate in more communicative situations than
others. In reality, however, they participate in fewer such situations. The
conversations they have are often with professional helpers, and a large
number of the communicative situations in which they participate are
routine. This is partly because motor-impaired children and adults spend
longer periods of time on routine activities, but it is also because parents
of speech-impaired children prefer to communicate in such situations – in
these settings they understand their children best (Culp, 1982).

A high degree of reliance on routine situations hinders participation in
new ones. One way of making the most of the environment is to find new
situations in which conversation may take place or form part of the activity.
The situations can, if necessary, be made easier for ordinary conversational
partners to follow, so that they experience success in the communicative
situation. At the same time, it is important that the situation is not
designed in such a way that too few demands are made on the aided
speaker, e.g. parents of disabled children use their knowledge about the
child in order to guess what they want. The children take part in few activities and their parents are familiar with most of them. It is easy for the
parents to guess the children's wishes, and the content of such conversations can quickly become repetitive and monotonous. Not everything in
the situation should be predictable. The conversational partner should
have a need to know what the individual is communicating, so that they
have a communicative responsibility. Lack of communicative responsibility
and genuine communication are common barriers to the development of
conversational skills (Glennen and Calculator, 1985; von Tetzchner and
Martinsen, 1996).

It is common practice to use an information booklet that is carried between home and nursery school or school. An information booklet can be useful in many situations, and is frequently used with individuals who belong to the supportive and alternative language groups. It ensures that practical information is systematically conveyed between home and school. However, it may also deprive the individuals of communicative responsibility, because, for example, they are unable to choose what is communicated from home or school. Only those topics mentioned in the book will be discussed. Many of the questions asked are not genuine because the conversational partner knows or can make a good guess at the answer. In this way, the individuals have few cues to tell them whether they are communicating well or poorly. Communicative setbacks may lead to positive learning and enhance language acquisition, provided that the individuals know what was wrong and what kind of strategies can be applied to make their communication more effective.

An increase in the number of different communicative situations implies an opening up of society for disabled individuals. Communication should occur not only at home, nursery school, school, work and in other familiar situations, but also with unknown people, on the street, in cafés, shops, meeting places, cinemas, etc. However, it is not always just a case of throwing the individuals into new situations. They are often apprehensive about being exposed to people who are not used to individuals who use communication aids, and may be fearful and reject new situations. It may therefore be necessary to begin by giving the individuals a good overview of the situation and what is likely to happen, so that they can feel more secure. Role-play may be one way of preparing for new situations and gaining confidence.

> Becky is a 9-year-old girl with cerebral palsy. She has some speech but it is almost unintelligible. She uses a communication book with 200 Rebus signs. The book contains mini-communication boards with different domains (art, snacks, assembly, etc.). She often goes to Burger King with her parents but has never ordered anything there herself. First, she talks with her teacher about what happens at Burger King. One must wait to be served, order exactly what one wants and pay. Becky and her teacher then make a domain board for Burger King. In the classroom, they make a model of Burger King, in which a schoolmate plays the role of waiter. When the 'waiter' asks what she wants, Becky answers with the Burger King signs in her book. She practises asking the waiter whether or not he has understood her correctly. When Becky goes to Burger King with her friend who played the role of waiter, she gets the hamburger she wants without any difficulties (Mills and Higgins, 1984).

Martin is a 12-year-old boy with cerebral palsy. He has several communication books with limited vocabularies and also uses an electronic writing instrument with which what he writes is printed on paper. However, the writing process is extremely slow. Martin likes to read but has never been to the library. First, he and his teacher talk about what it is like at the library, and they discuss the process of borrowing books. He practises writing a few sentences that he will find useful, such as <u>Where are the books about lions?</u> and <u>How many books can I borrow?</u> Then a friend from his class plays the role of librarian. He asks questions and Martin answers. The following day, they go to the library, where Martin easily masters the new situation (Higgins and Mills, 1986).

Participation in real situations gives the individuals authentic knowledge of the society in which they live and is a part of their enculturalization. It is therefore important to stress that role-playing should not be a replacement for real situations; it is precisely pretend situations that characterize many of the experiences of disabled individuals using aided communication. The role-playing is intended only as a means of making it easier for the individual to start to take part in the real situation. This objective of the role-playing should be clear from the outset, for both teacher and learner.

Generally speaking, aided speakers participate less in conversations than others. For children and adolescents, the vast majority of their conversations will be with adults (Harris, 1982). Interaction and communication with peers should therefore be increased. Situations in which children interact with adults differ from those in which children interact with one another. Children and adolescents who use communication aids also seem to have more varied conversations with their peers than with adults (Sutton, 1982). Conversations with peers also give the individuals access to a youth culture. Particular care should be taken to design activities that may take place without the help of an adult, e.g. role-playing and games. Sometimes adults have to be mediators between children who use communication aids, and it is important that the adults do not try to influence the messages that they relay.

A girl and a boy, both using communication aids and a few manual signs, were sitting together with their teacher, who was functioning as a mediator between them. The girl was listing the children she wanted for her birthday, but did not mention the boy, who eagerly indicated that he wanted to come. The teacher relayed the request. The girl indicated *NO* and the teacher relayed this message to the boy without interfering, i.e. without attempting to make her change her answer (Soro, Basil and von Tetzchner, 1992).

Adults should refrain from interrupting unnecessarily, even if conflicts and arguments arise. Just as other people do, users of communication aids should experience such situations and learn how to deal with them. Shielding disabled children more than others against such circumstances means that they do not have opportunities to gain commonplace experiences and learn to tackle everyday situations. A result of this may also be poorer emotional self-regulation. With regard to adolescents, schoolfriends or other peers may have some responsibility for helping the individuals and including them in leisure-time activities. As far as possible, these should be activities that are popular among young people, encouraging the individuals to play as equal a role as possible despite the fact that they are motor impaired. Visits to the cinema, sports events, homework, visits to cafés, listening to records and hanging around on street corners are examples of such activities.

Telecommunication

More communication does not necessarily mean that all of the communication *must* take place face to face. Telecommunications play an increasingly important role in modern societies, and it is important that language-impaired people also have the best possible access to these services. Furthermore, for people with motor impairment who have difficulty in moving, telecommunication is an important means to greater social participation. Conversations may take place directly via text telephone or computer, with written or synthetic speech output. In the last few years, electronic mail has become usual. For motor-impaired people, electronic writing is easier both to read and to write (McKinnon et al., 1995). It is also possible to have both telecommunication conversations and electronic mail with Blissymbols and other graphic signs (Tronconi, 1989; von Tetzchner, 1991; Gandell and Sutton, 1998).

The Internet, the highway of modern information and communication technology, also provides opportunities for 'conversations' in the form of electronic meeting places. A computer linked to the Internet via a modem or an ISDN card may be used to communicate with people anywhere in the world – somebody next door or someone on another continent. A similar system may be created with electronic mail and a list server. Internet meeting places and e-mail servers are usually established around common themes and interests. Those who participate in the meetings are not usually present at the same time but, because new comments build on previous ones, these communications resemble group conversations. The participants can see what the others have written, and write their own comments when it suits them. The advantage of electronic meeting places for people who use communication aids is that they need not communicate quickly. They can write what they want at their own speed, and are not dependent on others to interpret for them. However, at present participants must be able to use orthographic script in order to participate independently (Magnusson and Lundman, 1987; Cullen et al., 1995). There are systems that allow for the use of Blissymbols and other graphic signs in electronic letters, and it is only a matter of time before electronic meeting places will be established on the Internet.

Partner strategies

In addition to their own role, partners in a conversation with a communication aid user must often take an active part in formulating what the individuals want to say. The partners interpret elements as they are indicated by the aided speaker, assemble these elements and, to some extent, guess what the individuals are saying before they have finished forming the sentence. The conversational partners are therefore active participants when they are both speaking and listening. The conversational partners' strategies and degree of competence will vary, and they can both enhance and hinder the success of the individuals' communications. As the conversational partners have a double role, training family, peers and others as the conversational partners is an important means of providing communication aid users with better conversational skills.

In a typical conversation between an aided and a natural speaker, it is the natural speaker who takes the initiative to change subjects and control the conversation. This is done in a way that may best be described as a *simplification strategy*, i.e. the conversational partner limits the topic of conversation and what the aided speaker may say. This may make it easy for the individual to be part of the conversation, but difficult for him or her to make a contribution. In many instances, one gets the impression that the role of helper held by the conversational partner deludes him or her into underestimating the aided speaker. It is particularly among conversational partners who are not aware of their special role that one may find someone talking down to aided speakers and not taking into account what the individual actually knows and understands (Shane and Cohen, 1981; Blau, 1983; Sweidel, 1989).

The aided speakers' contributions to the conversation tend to consist of giving replies, and the conversational partners restrict the number of possible answers through the way in which they pose the questions. In spite of the fact that the communication takes time, the contributions made by the speech-impaired individuals are limited. It is the conversational partner who takes the initiative and chooses the topic of conversation. Sutton (1982) found that the natural speaker took the initiative 84 per cent of the time, whereas 10- to 27-year-old users of Blissymbols took the initiative to communicate only 16 per cent of the time. Similarly, Light (1985) found that the mothers of 3- to 6-year-old Blissymbol users took the initiative 85 per cent of the time.

Time to say something

A conversation always takes much longer if communication aids are used than if both participants are able to speak naturally. If a conversation has several turns and contains a mutual exchange of information and opinions, the time taken increases considerably. If individuals wish to say something that is outside the bounds of ordinary routines, it may take a long time, making it difficult to say things that are important. This is also the main reason for the asymmetrical conversational structure and the strategies generally used by conversational partners. Many conversational partners find it difficult to wait. Light (1985) found that mothers of 3- to 6-year-old children began to speak after 1–2 seconds. Pauses of more than 1 second were followed by speech from the mothers 92.5 per cent of the time. The children who needed longer time to use Blissymbols only had time to answer yes–no questions (see below), which they were able to answer quickly by vocalizing, nodding or shaking their heads. The importance of giving the individuals sufficient time was well demonstrated by the fact that the mother of the child who communicated the most also waited the longest – as much as 47 seconds. Although the average number of communicative initiatives on the part of the children in the course of 20 minutes was 11, this particular child had 45 initiatives. Similarly, Glennen and Calculator (1985) found an increase in communicative initiative for two children aged 9 and 12 years once the conversational partners had been taught to wait.

To give aided speakers the opportunity to control the course of conversation better and contribute to the conversation on a more equal footing, it is first and foremost important that they are given the time necessary for them to say what they want. This implies that the conversational partners must restrain themselves from the urge to get on with the conversation. They must wait long enough before they begin to interpret or guess at what the individuals are saying, or take the communicative initiative, be it a continuation of the conversation or a change of topic.

Guessing

To speed up the conversation, it is usual for the conversational partner to guess the word before it is fully spelled out, or whole sentences before all the signs are produced or pointed at. Most utterances made by children who use communication aids and graphic signs are single-sign utterances (Harris, 1982; von Tetzchner and Martinsen, 1996). This results partly from the fact that a large part of the children's utterances is a reply to a question, but partly from the fact that the conversational partners guess after the first sign. The listeners guess what the individuals wish to say, and express this for them. Guessing in this way may be a good strategy for making conversations more effective, but it may also lead to the individuals being unable to express themselves. The interpretation of words and sentences generally takes place one element at a time, which means that the listeners may have to remember the letters in the word that is being spelled out and the words or graphic signs that have already been produced. This can be quite difficult, especially if a conversational partner has to spend some time figuring out a sign analogy or spelling out a long word. The utterances need not be especially long before mistakes are made. If a conversational partner guesses wrongly, the result can be longer dialogues (Collins, 1996, p. 95):

Fay had no useful speech and uses a communication board with 200 Blissymbols. She is communicating with a carer, Conrad.

F: {*FATHER. Mmm mmm.*}
C: *Wanna tell your father.*
F: *HOLIDAY.*
C: Looks up at Fay, then down at communication board.
F: [continues pointing] {*HOLIDAY. Mm mm mm.*}
C: *Oh you're going . . . .* [Looks down at communication board]
F: Shakes head and vocalizes.
C: *. . . on holiday with your father.*
F: Leans forward over communication board.
C: *Right.* [Leans back a little and says something inaudible.]
F: *LIKE.*
C: *You like.*
F: {*FATHER. Mmm mmm.*}
C: *Your father.*
F: Moving finger to point to another Blissymbol.
C: *To go on holiday.*
F: {'Yes' [looks up at Conrad, nods]. *Mm.*}
C: *Right.*
C: [Sits back] *You'd like that to happen.*
F: *Mmm.* 'Yes' [nods].

In this example, Conrad tried to cover too much in one guess. When Fay pointed to *FATHER*, rather than just acknowledge the Blissymbol and wait for the next, he attempted to guess the whole of what Fay was beginning to say, assuming that Fay was the subject and her father the object. When this understanding was rejected (implicitly through continuing to point to *HOLIDAY* and providing no confirmation of Conrad's guess), Conrad proffered a second guess, again of the whole of what Fay was trying to say. This time Conrad understood Fay to be continuing the prior talk by saying something about what she would like to do for her next holiday. In reality, Fay was trying to talk about something new: that she would like her father to go on holiday. It demonstrates that the conversational partner must be patient and take care to get confirmation that the guess is correct. Such confirmation is part of taking the communication of the disabled individual seriously (von Tetzchner and Jensen, 1999). It is an essential part of a conversational partner's strategy in order to ensure that misunderstandings are not built on in the conversation.

In some instances, guessing may lead to dependency and hinder development of good conversational strategies.

> Larry is 26 years old and has cerebral palsy. He can speak, but his speech is difficult to understand. To make himself understood by people who have difficulty comprehending what he says, he uses a letter board. He spoke with a Swedish girl who did not know him, and who did not understand that he said the word hospital although this word is very similar in Norwegian and Swedish. Larry began to spell out the word, but gave up after h-o-s-p-i. As his conversational partner had not guessed the word, Larry began to spell the word from the beginning instead of spelling out the whole word. This caused great problems in the communicative situation and meant that it took him a long time to finish telling the joke he had started.

This discussion is not meant as an argument against employing guessing as a strategy. Many users of communication aids prefer the conversational partner to guess what they are trying to say before they have finished formulating the utterance. It can be a good strategy on the part of the conversational partner to guess what is being said before the utterance is fully produced, and people who know the user well are best able do this effectively. When graphic signs are used, this kind of guessing is natural because the conversational partner usually interprets in spoken language what the user is saying with the aid of the signs. Even though guessing is often expedient, it is essential to make sure that it is confirmed. It is also important that the individuals are able to master other strategies so that the guessing does not cause them to become dependent on the conversational partner, and that they learn to express themselves on occasions when the conversational partners do not guess or the guessing leads them nowhere.

Yes–no questions

It is typical of conversations between aided and natural speakers that the communication aid user has a responsive role, answering questions and requests from the conversational partner. In a study carried out by Sutton (1982), questions accounted for 2 per cent of the children's utterances and 34 per cent of the utterances of their conversational partners. In a study of adult communication aid users, Wexler and associates (1983) found that the aided speakers produced 8 requests and questions and 163 answers, whereas the conversational partners had 285 questions and challenges and 8 answers. One of the reasons may be that the normally speaking partners experience that the communication is more normal when they are asking questions than when the disabled individual is using a graphic system.

A large part of the communication from the natural to the aided speaker consists of yes–no questions. Sutton (1982) found that 16 per cent of the spoken utterances to 10- to 27-year-old Blissymbol users were yes–no questions. In a study carried out by Culp (1982), 40 per cent of the utterances made by aided speakers were answers to yes–no questions. In addition, a large number of the questions posed by conversational partners are about circumstances for which they already know the answer (Light, 1985; von Tetzchner and Martinsen, 1996). Often the aided speakers are aware of this, and the conversations may have little meaning besides them being together.

Moreover, questions may be followed up by more specific sub-questions before the individual has been given the chance to answer. In the following example, the teacher (T) begins by asking a question that could have been a good starting point for a conversation, but ruins a possible conversation with the pupil (P) before it has even begun (Harris, 1982).

T: *What did you do last night?*
P: [Begins to formulate an answer on the communication board]
T: *Did you go home?*
T: *Did you go to the cinema?*
T: *Did you watch television?*
T: *Did you watch Walt Disney?*
T: *Did your brother come?*

The dominant use of yes–no questions is particularly detrimental to children's communication because it hinders the acquisition of new expressive vocabulary and strategies for relaying more complex messages. To increase the number of contributions to the conversation on the part of the individual, the conversational partner should use fewer yes–no questions, when it is not necessary to use these, to find out what individuals mean – for example, because they do not have the necessary signs to be able to express what they want to say. As far as possible, questions should be open, starting with question words such as *what*, *who* and *where*, which will prompt other answers to 'yes' and 'no', but the general aim should be to reduce the number of questions.

Corrections

Many children and adolescents seldom use their communication aid spontaneously. To make them use the aid more frequently, professionals and parents often encourage the use of the aid in situations in which individuals have managed to make themselves understood in other ways (Harris, 1982).

T: *What do you want?*
P: [Points to the ball.]
T: *No, tell me with your board.*
P: Points to the ball again.]
T: *How can you tell me with your board?*
P: [Puts head down on lap tray.]

Functional intervention does not consist of teaching individuals new ways to express themselves in situations where they are already capable of communicating effectively. The aim is for them to learn to communicate in situations where their mastery is insufficient or they feel uncertain. Forcing individuals to use a communication aid when this is not functional, in the belief that they will become better at communicating because they are pointing at a graphic sign instead of an object, has little purpose. The individual in the example above mastered the use of the graphic sign, and the 'correction' is merely felt by the individual as unnecessary nagging. Such situations produce negative experiences, which may deprive the individuals of their motivation to communicate.

Partner styles

Communication partners often differ considerably in their use of strategies when communicating with people who use alternative communication systems. As a complement to teaching significant people in the environment to become better communication partners, it may facilitate communication if the communication-impaired individuals are helped to become aware of differences in the partners' competence and strategy use, e.g. between children and adults, and how they can take these differences into consideration when interacting with them (Buzolich and Lunger, 1995).

Conversational strategies

Basic conversational skills comprise the ability to start and end conversations, take turns, negotiate meaning and repair breakdowns. The focus of this part is on graphic communication, but most of the issues also apply to conversations with manual signs.

Starting and ending conversations

To begin a conversation, individuals must have ways of attracting a conversational partner's attention. If they are able to vocalize, make clicking noises with the tongue, say some words or have a communication aid that uses synthetic speech, this is usually not a major problem. However, for individuals who are dependent on visual contact, it can be extremely difficult to attract the conversational partner's attention. Attempts at communication are often overlooked, especially on occasions when it is the individual who takes the first initiative. To be successful, the potential conversational partner must be looking in the right direction. When the individual is responding to something from the communication partner, the situation is different. The person who has asked the question is usually attentive to the person who is going to answer.

Studies have shown that mothers of pre-school children who use Blissymbols may take the initiative to communicate 85 per cent of the time (Light, 1985). Conversational partners of adult communication users may take the initiative 79 per cent of the time (Wexler et al., 1983). Smith (1991) found no initiations and voluntary turns in a 9-year-old girl who used Blissymbols when she communicated with her teacher and peers. Calculator and Dollaghan (1982) found that 20–40 per cent of communicative initiatives on the part of motor-impaired individuals were overlooked in the classroom. One reason for this, among others, is that many people with extensive motor impairments produce involuntary sounds or movements that people around them become used to and ignore. Many individuals who are able to articulate sounds have difficulty in doing so when it is important for them to express themselves. It may be necessary for individuals to use a type of alarm system to ensure that they are able to attract a conversational partner's attention,. A form of buzzer or a bell can be practical, but a small speech machine that says 'Hello' or something similar is better. For people who use communication aids with speech output, ready-made opening phrases may make it easy to begin a conversation, e.g. 'Hi, I'd like to talk to you'. Touching may also be a way of attracting someone's attention, but, for people who do not know the individual, this may seem threatening (Yoder and Kraat, 1983).

It is not uncommon for a communication aid user always to use the same topic as a means of initiating a conversation (Shane, Lipshultz and Shane, 1982). This leads to dull conversations, and the conversational partner becomes bored. In such cases, it is useful to teach the individual to use different subjects to start conversations.

As the conversation is to a great extent dominated by the conversational partner, he or she will also generally decide when the conversation will end. This may happen either sooner or later than the individual would

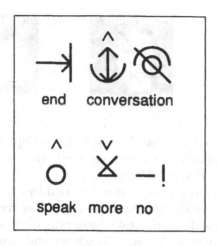

wish. It is not always easy for individuals to withdraw from the situation or demonstrate in one way or another that they wish to stop. It is therefore essential that they are given strategies for ending a conversation, e.g. to produce *END CONVERSATION* or some such phrase. If they have more to say, they must know how to signal this, e.g. by producing *SPEAK MORE* or *NO END.* Although the individuals use graphic signs, it is likely that they have suitable signs on their board; if not, they should be provided with the necessary signs. However, it is not very likely that the users have much experience with ending conversations, so they must also be taught how they can use the signs to do so.

Taking turns

To contribute to maintaining a conversation, individuals must be able to take their turns in it. Users of communication aids often lose their turn because they take so long getting started that the conversational partner does not wait. In the study by Light (1985), the mothers used almost all the opportunities they had to take their turn, whereas the children used only half of their chances. There are obligatory turns in a conversation, where the conversational partner prompts the other to say something, e.g. to answer a question. Aided speakers do not even always take these obligatory turns (Calculator and Luchko, 1983). Most of the opportunities that were used by the children in Light's study were answers to questions.

Part of the reason that users of communication aids do not enter the conversation is that the switching of turns is often signalled by non-verbal signals, which they do not master. These may take the form of intonation and facial expression. Among motor-impaired individuals, such signals are often misunderstood. An attempt at pointing may be regarded as a

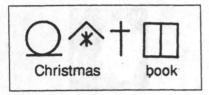

warding off. If the individual is unable to hold his or her head up, this may be perceived as an indication of a lack of interest and the conversation will be ended (Morris, 1981; Yoder and Kraat, 1983).

In addition, there is the imbalance in how much is said by each of the conversational partners. The naturally speaking partners may have long exchanges, whereas the aided speakers generally have only one exchange for each turn that they take (Light, 1985; von Tetzchner and Martinsen, 1996). This will result in children and adults in the expressive language group experiencing problems in conversing in an everyday, ordinary way. Conversing, making small comments while the conversational partner is speaking, and telling funny stories and cracking jokes are some of the most difficult things to do for an individual who depends on a communication board and a helper. The chances that individuals have of expressing more than they generally say every day in the same situations depend on plenty of time being available, and their conversational partners being attentive and careful not to decide too much of the conversation content.

Topic-comment

One possible way to improve conversations is if both individuals and their conversational partner learn to utilize a topic-comment structure in the conversation. This means that the individual and the conversational partner first decide on the topic of conversation, and that what is said later in the utterance or conversation is in the form of a comment on or a specification of the topic. Such a construction makes it easier for the conversational partner to understand and reduce the likelihood of misunderstanding. When it takes time to construct a sentence such as *CHRISTMAS BOOK*, the first sign *CHRISTMAS* functions to make the conversational partner aware that the individual is going to say something about Christmas. Thus, the next sign will lead the conversational partner to understand that the individual was given a book as a Christmas present. A topic-comment strategy increases the likelihood that the person who interprets or guesses what is being said will guess correctly.

The topic-comment structure is typical for language used by people who have different native languages and therefore have difficulty in communicating with one another. When they communicate regularly with one another, they may develop a common language. These languages, which are generally used for trading, are called pidgin languages (Romaine, 1988). As a topic-comment structure is used in situations where people have difficulty in communicating, there is reason to believe that this strategy is also well suited to people who use communication aids. It represents both a strategy for initiating a conversation or introducing a new subject, and a means of gaining control over the content of the conversation. At the same time, it is an economical strategy – enabling the use of fewer words, which also makes the strategy useful (Woll and Barnett, 1998).

The teaching of individuals who use communication aids has often been characterized by a normative attitude which requires the 'correct' use of language. The use of a topic-comment construction of sentences and conversations will differ from common notions of how language should be. To use a topic-comment structure with graphic signs or whole written words, it is necessary consciously to break with the normative conception of 'correct' language based on the culture's spoken language. This may be necessary in order to ensure that individuals who use communication aids have the most effective communication feasible in as many situations and settings as possible. In conversations with people who are unfamiliar with communication aids, it may nevertheless be necessary for users of communication aids to adapt linguistically. This is generally done by using a more elaborate or 'correct' language (Morningstar, 1981).

Breakdowns and repairs

Misunderstandings or lack of understanding may occur during conversations. Requests for repetitions and other attempts to clarify the meaning during conversations inform a speaker that what he or she has said was unclear in some way. In the course of language acquisition, it is important that children get feedback with regard to whether they are understood (Pinker, 1990). Such feedback often takes the form of negotiations about meaning.

A large proportion of the utterances produced in aided communication is misunderstood and leads to a breakdown in communication (Kraat, 1985; Collins, 1996; Hjelmquist and Sandberg, 1996). The breakdowns are often caused by the fact that the amount of time that the individuals spend expressing themselves make the listener lose concentration and thereby lose track of what is being said, although imprecise pointing and faults on the part of the user may also cause misunderstandings. To ensure that these breakdowns do not lead to the whole conversation breaking down, it is essential that the individuals have strategies to signal that a misunderstanding has occurred and for remedying this. Breakdowns in communication may also be the result of problems encountered by individuals who attempt to express themselves with a limited number of signs or words.

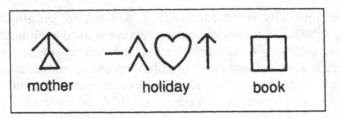

A 12-year-old girl with cerebral palsy was going home for her Christmas holidays and produced *MOTHER HOLIDAY BOOK* in Blissymbols. She refused to leave the school and continued to repeat the same three Blissymbols. After an hour, her teacher discovered that the girl wanted to take home the 'report card' that he had read aloud for her, where it said that she had made great progress.

It is not uncommon that people with limited means of expressing themselves allow a misunderstanding to pass because they do not know how to repair or remedy it or because it would take too long to rectify (Yoder and Kraat, 1983). Moreover, young normally developing children have few reparation strategies, which is also evident in young aided speakers (Light, 1985). In the above example, it was the girl's persistence that led to her finally taking her report card home with her. However, she was unable to rephrase what she wanted to say, and it is unlikely that she had received sufficient teaching of how to clarify situations that were not understood.

It is important that children are taught to use repair strategies, and also receive teaching in how they can make conversational partners aware that they have misconstrued or misunderstood what was said. The most common strategy used when repairing misunderstandings is to point at the same graphic sign once more or spell the word again. This is a good strategy to use if the listener did not see which sign the aided speaker used or lost track of the spelling the first time. Another strategy is to reformulate what was expressed. This is especially important when using graphic signs where it is often necessary for individuals to paraphrase in order to make clear what they want to say. Repetition might be construed as the next word or utterance, and conversational partners might be uncertain about where the misunderstanding lies. *MISUNDERSTANDING* should therefore be on the board, to indicate that the interpretation or perception of what has been said is incorrect. In synthetic speech an utterance such as '*That wasn't exactly what I meant*' may be used. Individuals should learn to use this sign before they begin to repeat signs or words or try to clarify or paraphrase what they intended to say.

The expressions of the aided speaker are not the only cause of communication breakdowns. The ability to understand and use clarification

questions appears quite late, however, indicating that this is an advanced linguistic skill. Before 5 years of age, normally speaking children are not very attentive to expressions of confusion or surprise in their conversation partners, which may indicate that they have not understood what was said. Children often fail to indicate lack of understanding (Garvey, 1977; Lloyd, Camaioni and Ercolani, 1995). As soon as their comprehension allows, aided speakers should be taught to look for clues to misunderstanding in the normally speaking partner, and it should be made certain that they have graphic signs that can be used in clarification questions, e.g. *WHAT YOU SAY* and *WHAT YOU MEAN*. True clarification questions from aided speakers may inform the communication partner about their comprehension of spoken language. The clarifications provided may also help develop the clarification strategies of the aided speaker.

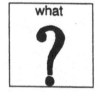

Finally, it is important to distinguish between corrections and requests for clarification. In graphic communication, the speaking partner typically interprets and articulates the utterance of children, who may then acknowledge that the formulation or interpretation is correct. However, it is quite usual that people ask disabled children to repeat a graphic utterance, even when it has been well understood. A request for repetition usually signals an error, and children typically vary their answers when asked again, and thus create changes in expression when this is not appropriate or needed. Moreover, if children experience corrections as rejections of their attempt to communicate, this may have a negative influence on their language development. True negotiations about meaning, on the other hand, do not seem to make children feel rejected, but rather to influence language development in a positive manner (Barnes et al., 1983).

Narratives

Narratives are descriptions of past events, often sequences of personal experiences, and constitute an important basis for children's language development and learning about the world (Nelson, 1996). The co-construction of narratives with an adult also represents crucial opportunities for learning about oneself and others.

Narratives may contain sentences but, in the early phases of language development, they may also consist of single-word utterances that indicate only the time sequence of events. However, the use of single-sign utterances is typical of the narratives of children with good comprehension of speech using communication aids also at more advanced age levels, as in this example from von Tetzchner and Martinsen (1996, pp. 81–82).

Eva, aged 5;4 years, was using direct selection and a communication book with 285 PIC signs and photographs. She and her mother were communicating about a visit to an aunt.

M: *When we went to aunt Kari, what did you bring?*
E: *BICYCLE.*
M: *You brought that bicycle when we went to aunt Kari.*
E: *BICYCLE.* [TO] BICYCLE [lifts the arm up and down, which is a manual home sign for 'to bicycle'].
M: *Yes, you did bicycle there.*
M: *Hm?*
E: *SANDBOX.*
M: *Were you also in the sandbox?*
E: 'Yes' [nods].
M: *Hm.*
E: *SWING.*
M: *And then you used the swing.*
E: 'Yes' [nods].
M: *Hm.*
E: *SWITCHBACK.*
M: *And the switchback was there. Eva was in a playground when we visited aunt Kari.*

In this dialogue, the mother had prompted Eva to indicate *BICYCLE* with the request: *What did you bring?* Thereafter, however, Eva took control of the dialogue, directing the mother to create a narrative where [TO] BICYCLE, *SANDBOX, SWING* and *SWITCHBACK* were parts. Eva made references to events that were known beforehand to both herself and her mother, and the dialogue became a retelling of what she did at that specific time. The mother replied to Eva's single-sign utterances, but did not ask her to comment or expand on them, taking that role upon herself. Eva did not herself attempt to make a comment.

This dialogue structure is typical of interactions between young communication aid users and normally speaking adults. The children typically use a few graphic signs to prompt an adult partner to tell a story, saying something like: 'Tell me something that is connected with the following topic.' This particular pragmatic use of signs in dialogues may be coined *directive*, because the signs are used to direct the attention of the speaking partner towards a topic, on which the users want the partner to comment on their own behalf. It is not a true dialogue skill because it does not promote the continuation of conversational exchanges.

The ability to relay narratives that comprise more than one event is an important skill that needs to be promoted among individuals using manual and graphic communication, including those who belong to the alternative language group. In addition, although narratives do not require relational utterances, they still represent useful opportunities for promoting sentence construction. To relay the content of an event involving people, objects, attributes, events, activities, etc., there is very often a need to know about more than one semantic role. The narrative structure may link different semantic elements and thus the child's use of vertically and horizontally structured sentences. To facilitate this development, the adult has to adapt the events to be narrated in such a manner that people, actions, objects and locations need to be mentioned.

As part of this strategy, adults may create situations and events that the children are encouraged to describe, freely or within a framework, in which they provide information by filling in missing parts of an utterance. It is more fun for children to describe unusual or humorous events than everyday routines, such as when a teacher stands on the head or starts to eat from an empty plate, or a cat visits the classroom. Even children with profound learning disability may enjoy such events and be motivated to describe and tell about them in a simple manner. On the other hand, it is necessary to take into account that some children, particularly those with autism, may have difficulties learning words that reflect their own experiences.

Finally, the narratives of even individuals with severe and profound learning disabilities do not need to relate only to their immediate surroundings and personal experiences. Tales of fantasy and adventure are central to human communication and culture. Both simple stories such as *Three little pigs* and classic works such as *The Odyssey*, *The Hobbit* and *Gulliver's Travels* may be adapted for this group and used in communication intervention (Grove, 1998; Park, 2000).

Chapter 12
The language environment

Individuals who learn alternative communication systems spend little time in teaching situations compared with the time that they spend in their natural environment. If teaching is to have any purpose, it must help the individual to be able to use and develop communication skills in everyday situations. However, the alternative language mode is often little used outside educational settings. A lack of knowledge about the system and insensitive communicative strategies on the part of the conversational partners result in few truly communicative opportunities (Murphy et al., 1996). Many users of alternative communication systems become *communicative under-achievers*. They are often not credited with an ability to communicate or with having anything about which to communicate. This means that the people in the individuals' environment must learn how they communicate, and be given opportunities to communicate with them to find out what they are capable of. All too often, people in the environment do not master the alternative language form well enough. Communication partners often do not appear to see the need to learn the individuals' language form, particularly when the individuals have a comparatively good comprehension of spoken language, which is often the case for people with Down's syndrome who use manual signs. The result is a communicative one-way road: from the speaking communication partners to the communication-impaired individuals.

Improved knowledge about alternative communication systems among people in the environment is most efficiently obtained through systematic training and guidance of family, friends and professionals. As the process of acquiring alternative language modes tends to be slow and laborious, training and support for family, friends and staff should also have a long-term perspective. The training of family and staff makes them better communicators, which contributes to making the individuals better communicators, in turn creating new needs for family and staff training, etc.

Children who learn to speak normally do so through interaction with a supportive language environment. An ordinary language environment consists of family members, nursery school and school staff, and other adults and children in the child's immediate surroundings. Individuals who are taught alternative communication systems have also grown up in normal language environments, but they have been unable to acquire language within the ordinary framework. It is therefore necessary to adapt the environment specially for them. Being able to communicate with people in the environment is an important aspect of the quality of life. The adaptation should therefore include as many as possible of those in close contact with the individual, and this entails teaching the family and nursery school, school and institution staff, as well as significant others.

Adapting the environment

Intervention with infants and young disabled children is usually aimed at encouraging interaction and communication. The intervention measures are directed at how the parents and others react to the child. Intervention involving alternative communication systems does not generally begin during the first year of life. The use of graphic and manual signs is generally discussed only if the parents broach the subject, and is then considered a possibility only if the child does not begin to speak normally.

For children who are known to be *at risk* of developing inadequate speech, discussion about alternative communication may begin when the child is only a few months old (le Prevost, 1983; Launonen, 1996, 1998). The use of manual signs requires some teaching and it is an advantage if key people in the environment have learned some signs before the child is expected to start using them. It may also be useful to prepare both staff and older children in the nursery school where the child attends, or will soon attend, by teaching them some signs. From very early on, parents and other adults may perform manual signs when the child shows interest in objects and activities in the environment.

Graphic signs can also be introduced in the same gradual way, so that the signs become a part of the language environment before the child is expected to use them. In this way, people in the environment become familiar with the graphic signs, and the child may experience less pressure from expectations when they are introduced.

The consequences of the environmental adaptation for older children, adolescents and adults depend on their linguistic abilities. For people with little language comprehension and a poor ability to express themselves, overinterpretation will still play an important role. One of the aims of an adapted environment is to get the people in contact with individuals in the alternative language group to react to a greater part of their behaviour as though it was communicative. On the whole, people are particularly aware of the vocal sounds made by the individuals, but often overlook communicative efforts where individuals use, for example, arm movements or posture. An adapted environment may make it easier to (over)interpret the individual's movements, facial expressions and posture. This increases the likelihood that the individual will be reacted to, which in turn fosters self-initiated activity.

For individuals with better spoken language skills, it is most important to ensure that they are able to converse with people who understand them. This may, for example, be done by teaching potential communication partners through planned 'incidental learning', and by making people in the environment aware of the individual's capabilities.

Individuals with extensive motor impairment often have such fixed routines that they have few opportunities to communicate. An important objective of the environmental adaptation for these individuals is to create more varied everyday situations and to produce communicative situations in which the conversational partners do not always know in advance what will be said.

The simultaneous use of speech and signs

One should always speak while performing manual, graphic and tangible signs, so that sign learners have the opportunity to relate the signs to spoken words if they have the ability to do so. Intervention with simultaneous use of speech and signs has improved the comprehension of spoken language for many individuals. For others, the accompanying speech seems to have neither a positive nor a negative effect (Clark, Remington and Light, 1986; Romski and Sevcik, 1996). Thus, the conclusion in terms of whether speech should be used seems to be quite clear: it is always correct to use speech in association with signs. In fact, it is not possible to omit speech. With the possible exception of a few small communities of deaf signers, spoken language will always be the most common communication form in the environment. However, not all the individuals will benefit from it.

To ensure optimal conditions for the acquisition of an alternative language form, it is necessary that the people in the environment support the individual's possibilities of learning in social interaction with those people. These people may adopt an alternative mode and use this fully in all communication with the individual, thus creating an enclave of alternative communication use within an environment of natural speakers. Such enclaves may consist of the school, day centre, home, institution and similarly restricted environments. Although this may be the optimal learning condition for people with little or no comprehension of spoken language, it has proved difficult in practice to make this kind of overall adaptation (Martinsen and von Tetzchner, 1996).

People in the environment may also speak normally without simultaneous sign use when responding to an individual using an alternative communication form. In these interchanges, both the communication-impaired individuals and their communication partners use different modes for comprehension and production. This is the typical environment of people belonging to the expressive group, but it is also common among people in the other two groups. The efficiency of this adaptation depends on both the individuals' comprehension of spoken language and on how the connections between the alternative communication form and speech are made apparent by people in the environment.

Finally, people in the environment may speak normally and support their speech with manual or graphic signs (key word sign use). This is probably the most common adaptation of the environment for people belonging to the supportive and alternative language groups. However, possibilities for communication-impaired individuals to utilize the environment will, to a large degree, depend on their understanding of spoken language, and such adaptations are probably, in most cases, insufficient for people with comprehension problems (compare Grove, Dockrell and Woll, 1996; Romski and Sevcik, 1996).

Simplified language

People who communicate with a language-impaired individual should simplify their speech and avoid complex sentences. However, there may be limits to how much the spoken language should be changed. Ungrammatically shortened sentences do not appear to lead to improved comprehension on the part of learning-disabled individuals, who themselves generally produce one-word utterances. Experimental studies of children with normal language development have produced mixed results. In one study in which children with an average utterance length of under two words were required to follow more or less linguistically well-formulated instructions, Petretic and Tweeney (1977) found that the well-formulated sentences were more likely to lead to the correct action. Shortening sentences and omitting function words did not lead to improved comprehension. In a similar study, Shipley, Gleitman and Smith (1969) found that children who themselves chiefly used one-word utterances reacted more frequently to shortened and simplified utterances than to utterances that were well formulated.

As it is unnatural to speak in 'telegraphese', it seems best to use complete but simple sentences. The comprehension and use of passive sentences and utterances containing long subordinate clauses appear at a late stage in normal development, and are probably so difficult that it is best to avoid using them. It is essential that the spoken language is natural, so that the adults feel comfortable and can direct their attention to the individual instead of being preoccupied with speaking correctly.

It is common that signs serve as a support for speech rather than being used to express whole sentences. When manual signs are used, small words and function words are generally omitted (Grove, Dockrell and Woll, 1996). This makes it easier to use manual signs, but individuals who learn alternative communication modes should also be given the opportunity to learn prepositions and other function words, once they have reached the appropriate linguistic level.

The way in which the conversational partner speaks determines which role the individual will play in the conversation. Even motor-impaired individuals with good comprehension of spoken language and a communication board with a reasonable number of signs receive a disproportionate number of yes–no questions (Basil, 1986; von Tetzchner and Martinsen, 1996). To provide individuals with the opportunity to use a greater number of signs and a more varied language, the people with whom they are in contact must be aware of the way in which they themselves use spoken and graphic language. This means that they should vary their language and, for example, increase the number of comments that they make and ask open questions when speaking with aided speakers.

Models

A good language environment consists of people who use the alternative communication form and act as language models. It is natural to use manual signs as a means of support when speaking to individuals who are learning manual signs. However, people in the environment rarely use a board of their own, or the individuals' board, as a means of helping them to understand speech when they converse with communication aid users (Bruno and Bryen, 1986; Romski and Sevcik, 1996). One result of this is that new graphic signs are not introduced 'naturally' in the same way as manual signs.

It is quite common that other children in the school or nursery school learn some manual signs. They generally use these to tell the sign user that they are going to eat, go for a walk, etc. Graphic signs may be used by naturally speaking children in the same way as manual signs, but some training may be necessary to support this. Although most graphic sign systems are easy to understand, it is still possible for children who cannot read to misunderstand them (see Smith, 1996). The fact that the graphic signs are something that the children have to learn, and that they are not merely incidental pictures, makes them more interesting for the other children. In this way, the status of the sign system is enhanced, as is that of the child who uses it.

When people in the individuals' environment use their communication form and show that they take it seriously, this may boost the individuals' status (compare Woll and Barnett, 1998).

> At a day centre for learning-disabled individuals, a youth meeting was held once a week. One of the adolescents used manual signs, while the others were able to speak. The youth who used signs had a good understanding of spoken language and used 200 manual signs actively. The other youths did not use signs and had trouble understanding him at the meetings. One of the teachers therefore had to interpret for him. This led to the other youths taking what he expressed seriously, and his esteem in the group was boosted (Steindal K, personal communication, 1990).

To create awareness of graphic signs among people in the environment, one may also use graphic signs as labels on objects in the environment, e.g. *DOOR*, *TOILET*, *CHAIR*, *GLASS*, *TELEVISION*, *RADIO* and *BED*. It may help the individuals to learn the names of things; graphic signs become part of the environment but, more importantly, make it easier for people to use graphic signs when they speak with them. It is also useful to label cupboards and drawers containing the individuals' belongings and other relevant objects. The graphic signs that are used in this manner are typically the ones that the individuals are in the process of learning.

Teaching families

Children's parents and siblings are central people in their lives, and hence also important partners in any intervention. Children will not become competent users of graphic, manual and tangible signs unless the members of their family understand and support the effort. Thus, families need knowledge about the communicative possibilities of the children and how to communicate with them, i.e. to learn, develop and use strategies that provide them with opportunities for taking communicative initiative and participating in dialogues with real content. If families are not given sufficient knowledge, a lack of understanding may negatively influence the children's communication opportunities and possibilities for participation in activities that they like.

> Margarida has no speech and is unable to produce vocalisations loud enough to be heard. Until she was 8 years old, she did not have opportunities to show her basic needs, wants and feelings in an efficient way. When she arrived from school, she was seated on the sofa with the television in front of her, her parents occupying themselves with their daily duties. Unable to walk and vocalise, she could not move away or even change the station of her own volition. The parents said that she loved to watch television because she stayed still for 2 or 3 hours without giving them trouble (Lourenço et al., 1996, p. 312).

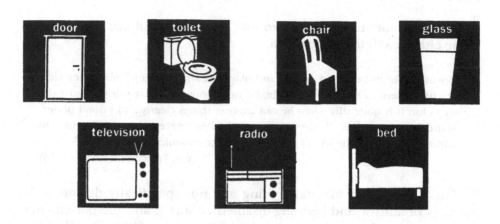

Intervention has a greater and more lasting effect when the families are included as active participants, receive proper training and share the 'ownership' of the intervention (Berry, 1987; Angelo, Jones and Kokoska, 1995). This requires a co-operative effort, but in many instances either the parents are not consulted or else it is left entirely up to them to put such measures into effect. However, active participation by parents does not mean that they should act as teachers for their children or assume the responsibilities of professionals. The role of parents is first and foremost to be parents and, in the case of a severely disabled child, this is a demanding enough task in itself. It may take the parents of a disabled child a considerable amount of time and resources to perform such common-place activities with the child as dressing, washing and eating. There is often little time left for the parents and child to participate in more pleasant activities together. The parents' training should aim at facilitating joint activities and communication, and to make everyday activities and routines as smooth, varied and interesting as possible.

A parent-teaching programme typically consists of three elements: general courses, individual sessions and parent–child interactions with guidance and follow-up discussions, which usually include video record-ings. If they are old enough, siblings may be included in all three elements, or they may receive all their information and support from the parents. Parents should be informed about what augmentative and alter-native communication is, and of research and clinical experiences with it. It is especially important to emphasize that one has not given up hope that the child will start to speak and that the aim is to enhance the possible development of speech. An important part of the discussions about the child's interactions is to point out the child's progress to the family.

Professionals sometimes want to spare parents the effort that thorough learning of their children's communication imply, but thereby the profes-sionals in fact 'protect' the parents from communicating optimally with their own children. It is a natural part of the intervention to teach the family the communication system that their child will use. This is often done either too little or too much.

> 'I would like to be ahead of him and maybe learn his signs before they start teaching them to him. For example, he now knows colours I don't know the signs for. It is quite silly when he can express things clearly and I don't under-stand because I don't know the signs. It is not necessary to teach him to communicate when he hasn't got anybody to communicate with.'
>
> von Tetzchner (1996b, p. 14)

Most courses in manual signing are not specifically designed for parents of autistic and learning-disabled children, and the parents may feel that many of the signs that they have learned are of little use. They may spend the only free evening that they have each week in order to attend a manual sign course, struggling to find baby-sitters, etc., and learn several hundred signs at the end of 1 year. If, during the same period of time, the child has learned only 10 signs, the parents may feel that this is a poor result and be disappointed with the intervention for which they had had great hopes and in which they had invested a lot of time. It may be better if the family is taught by professionals who are responsible for teaching language-impaired individuals. There are also course books with manual sign vocabularies designed especially for children. It is unnecessary for the family to learn a much greater number of signs than those the child is in the process of learning. If the child's development turns out to be rapid, this will motivate the family to learn new signs. If the child learns to use 10 manual signs and the members of the family are able to use 20, the result will be good in terms of time and energy invested.

Families of children who learn graphic signs also need to have the system explained to them thoroughly. They need to see how the signs should be used, and preferably participate in teaching sessions at the nursery school or school. It should be emphasized that graphic signs are not merely a collection of incidental pictures but a communication system. They are the child's words and replace or supplement spoken language for the time being. This is especially important with simple systems such as PIC and PCS. Some parents begin to talk about what they see on the signs the child points to in much the same way that they comment about ordinary pictures (C. Basil, personal communication, 1989). This undermines the intended linguistic function of these pictures. The family should therefore be taught how the actual communicative process takes place, and be guided in how they should use graphic signs, for example, to comment on ordinary pictures.

For the more complex system, Blissymbolics, it appears that many parents sabotage the use of the communication board, and this is probably the result of inadequate teaching. As a result of their own uncertainty and limited ability to support the children's use of the system, they feel that they do not understand their children any better than before. They choose instead to continue to use an established pictographic system such as PIC signs or PCS and ask their child yes–no questions until the child learns to read, in spite of the fact that this may take a long time and sometimes fail (von Tetzchner, 1997a).

Family relationships will influence how the children communicate, and the family therefore needs to sustain their acquisition of an alternative language form. A negative attitude on the part of the parents may rub off on the children, and lead to them not learning to make full use of the linguistic tool that they have at their disposal.

It is essential that the child learns to use new signs not only at nursery school or school, but also at home. Thus, the parents should follow up the child's teaching. This may be supported by giving the child 'homework', i.e. tasks that the parents and child are to perform at home. Similarly, signs learned first at home should be included in the activities at school as much as possible. However, it is important that professionals do not regard communication at home as simply a follow-up of school and doing homework. Parents should be helped to communicate as well as possible with their child at home. They do not need teacher skills in the home – they need parent skills, enhanced and adapted to the child with the help of teachers and other professionals. This means that it is not enough to tell parents what is being done at school or pre-school. Professionals must base their help and guidance on true knowledge about the home situation, and how best this can be adapted to support the child's development of language and communication, while at the same time taking the family's total needs, potentials and limitations into consideration.

General teaching and discussion of intervention and teaching methods will not guarantee that training and the use of alternative communication modes are well implemented at home (Casey, 1978; Basil, 1986). Role-playing may be used to a certain extent, and video recordings may also be useful. A good strategy is that parents observe professionals teaching and giving practical instruction. The parents will be able to see how the children indicate and perform signs, which will help them to recognize their children's attempts to communicate in the home. Some of the child–teacher sessions should take place regularly in the child's home, with comments from parents and siblings, and alternate with child–parent and child–sibling sessions, with comments from the teacher (Basil and Soro-Camats, 1996). This will also serve to adapt the intervention better to the children's communication opportunities in the home, and make it more likely that the family members are able to make use of these opportunities.

However, the training that takes place at home should not be so exten-sive that it encroaches on all other activities enjoyed by the family. Their function should be to ensure good communication strategies in everyday family activities, not to turn the home into a classroom. Parents may be given tasks that are too extensive, and it is not uncommon to hear criticism from professionals who do not think that the parents follow up properly. If the parents are given special training assignments at home, these should be the child's homework and take the family's whole situation into account. Professionals tend to forget that, although they can leave their work at the office, parents have the responsibility for the whole time.

Although it is important that part of the family training takes place in the child's home, courses and workshops where families are together for 1–3 weeks also have important advantages. The children's and the parents' programmes should be partly overlapping and partly in parallel. The children may get intensive training in which the family participates some of the time, to promote good joint interaction and communication skills. The parents (and siblings) should receive high-quality lectures with theoretical and practical issues related to augmentative and alternative communication, and participate in discussions about how to chose vocabu-lary and promote multi-sign utterances, role-playing and other forms of group activities. It is of particular significance that, in such workshops, the parents are relieved of their daily duties and have time to focus in depth on the relevant issues, get to know each other and build up a network, and have the opportunities to exchange experiences, problems and solutions. Such courses have been demonstrated to change both parent and child performance (Bruno and Dribbon, 1998).

Finally, fathers of children with alternative communication systems often have poor knowledge of the system and little training in communi-cating with the child (Sweeney, 1999). Although intervention is not the time or place for focusing on sex roles, the sharing of responsibilities by parents should be encouraged. Fathers and mothers often have different interests. These may be used by professionals in a constructive manner to widen the individual's experiences and enhance language learning, e.g. by giving a technically interested father special computer training and responsibility for maintaining high technology aids, or introducing sports terms so that the father and child can enjoy sports events together.

Teaching peers and friends

Classmates and other peers are important parts of children's language environment and an invaluable resource when adapting the environment for children who use manual, graphic and tangible signs; a number of studies have shown increased communication and more balanced dialogues as a result of peer training (Hunt, Alwell and Goetz, 1991;

Romski and Sevcik, 1996). For children in the expressive language group, peers may be better informed about the communication-impaired child's interests and preferences because these typically correspond to those of other children of the same age. Moreover, disabled children have been found to feel less dependent when being helped by other children instead of adults (Madge and Fassam, 1982). In addition, for children with autism and learning disability, training peers how to react to their communication attempts and initiate interaction with them may improve their communicative environment considerably, and thereby reduce frustration and anger and increase positive experiences for both parties (Goldstein et al., 1992).

Individual differences in communicative style influence conversations, and existing habits and strategies should be taken into account when training peers. Older children in the expressive group may themselves be able to observe partner styles. Buzolich and Lunger (1995) let Vivian, a 12-year-old motor-impaired girl who used a communication aid, assess the styles of three class mates who were singled out for special training as communication partners. The result was that both Vivian and the class-mates changed strategies as they became aware of each other's style of communication. The result was that their communication became better adapted to each other.

The use of significant others in the environment is not limited to children. Communication-impaired adults also have friends and other people who are close to them, who are important communication partners and who may function as models in the environment. By giving these people sufficient insight into the individuals' communication and access to good partner strategies, the language environment may become more inviting and increase both the quantity and the quality of the individuals' everyday communication. Light and her associates (1992) demonstrate increased turn-taking and initiation by two communication-impaired adults, and reduced turn-taking and initiation by their aides and friends, following a short instructional programme. However, it is important to ensure that these people do not start to behave like teachers in a classroom.

Finally, it is an important objective to promote interaction between those learning-disabled people who speak and those who use alternative communication forms. Learning-disabled people tend to communicate little among themselves, even when they spend much time together in day centres and supported houses. Their communication is mainly directed at staff, who for their part often have limited time to respond to their initiatives. Many of the learning-disabled people are able to speak and motivated to communicate more but, as other normally speaking people, they need to be given the necessary training to become good communication partners for people who use manual, tangible and graphic signs. This may take the form of specially adapted courses and practical guidance.

The result may be a significant extension of the communicative environment. This form of training is also a signal from the professionals to the learning-disabled people that their communication – also the non-speech one – is important and that they are willing to invest in increasing staff-independent use of it.

Teaching staff

Staff training is an essential part of any intervention involving alternative communication systems. Although the use of such systems has become more usual, most professionals have limited experience of working with people who use these systems and hence have no or limited knowledge about the systems. One of the primary objectives will be to make professionals realize that the individuals are actually using a form of language, not only some more or less 'natural' gestures and pictures.

If the intervention is to be successful, all the people who work with or around the individuals must be given information and helped to develop the necessary skills. On many occasions, it is only those who show most interest, have a flair for manual, graphic and tangible communication, or are singled out for one reason or another, who are taught about augmentative and alternative communication (compare Sweeney, 1999). It is typically only these people who are able to use manual signs, feel comfortable with graphic communication, and know how they should react to the individual's attempts at communication. Staff training should include *everyone* who is in contact with the individual, including relief care staff. Assistants often have the most opportunities to communicate with the individuals, but rarely receive training and systematic supervision.

Staff training should take place on a regular basis, and be aimed at all aspects of the intervention. Staff who receive intensive training from external specialists should be responsible for training the other members of the staff, thus increasing the total impact of the training on the environment (Granlund, Terneby and Olsson, 1992). This will also increase the awareness and thus the competence of the staff members who received the intensive training.

Staff training is often inadequate, typically limited to the teaching of a few manual signs or to a demonstration of what the graphic signs look like. In fact, this is the easiest part. The staff should be told about the individuals' assessment and the implications that the individuals' skills and problems may have for interactions with them. The staff should learn about the basis for the formation of the manual, graphic and tangible signs, how the systems are constructed, and the theoretical foundation of the communication intervention in general. A professional explained the need for this kind of training in this manner:

'To study the theoretical background and the research on intervention method-
ologies was essential for me in order to understand the disabled child. It made
me regard and treat the child in a totally different way.'

Mendes and Rato (1996, p. 351)

Although many people feel both awkward and silly pointing at graphic
signs or performing manual signs, this is the easiest part of the training. It
may in fact be an advantage that staff members do not have much prior
experience with manual signs, because this makes them perform the signs
more slowly and clearly, making them easier for the individual to perceive.

With manual sign, it is considerably more difficult to read other
people's signs than it is to produce signs oneself. A significant part of the
teaching should therefore be aimed at understanding other people's
manual sign use. Understanding manual signs produced by others can be
particularly difficult in everyday situations. In a defined teaching situation,
the teacher usually knows which manual sign the individual is trying to
perform, and is able to respond to the sign even when it is poorly articulated. In a spontaneous communication in the ordinary environment, the
same sign may never be understood.

Associations for deaf people usually have a number of videos that may
be rented for teaching purposes. It is also possible to make one's own
video, or perform signs that the others are supposed to guess. It is particularly useful to make video recordings of the individuals in question
performing signs, so that the members of staff can learn what the signs
look like when particular individuals perform them. It can be good
training to try to guess from the video which sign an individual is
attempting to perform, without giving any extra clues, i.e. by turning the
volume down so it is impossible to hear what the teacher is saying, by
making sure that the picture is not showing the object or activity about
which the person is communicating, and taking care that the teacher does
not perform the sign first.

With some communication aid users, it can be difficult to understand
where and how they are pointing. Video recordings can be a useful means
of demonstrating which method of pointing is best suited to particular
individuals, and thus help reduce the likelihood that people in the
environment will misunderstand their pointing.

In the case of graphic signs, the gloss is usually written above the sign
so it is not necessary for people in the environment who can read to learn
the design of each of the separate signs. All members of staff should nevertheless be given an introduction to how the system is constructed, and the
reasons why specific signs are included on the individual's communication board. It is good practice for the staff members to try to use the signs
to communicate with one another, so that they gain an insight into the

system's potential and limitations. The staff should also be introduced to the more general reasons for choosing the system, and be informed about the individual's expected development. This will help them to react correctly in new situations, and to take note of any significant developments.

The staff members also need to know how the individuals wish the communication to take place, e.g. whether they should guess or interpret the communication before the individuals are finished saying what they want to say. To promote spontaneous communication, it is important that the staff members are taught not to take the communicative initiative all the time, but to be sensitive and respond to the individual's own attempts at communicating. The staff members must learn to become aware of their role as communication partners. Kaiser, Ostrosky and Alpert (1993) found that, when pre-school staff were trained to be better communication partners and given strategies for promoting the use of communication aids in ordinary settings, the total communication of children using communication aids increased. After a long training course including a video of interactions between individuals and staff, some participants reported:

'I started to become aware of all the attempts, ways and possibilities used by the girl to communicate, allowing her time to take her turn, avoiding a situation where her every effort ended with the frustration of being misunderstood.'
'The most important factor was the development of my skills as an interlocutor. I learned to observe, to be attentive and to react better to the child's behaviour. I started to adapt my speech to my communication partner.'

Mendes and Rato (1996, p. 349)

When graphic signs are used, the communication partner can easily lose track of what is being said and forget to answer a question or a comment that an individual has spent a long time producing. The difficulties that may arise from using the system should be emphasised, as well as how misunderstandings can be rectified. If the staff members know about the problems that the users may encounter, it will be considerably easier for them to help solve such problems.

For users of Blissymbols, it is essential that the staff members are familiar with individual signs, the use of analogies, sentence formation and basic conversational strategies. This will enable the individuals to use the system as effectively as possible, and prevent them from having to adapt their communication to a more elementary level in order to communicate with the staff members.

In addition to direct teaching and instruction, the people who are responsible for staff training should act as models for the rest of the staff members in natural, unplanned situations. For many of the staff members, using signs will be a new experience, and a model may make it easier for them to try using what they have learned.

Individuals who use alternative communication forms are often met with indifference, rejection or fear. Staff training should therefore emphasize the importance of staff being available for communication and showing that they give priority, over other tasks, to communicative interactions. When staff members show an interest in and an understanding of the individual's communication system, this signals a positive attitude to and respect for both the communicative form and the individual. For people belonging to the expressive language group, in particular, this may heighten their self-esteem. It will do no harm if members of staff tell individuals with good comprehension of spoken language that they find it difficult to master the individuals' system, and that they admire their skills and proficiency. An admission of this kind may make the users feel more competent, and perhaps less despairing of other people's misunderstandings and faults.

Cost and benefit

The benefits of family and staff training are high. In fact, without a competent and supportive environment, intervention is likely to fail in its objectives. The training of families and staff members will necessarily take time and resources, but this will be money and time well spent. Moreover, the willingness to use resources on families and staff signals the urgency of developing the individuals' language and communication skills to their maximum.

However, some training programmes focus too much on providing staff training that does not take too long or encroach on the time spent performing other tasks (compare McNaughton and Light, 1989). We believe that it is bad policy to save on staff training. A good educational programme helps to produce competent staff who understand and master their work. These professionals will produce the best language environment for individuals in the process of learning alternative communication modes.

Chapter 13
Overview of case studies

This chapter contains an overview of articles with descriptions of individuals with developmental disorders who receive intervention, including alternative communication systems. The aim of this chapter is to give parents and professionals access to more detailed descriptions of such intervention and only published articles are included. The overview contains information about the individuals' ages and impairments (based on the classification made in the article), and about the communication systems that have been utilized. The full reference may be found in 'References' on p. 318.

A considerable number of articles containing descriptions of individuals have been published, and this list must in no way be considered complete. However, it contains descriptions of the most common groups with developmental disorders and a need for augmentative communication, and examples of the most commonly used communication systems and teaching strategies.

Impairment groups
Autism (A)
Learning disability (LD)
Motor impairment (M)
Multiple impairment (MI)
Specific language disorders (S)
Other (Oth)
Unspecified (?)
Communication systems
Blissymbols (B)
Computer-technology aids (C)
Gestures (G)
Lexigrams (L)
Manual signs (MS)
Morse (MO)

Other (Oth)
Pictures/photographs (P)
Picture Communication System (PCS)
Pictogram Ideogram Communication (PIC)
Picsym (PS)
Premack's word bricks (PWB)
Rebus (R)
Script (S)
Sigsym (SG)
Unspecified (?)

Descriptions

Authors	Impairments	Age (years)	System
Barrera et al. (1980)	A	4	MS
Barrera and Sulzer-Azaroff (1983)	A	6, 7, 9	MS
Basil (1992)	M	17–18	PCS
Basil and Soro-Camats (1996)	M	17	PCS
Baumgart, Johnson and Helmstetter (1990)	M, LD, MI, A	3–37	Oth, P, B
Bedwinek (1983)	LD	5	G
Bennet et al. (1986)	MI	14, 14, 17	MS
Blischak and Lloyd (1996)	MI	38	R, S, R, MS, C
Bonvillian and Nelson (1976)	A	5	MS
Bonvillian and Nelson (1978)	A	12	MS
Booth (1978)	LD	15	MS
Brady and Smouse (1978)	A	6	Oth
Brookner and Murphy (1975)	LD, S	13	MS, S
Bruno (1989)	M	4	P
Buffington et al. (1998)	A	4–6	G
Buzolich (1987)	M, LD	7, 9, 15	MS, B, C
Buzolich and Lunger (1995)	M	12	S, C
Carr et al. (1978)	A	10–15	MS
Carr, Kologinsky and Leff-Simon (1987)	A	11–16	MS
Casey (1978)	A	6, 7	MS
Clarke, Remington and Light (1986)	LD	6, 11, 11	MS
Clarke, Remington and Light (1988)	LD	5–12	MS
Coleman, Cook and Meyers (1980)	M	44	C
Cook and Coleman (1987)	M, LD	14	B, P
Cregan (1993)	LD	14	SG
Culatta and Blackstone (1980)	LD, MI	3, 5, 5	MS
Culp (1989)	S	8	MS
Cumley and Swanson (1999)	S	3, 8, 12	PCS, S, C
Dattillo and Camarata (1991)	M, MI	21, 36	P, S, C
Deich and Hodges (1977)	A, LD	2–20	MS, PWB
Dixon (1996)	M	2	P, B, S, C

Authors	Impairments	Age (years)	System
Duker and Michielsen (1983)	LD	8, 12, 16	MS
Duker and Moonen (1985)	LD	11, 13, 14	MS
Duker and Moonen (1986)	LD	10, 12, 14	MS
Duker and Morsink (1984)	A, LD	8–23	MS
Durand (1993)	MI, LD	3, 5, 15	?, C
Elder and Bergman (1978)	LD	3–17	B
English and Prutting (1975)	Oth	1	MS
Everson and Goodwyn (1987)	M	16–19	C
Faulk (1988)	MI	9	MS, S, P, C
Fay (1993)	MI	35	S, C
Fenn and Rowe (1975)	LD	10–13	MS
Ferrier (1991)	M	47	S, C
Flensborg (1988)	M	12, 12	B, S, C
Foss (1981)	A, Oth	25, 39	MS
Foxx et al. (1988)	LD, MI	18, 20	MS
Fuller, Newcombe and Ounsted (1983)	MI	6	MS
Fulwiler and Fouts (1976)	A	5	MS
Gangkofer and von Tetzchner (1996)	LD	13	MS, B
Gee et al. (1991)	MI	5, 7, 10	Oth
Glennen and Calculator (1985)	M, MI	15, 12	P, R, S
Goodman and Remington (1993)	LD	4–6	MS
Goosens' (1989)	M	6	PCS
Goosens' and Kraat (1985)	M, MR	3, 5, 7	P, S, C
Hamilton and Snell (1993)	A	15	P
Hansen (1986)	A	6	MS
Harris (1982)	M	6, 6, 7	S, C
Harris, Doyle and Haaf (1996)	S	5	PCS, C
Healy (1994)	M, LD	?	Oth, C
Heim and Baker-Mills (1996)	MI	2	B, G
Heller at al. (1996)	MI	19, 19, 20	MS, PCS, Oth
Hill et al. (1968)	M	6	S
Hind (1989)	M	3	B, C
Hinderscheit and Reichle (1987)	MI	18	R
Hinerman et al. (1982)	A	5	MS
Hobson and Duncan (1979)	LD	16–57	MS
Hooper, Connell and Flett (1987)	M	17	MS, B
Horner and Budd (1985)	A, LD	11	MS
Hsieh and Luo (1999)	M	14	C, MO
Hughes (1974–75)	S	7–11	PWB
Hunt, Alwell and Goetz (1991)	LD, MI	15, 15, 17	P
Hurlbut, Iwata and Green (1982)	M, LD	14, 16, 18	P, B
Iacono, Mirenda and Beukelman (1993)	LD	3, 4	MS, PCS
Iacono and Duncom (1995)	MI	2	MS, PS, C

Authors	Impairments	Age (years)	System
Iacono and Parsons (1986)	LD	11, 13, 15	MS
Kahn (1981)	LD	5–8	MS
Karlan et al. (1982)	S	6–7	MS
Keogh et al. (1987)	A, LD	14, 25	MS
Koerselman (1996)	S	7	B
Kollinzas (1984)	LD	20	MS
Konstantareas, Oxman and Webster (1977)	A, LD	5–9	MS
Konstantareas, Webster and Oxman (1979)	A, LD	8–10	MS
Kotkin, Simpson and Desanto (1978)	LD	6, 7	MS
Kouri (1989)	LD	2	MS
Kozleski (1991)	A	7–13	B, PWB, R, P, S
Kristen (1997)	M	17	P, PCS
Lagerman and Höök (1982)	M	11	S, C
Layton and Baker (1981)	A	8	MS
le Prevost (1983)	LD	1	MS
Leber (1994)	MI	12	P, S, Oth
Light et al. (1992)	MI	26	Oth, C
Light et al. (1998)	A	6	S, C
Light et al. (1999)	M, LD	10–44	G, P, S, C
Light, Remington and Porter (1982)	A, LD	14, 14, 14	PWB
Locke and Mirenda (1988)	LD	11	Oth
Luetke-Stahlman (1985)	S	5	MS
Marshall and Hegrenes (1972)	A	7	S
Mathy-Laikko et al. (1989)	MI	8	Oth
McDonald and Schultz (1973)	M	6	B
McEwen and Karlan (1989)	MI	3, 4	Oth
McGregor et al. (1992)	MI	20	P, S, C
McIlvane et al. (1984)	A, LD	18, 27	MS
McLean and McLean (1973)	A	8, 8, 10	Oth
McNaughton and Light (1989)	M, LD	27	G
Mills and Higgins (1984)	M	9	R, S
Mirenda and Dattilo (1987)	LD	10, 11, 12	P
Mirenda and Santogrossi (1985)	LD	8	PCS
Murdock (1978)	LD	15	S
Møller and von Tetzchner (1996)	MI	42	MS, PCS, PIC
Nelms (1996)	MI	11	Oth, C
Odom and Upthegrove (1997)	M	29	S, C
O'Keefe and Datillo (1992)	LD, MI	24, 38, 60	R, P, C
Oliver and Halle (1982)	LD	7	MS
Osguthorpe and Chang (1987)	M, LD	11–14	R
Parkinson, Royal and Darvil (1995)	MI	15, 15	MS, C
Pecyna (1988)	LD	4	R
Peters (1973)	M, MI	13	MS

Authors	Impairments	Age (years)	System
Peterson et al. (1995)	A	7, 9	MS, G, P
Ratusnik and Ratusnik (1974)	A	10	S
Reichle and Brown (1986)	A	23	R, PIC
Reichle, Rogers and Barrett (1984)	LD	15	MS
Reichle et al. (1987)	A, MI	18, 18	P
Reichle and Ward (1985)	LD	13	MS, S, C
Reichle and Yoder (1985)	MI	3–4	PIC
Reid and Hurlbut (1977)	M, MI	31–34	P
Remington and Clarke (1983)	A	10, 15	MS
Remington and Clarke (1993a)	LD	6–12	MS
Remington and Clarke (1993b)	LD	4–11	MS
Robinson and Owens (1995)	LD	27	P
Romski and Ruder (1984)	LD	3–7	MS
Romski and Sevcik (1989)	LD	18 (19	L
Romski et al. (1984)	LD	11–18	L
Romski, Sevcik and Pate (1988)	M, LD	14–9	L
Rotholz, Berkowitz and Burberry (1989)	A1	7, 18	MS, PCS
Rowe and Rapp (1980)	M, S	6, 13	MS
Salvin et al. (1977)	A	5	MS
Schaeffer et al. (1977)	A	4, 5, 5	MS
Schepis et al. (1982)	A, LD	18–21	MS
Schepis, Reid and Berman (1996)	MI	23, 38, 42	C
Schepis et al. (1998)	A, LD	3–5	P, C
Schlosser et al. (1998)	A	10	PCS, S, C
Sigafoos, Laurie and Pennell (1996)	MI	7–15	P, C
Sigafoos and Roberts-Pennell (1999)	LD	6	G, C
Sisson and Barrett (1984)	LD	4, 7, 8	MS
Smeets and Striefel (1976)	LD	16	MS
Smith-Lewis and Ford (1987)	M	25	MS
Smith (1991)	M	19	P, B, S
Smith (1992)	M	7–9	G, PCS, C
Smith (1994)	M	7–9	G, PCS, C
Sommer, Whitman and Keogh (1988)	A, MI, LD	8–25	MS
Soto et al. (1993)	LD	22	SG, C
Spiegel, Benjamin and Spiegel (1993)	MI	19	S, P, C
Topper (1975)	LD	28	MS
Trefler and Crislip (1985)	M	18	S, C
Trevinarus and Tannock (1987)	M	7, 8	B, P, S, C
Vanderheiden et al. (1975)	M	11–16	B
Vanderheiden and Lloyd (1986)	M	7	S, C, ?
Vaughn and Horner (1995)	A	21	P
Villiers and McNaughton (1974)	A	6, 9	S
von Tetzchner (1984a)	S	3	MS

Authors	Impairments	Age (years)	System
von Tetzchner (1984b)	A	5	MS
Watson and Leahy (1995)	S	3	MS
Webster et al. (1973)	A, LD	6	MS
Wells (1981)	LD	18, 25, 26	MS
Wherry and Edwards (1983)	A	5	MS
Wilken-Timm (1997)	M	5	PCS, C
Yorkston et al. (1989)	M	36	B, PS

List of sign illustrations

Manual signs

AEROPLANE, 159
AFTERWARDS, 259
ANGRY, 179
APPLE, 127, 200, 233, 246
BALL, 145, 184, 247, 263
BANANA, 127, 200, 247
BEAK, 208
BED, 233
BIRD, 208
BISCUIT, 156, 174
BOAT, 184
BOOK, 186, 261
BOOTS, 120
BREAD, 247
BUTTER, 233
CAKE, 212
CAR, 31, 152, 188, 250, 258
CAT, 232
CHAIR, 120
CHOCOLATE, 204
CLEAN, 235, 259
CLOTHES, 233
COFFEE, 152, 182, 268
COLD, 235
COME, 185

CRY, 179
CUP, 129
CUT, 153
DADDY/FATHER, 199
DANCE, 154
DINNER, 201
DOCTOR, 232
DOG, 232
DOLL, 186
DOOR, 120
DRAW, 153
DRESS, 233
DRINK, 172, 182, 188, 200, 212
DRIVE, 188
DUCK, 208
EAT, 117, 246, 248
EGG, 212
FATHER/DADDY, 139
FETCH, 245
FINISHED, 32, 134, 244, 272
FIRST, 179, 259
FLY, 208
FOOD, 143, 184, 188, 201
FORK, 210
FRUIT, 200
GET, 148, 205, 247

GIVE, 205, 208
GLASS, 210
GLUE, 153
GONE, 205
GRAPE, 203
HELICOPTER, 216
HELLO, 129
HELP, 162, 205, 213
HERE, 235
HORSE, 120
HOT, 235
I, 270
ICE-CREAM, 203
JUICE/SQUASH, 156, 157, 182, 200, 215
JUMP, 170, 203
KNIFE, 210
LAMP, 233
LARGE, 31, 249, 250
LEFT, 222
MAGAZINE, 153
MEAT, 212
MILK, 156, 188, 193, 200
MINERAL WATER, 245
MORE, 270
MOTHER/MUMMY, 9, 199
MUSIC, 141, 184, 260

NAPPY, 233
NEST, 208
NO, 204
NOW, 260
NURSE, 232
OUT, 211, 258, 275
PAPER, 153
PIECE, 149
PLATE, 215
PLAY, 185, 210, 258, 270
POTATO, 201
PUSH, 162
QUIET, 169
RAILS, 245
RAISIN, 181
READ, 159
RED, 201, 249
REINDEER, 153
RIDE, 187
RIGHT, 222
ROLL, 248
SAUSAGE, 156, 201
SCARF, 120
SCISSORS, 184
SEE/LOOK, 185
SEW, 182
SHIRT, 201
SHOP, 6
SIT, 169
SLEEP, 233
SMALL, 31, 249, 250
SPOON, 210
SPORT, 184, 260
STILL, 169
STOP, 140
STRAIGHT-AHEAD, 222
SUGAR, 232
SWIM, 187
SWING, 211, 258
TABLE, 120
TEAR, 159
THIRSTY, 188
THROW, 263, 270

TIDY, 235, 259
TOILET, 117, 120, 233
TRAIN, 245
TREE, 9
TROUSERS, 201
WAIT, 139
WALK, 117, 142, 203, 258, 260, 274
WANT, 270
WE-TWO, 6
WHAT, 163, 183, 216, 274
WING, 208
WORK, 151, 182, 244
WRITE, 272
YES, 270
YOU, 268, 270

Blissymbols

ACTION, 227
ALMOST-SAME-AS, 15
ANIMAL, 13, 225
BABY, 225
BAG, 163
BED, 196
BEHIND, 222
BICYCLE, 196
BIRD, 194
BOOK, 290, 292
CAR, 225
CAT, 238
CHAIR, 13
CHRISTMAS, 290
COLD, 196, 221
COMPUTER, 225
CONVERSATION, 289
CUP, 129
CYCLE, 227
DOCTOR, 225
DOLL, 225
DOOR, 196
ELEPHANT, 238
END, 289

ENTRANCE, 11
EXIT, 11
FALL, 196
FATHER CHRISTMAS, 12
FEELING, 13, 194
FILM STAR, 225
FUNNY, 196
GAME, 227
GIVE, 13
HAPPY, 13
HEAVY, 227
HELLO, 129
HELP, 196
HER, 179
HIS, 179
HISTORY, 225
HOLIDAY, 292
HOME, 13
HOT, 221
HOUSE, 13, 194
IN FRONT OF, 222
LARGE, 227
LIGHT, 227
LIKE, 196
LONG, 13
LOO, 13
MAN, 11, 113, 194
MATHEMATICS, 225
MEN, 13
MONEY, 13
MORE, 221, 289
MOTHER, 15, 192
MY/MINE, 179
NOSE, 13
NOT, 289
OPPOSITE-MEANING, 13, 194, 227
PAID, 13
PAST TENSE, 13
PLURAL, 13
PROTECTION, 194
RAIN, 11
SAIL, 227

SCHOOL, 225
SHOP, 6, 225
SHOWER, 221
SMALL, 196, 227
SPORT, 225
SQUARE, 227
STAMP, 225
STUPID, 13
TALK, 289
TELEPHONE, 163
TELEVISION, 163
TOILET, 13
TREE, 194
UNDER/BELOW, 196
UP, 13
WATER, 13
WE, 6
WHAT, 163
WISE, 13
WORK, 225
WRONG, 293
YOUR/YOURS, 179

Pictogram Ideogram Communication (PIC)

AEROPLANE, 159
APPLE, 126, 201, 247
BALL, 145, 185, 248, 263
BANANA, 126, 191, 201, 247
BED, 196, 303
BICYCLE, 196, 274, 295
BIG, 249
BIRD, 209
BOOK, 186, 261, 290
BREAD, 247
CAR, 23
CARROT, 191
CHAIR, 303
CHOCOLATE, 204
CHRISTMAS, 209

CLIMB, 170
COFFEE, 152, 182, 268
COLD, 196, 221
COMPUTER, 186
CRISPS, 212
CUP, 129
DANCE, 154
DENTIST, 142
DOLL, 186
DOOR, 196, 303
DOWN, 17
DRAW, 155
DRINK, 182, 201, 212
DUCK, 209
EAT, 118, 247
EGG, 212
FALL, 196
FATHER, 139, 199
FERRY/BOAT, 185
FINISHED, 32, 139, 232, 272
FOOD, 143, 184, 201
FORK, 210
FRIENDS, 195
FUNNY, 196
GAME, 271
GIVE, 148, 205, 248
GLASS, 210, 303
GRAPES, 203
HANDBAG, 148
HEAVY, 17
HELLO, 129
HELP, 162, 195, 196, 205, 213
HOME, 195
HORSE, 256, 17
HOT, 221
HOT DOG, 155, 201
HOUSE, 227
I, 6, 271
ICE-CREAM, 203
JACKET, 275
JUMP, 170, 197, 203, 256

KICK, 121, 248
KIND, 17
KNIFE, 191, 210
KNIT, 211
LEFT, 222
LETTER, 227
LIKE, 196
MEAT, 212
MILK, 155, 201
MINERAL WATER, 245
MOTHER, 199
MUSIC, 141, 184, 260
NO, 204
ORANGE, 126
OUT, 211, 259, 274
OVER, 249
PEN/PENCIL, 191
PLATE, 215
PLAY, 185, 259, 271
POTATO, 201
POTATO CHIPS, 212
PUSH, 162
QUIET, 139
RADIO, 303
READ, 159
RIDE, 187
RIGHT, 222
RUN, 170, 197
SAW, 191
SEE/LOOK, 185
SEW, 182
SHIRT/BLOUSE, 201
SHOP, 6
SHOWER, 221
SIT, 169
SLEEP, 17
SMALL, 196, 249
SPOON, 210
SPORT, 184, 227
SQUASH, 155, 157, 182
STAIRS, 191
STAND, 197
STILL, 169
SWIM, 187

SWING, 211, 259
TALK, 185, 289, 293
TEA, 233
TEAR, 159
TELEVISION, 121, 303
THROW, 248, 263, 271
TOILET, 118, 303
TOOTHBRUSH, 191
TRAIN, 245
TROUSERS, 201
UNDER, 196, 249, 256
UP, 17
VISIT, 259
WALK, 118, 142, 203,
    260, 274
WEAVE, 182
WORK, 151, 182, 211,
    244
WRITE, 272
YES, 271
YOU, 6, 268, 271, 293

**Picture
Communication
Symbols (PCS)**

BED, 196
BICYCLE, 18, 196
BISCUIT, 174,
CIRCUS, 18
COLD, 196
CUP, 18
DOOR, 196
DRINK, 172
EAT, 18
FALL, 196
FORK, 18, 197
FROM, 18
FUNNY, 196
GIVE, 18
GLASS, 18
(TO) HELP, 18
HELP, 18, 195, 196

JUMP, 18
KNIFE, 18
LIKE, 196
LOLLIPOP, 174
LORRY, 186
MORE, 221, 271
NO, 198
RAISINS, 181
RING, 209
SANDBOX, 295
SCHOOL, 18
SMALL, 18
TOOTHBRUSH, 197
UNDER, 196
WANT, 271
WHAT, 193, 275, 293
YES, 198

References and Citation Index

Adamson, L.B. and Dunbar, B. (1991). Communication development of young children with tracheostomies. *Augmentative and Alternative Communication* 7: 275–283. **p.64**.

Alm, N. and Newell, A.F. (1996). Being an interesting communication partner. In: von Tetzchner, S. and Jensen, M.H. (Eds) *Augmentative and Alternative Communication: European perspectives*. London: Whurr, pp. 171–181. **p.43**.

Amir, R.E., Van den Veyer, I.B., Wan, M., Tran, C.Q., Franckr, U. and Zoghbi, H.Y. (1999). Rett syndrome is caused by mutations in X-linked MECP2, encoding methyl-CpG-binding protein 2. *Nature Genetics* 23: 185–188. **p.82**.

Angelo, D.H., Jones, S.D. and Kokoska, S.M. (1995). Family perspective on augmentative and alternative communication: Families of young children. *Augmentative and Alternative Communication* 11: 193–201. **p.303**.

Armstrong, D. (1997). Recent developments in neuropathology – electron microscopy – brain pathology. *European Child and Adolescent Psychiatry* 6(suppl 1): 69–70. **p.84**.

Baker, B. (1982). Minspeak: A semantic compaction system that makes self-expression easier for communicatively disabled individuals. *Byte* 7: 186–202. **p.43**.

Baker, B. (1986). Using images to generate speech. *Byte* 11: 160–168. **p.43**.

Baker, L. and Cantwell, D.P. (1982). Language acquisition, cognitive development, and emotional disorder in childhood. In: Nelson, K.E. (Ed.), *Children's Language*, Volume 3. London: Lawrence Erlbaum, pp. 286–321. **p.65**.

Balandin, S. and Iacono, T. (1998). Topics of meal-break conversations. *Augmentative and Alternative Communication* 14: 131–146. **p.220**.

Barnes, S., Gutfreund, M., Scatterly, D. and Wells, G. (1983). Characteristics of adult speech which predict children's language development. *Journal of Child Language* 10: 65–84. **p.293**.

Barrera, R.D., Lobato-Barrera, D. and Sulzer-Azaroff, B. (1980). A simultaneous treatment comparison of three expressive language training programs with a mute autistic child. *Journal of Autism and Developmental Disorders* 10: 21–37. **p.313**.

Barrera, R.D. and Sulzer-Azaroff, B. (1983). An alternating treatment comparison of oral and total communication training programs with echolalic autistic children. *Journal of Applied Behavior Analysis* 16: 379–394. **p.313**.

Basil, C. (1986). Social interaction and learned helplessness in nonvocal severely handicapped children. Presented at The 2nd Biennial Conference on Augmentative and Alternative Communication, Cardiff, August 1986. **pp.301, 305**.

Basil, C. (1992). Social interaction and learned helplessness in severely disabled children. *Augmentative and Alternative Communication*, 8, 188–199. **pp.271, 313.**

Basil, C. and Soro-Camats, E. (1996). Supporting graphic language acquisition by a girl with multiple impairments. In: von Tetzchner, S. and Jensen, M.H. (Eds) *Augmentative and Alternative Communication: European perspectives*. London: Whurr. pp. 270–291. **pp.305, 313.**

Bates, E. (1979). *The Emergence of Symbols*. New York: Academic Press. **p.168.**

Bates, E., Bretherton, I. and Snyder, L. (1988). *From First Words to Grammar: Individual differences and dissociable mechanisms*. Cambridge: Cambridge University Press. **pp.156, 240.**

Bates, E., Dale, P.S. and Thal, D. (1995). Individual differences and their implications for theories of language development. In: Fletcher, P. and MacWhinney, B. (Eds) *The Handbook of Child Language*. Cambridge: Cambridge University Press, pp. 96–151. **p.217.**

Baumgart, D., Johnson, J. and Helmstetter, E. (1990). *Augmentative and Alternative Communication Systems for Persons with Moderate and Severe Disabilities*. Baltimore: Paul H. Brookes. **p.313.**

Bedwinek, A.P. (1983). The use of PACE to facilitate gestural and verbal communication in a language-impaired child. *Language, Speech, and Hearing Services in Schools* 14: 2–6. **p.313.**

Bennet, D.L., Gast, D.L., Wolery, M. and Schuster, J. (1986). Time delay and system of least prompts in teaching manual sign production. *Education and Training of the Mentally Retarded* 21: 117–129. **pp.161, 313.**

Berg, M.H. (1998). Children's use of pointing cues in aided language intervention. Presented at The 8th Biennial Conference on Augmentative and Alternative Communication, Dublin, August 1998. **p.169.**

Berry, D.C. and Dienes, Z. (1993a). Towards a working characterisation of implicit learning. In Berry, D.C. and Dienes, Z. (Eds) *Implicit Learning. Theoretical and Empirical Issues*. Hove: Lawrence Erlbaum, pp. 1–18. **p.136.**

Berry, D.C. and Dienes, Z. (1993b). Practical implications. In: Berry, D.C. and Dienes, Z. (Eds) *Implicit Learning. Theoretical and empirical issues*. Hove: Lawrence Erlbaum, pp. 129–143. **p.137.**

Berry, J.O. (1987). Strategies for involving parents in programs for young children using augmentative and alternative communication. *Augmentative and Alternative Communication* 3: 90–93. **p.303.**

Beukelman, D.R. and Mirenda, P. (1998). *Augmentative and Alternative Communication: Management of severe communication d:sorders in children and adults*, 2nd edn. London: Paul H. Brookes. **p.126.**

Beukelman, D.R. and Yorkston, K.M. (1984). Computer enhancement of message formulation and presentation for communication system users. *Seminars in Speech and Language* 5: 1–10. **p.218.**

Beukelman, D.R., Yorkston, K.M., Poblete, M. and Naranjo, C. (1984). Frequency of word occurrence in communication samples produced by adult communication aid users. *Journal of Speech and Hearing Disorders* 49: 360–367. **p.59.**

Biklen, D. (1990). Communication unbound: Autism and praxis. *Harvard Educational Review* 60: 291–314. **p.176.**

Biklen, D. (1993). *Communication Unbound*. New York: Teachers College Press. **p.177.**

Bishop, D.V.M. (1994). Grammatical errors in specific language impairment: Competence or performance limitations. *Applied Psycholinguistics* 15: 507–550. **p.72.**

Bishop, K., Rankin, J. and Mirenda, P. (1994). Impact of graphic symbol use on reading acquisition. *Augmentative and Alternative Communication* 10: 113–125. **p.237.**

Bjerkan, B. (1975). En re-definering av stamming og en analyse av stammingens situasjonsvariabilitet (A redefinition of stuttering and an analysis of the situational variability of stuttering). Thesis, University of Oslo. **p.253.**

Blackstone, S. and Painter, M. (1985). Speech problems in multihandicapped children. In: Darby, J. (Ed.) *Speech and Language Evaluation in Neurology: Childhood Disorders.* Orlando: Grune & Stratton, pp. 219–242. **p.62.**

Blau, A. (1983). On interaction. *Communicating Together* 1: 10–12. **p.282.**

Blischak, D.M. (1994). Phonological awareness: Implications for individuals with little or no functional speech. *Augmentative and Alternative Communication* 10: 245–254. **p.236.**

Blischak, D.M. and Lloyd, L.L. (1996). Multimodal augmentative and alternative communication: A case study. *Augmentative and Alternative Communication* 12: 37–46. **p.313.**

Blischak, D.M. and McDaniels, M.A. (1995). Effects of picture size and placement on memory for written words. *Journal of Speech and Hearing Research* 38: 1356–1362. **p.237.**

Bliss, C. (1965). *Semantography (Blissymbolics).* Sydney: Semantography Publications. **pp.11, 12.**

Bloom, L. (1973). *One Word at a Time.* The Hague: Mouton. **pp.158, 250.**

Bloom, L. (1998). Language acquisition in its developmental context. In: Damon ,W., Kuhn, D. and Siegler, R.S. (Eds) *Handbook of Child Psychology,* Volume 2. New York: Wiley, pp. 309–420. **pp.256, 261.**

Bloom, L. and Lahey, M. (1978). *Language Development and Language Disorders.* New York: John Wiley & Sons. **p.241.**

Bloom, Y. (1990). *Object Symbols: A communication option.* North Rocks, Australia: North Rocks Press. **pp.24, 33.**

Bloomberg, K. and Johnson, H. (1990). A statewide demographic survey of people with severe communication impairments. *Augmentative and Alternative Communication* 6: 50–60. **p.62.**

Bloomberg, K.P. and Lloyd, L.L. (1986). Graphic/aided symbols and systems: resource information. *Communication Outlook* 7: 24–30. **p.10.**

Bo-enheden M-huset. (1986). *Hva sker der i M-Huset???* København: Københavns Amtskommune. **p.175.**

Bondurant, J.L., Romeo, D.J. and Kretschmer, R. (1983). Language behaviors of mothers of children with normal and delayed language. *Language, Speech, and Hearing Services in Schools* 14: 233–242. **p.71.**

Bondy, A.S. and Frost, L.A. (1998). The Picture Exchange Communication System. *Seminars in Speech and Language* 19: 373–424. **pp.47, 134, 172.**

Bonvillian, J.D. and Blackburn, D.W. (1991). Manual communication and autism: Factors relating to sign language acquisition. In: Siple, P. and Fischer, S.D. (Eds) *Theoretical Issues in Sign Language Research,* Volume 2: *Psychology.* Chicago: Chicago University Press, pp. 255–277. **pp.81, 243.**

Bonvillian, J.D. and Nelson, K.E. (1976). Sign language acquisition in a mute autistic boy. *Journal of Speech and Hearing Disorders* 41: 339–347. **p.313.**

Bonvillian, J.D. and Nelson, K.E. (1978). Development of sign language in language-handicapped individuals. In: Siple, P. (Ed.) *Understanding Language through Sign Language Research*. New York: Academic Press, pp. 187–212. **p.313.**

Bonvillian, J.D., Orlansky, M.D. and Novack, L.L. (1981). Early sign language acquisition and its relation to cognitive and motor development. Presented at the 2nd International Symposium on Sign Language Research, Bristol, July 1981. **pp.167, 192.**

Booth, T. (1978). Early receptive language training for the severely and profoundly retarded. *Language, Speech, and Hearing Services in Schools* 9: 142–150. **pp.145, 313.**

Bottorf, L. and DePape, D. (1982). Initiating communication systems for severely speech-impaired persons. *Topics in Language Disorders* 2: 55–71. **p.68.**

Brady, D.O. and Smouse, A.D. (1978). A simultaneous comparison of three methods for language training with an autistic child. *Journal of Autism and Childhood Schizophrenia* 8: 271–279. **p.313.**

Brady, N.C. and McLean, L.K. (1995). Arbitrary symbols learning by adults with severe mental retardation: Comparison of Lexigrams and printed words. *American Journal of Mental Retardation* 100: 423–427. **p.31.**

Braine, M.D.S. (1963). The ontogeny of English phrase structure: The first phase. *Language* 39: 1–14. **p.245.**

Braun, U. and Stuckenschneider-Braun, M. (1990). Adapting 'Words Strategy' to the German culture and language. *Augmentative and Alternative Communication* 6: 115. **p.227.**

Brodin, J. and von Tetzchner, S. (1996). Augmentative and alternative telecommunication for people with intellectual impairment – a preview. In: von Tetzchner. S. and Jensen. M.H. (Eds) *Augmentative and Alternative Communication: European perspectives*. London: Whurr, pp. 195–212. **p.45.**

Brookner, S.P. and Murphy, N.O. (1975). The use of a total communication approach with a nondeaf child: A case study. *Language, Speech, and Hearing Services in Schools* 6: 313–319. **p.313.**

Brown, R. (1977). Why are signed languages easier to learn than spoken languages? Presented at the National Symposium on Sign Language Research and Teaching, Chicago, 1977. **p.192.**

Bruno, J. (1989). Customizing a Minspeak system for a preliterate child: A case example. *Augmentative and Alternative Communication* 5: 89–100. **p.313.**

Bruno, J. and Bryen, D.N. (1986). The impact of modelling on physically disabled nonspeaking children's communication. Presented at the 2nd Biennial Conference on Augmentative and Alternative Communication, Cardiff, September 1986. **pp.244, 301.**

Bruno, J. and Dribbon, M. (1998). Outcomes in AAC: Evaluating the effectiveness of a parent training program. *Augmentative and Alternative Communication* 14: 59–70. **p.306.**

Bryen, D.N. and Joyce, D.G. (1985). Language intervention with the severely handicapped: A decade of research. *Journal of Special Education* 19: 7–39. **p.167.**

Buffington, D.M., Krantz, P.J., McClannahan, L.E. and Poulson, C.L. (1998). Procedures for teaching appropriate gestural communication skills to children with autism. *Journal of Autism and Developmental Disorders* 28: 535–545. **p.313.**

Burd, L., Hamnes, K., Boernhoeft, D.M. and Fosher, W. (1988). A North-Dakota prevalence study of nonverbal school-age children. *Language, Speech and Hearing Services in Schools* 19: 371–383. **p.62.**

Burkhart, L.J. (1987). *Using Computers and Speech Synthesis to Facilitate Communicative Interaction with Young and/or Severely Handicapped Children.* College Park: Burkhart. **p.68.**

Burr, D.B. and Rohr, A. (1978). Patterns of psycholinguistic development in the severely retarded: A hypothesis. *Social Biology* 25: 15–22. **p.94.**

Buzolich, M.J. (1987). Children in transition: Implementing augmentative communication systems with severely speech-handicapped children. *Seminars in Speech and Language* 8: 199–213. **p.313.**

Buzolich, M.J. and Lunger, J. (1995). Empowering system users in peer training. *Augmentative and Alternative Communication* 11: 37–48. **pp.287, 307, 313.**

Byler, J.K. (1985). The Makaton vocabulary: An analysis based on recent research. *British Journal of Special Education* 12: 113–129. **p.229.**

Calculator, S. and Dollaghan, C. (1982). The use of communication boards in a residential setting: An evaluation. *Journal of Speech and Hearing Disorders* 47: 281–287. **p.288.**

Calculator, S. and Luchko, C.D.A. (1983). Evaluating the effectiveness of a communication board training program. *Journal of Speech and Hearing Disorders* 48: 185–191. **p.289.**

Caparulo, B.K. and Cohen, D.J. (1977). Cognitive structures, language, and emerging social competence in autistic and aphasic children. *Journal of the American Academy of Child Psychiatry* 16: 620–645. **p.72.**

Capute, A.J. and Accardo, P.J. (1991). Cerebral palsy. In: Capute, A.J. and Accardo, P.J. (Eds) *Developmental Disabilities in Infancy and Childhood.* Baltimore: Paul H. Brookes, pp. 335–348. **p.67.**

Carey, S. (1978). The child as word learner. In: Halle, M., Bresnan, J. and Miller, G.A. (Eds) *Linguistic Theory and Psychological Reality.* Cambridge, MA: MIT Press, pp. 264–293. **p.217.**

Carlson, F. (1981). A format for selecting vocabulary for the nonspeaking child. *Language, Speech, and Hearing Services in Schools* 12: 240–145. **p.223.**

Carr, E.G. (1985). Language acquisition in developmentally disabled children. *Annals of Child Development* 2: 49–76. **p.160.**

Carr, E.G. (1988). Tegnspråk (Sign language). In: Løvaas, O.I. (Ed.) *Opplæring av utviklingshemmede barn.* Oslo: Gyldendal, pp. 177–186. **p.134.**

Carr, E.G., Binkoff, J.A., Kologinsky, E. and Eddy, M. (1978). Acquisition of sign language by autistic children. I: Expressive labelling. *Journal of Applied Behavior Analysis* 11: 489–501. **p.313.**

Carr, E.G. and Durand, V.M. (1987). See me, help me. *Psychology Today* 21(11): 62–65. **p.107.**

Carr, E.G., Kologinsky, E. and Leff-Simon, S. (1987). Acquisition of sign language by autistic children. III: Generalized descriptive phrases. *Journal of Autism and Developmental Disorders* 17: 217–229. **p.313.**

Carr, E.G., Levin, L., McConnachie, G., Carlson, J.I., Kemp, D.C. and Smith, C.E. (1994). *Communication Intervention for Problem Behavior: A user's guide for producing positive change.* Baltimore: Paul H. Brookes. **p.89.**

Carrier, J.K. (1974). Nonspeech noun usage training with severely and profoundly retarded children. *Journal of Speech and Hearing Research* 17: 510–517. **p.25.**

Carrier, J.K. and Peak, T. (1975). *NONSLIP (Non-Speech Language Initiation Program)*. Kansas City: H. & H. Enterprise. **pp.25, 28.**

Casey, L.O. (1978). Development of communicative behavior in autistic children: A parent program using manual signs. *Journal of Autism and Childhood Schizophrenia* 8: 45–59. **pp.134, 305, 313.**

Chapman, R.S. and Miller, J.F. (1980). Analyzing language and communication in the child. In: Schiefelbusch, R.L. (Ed.) *Nonspeech Language and Communication*. Baltimore: University Park Press, pp. 159–196. **p.167.**

Cicchetti, D. and Beeghly, M. (Eds) (1990). *Children with Down Syndrome: A developmental perspective*. Cambridge: Cambridge University Press. **p.74.**

Clark, C.R. (1981). Learning words using traditional orthography and the symbols of Rebus, Bliss and Carrier. *Journal of Speech and Hearing Disorders* 46: 191–196. **pp.27, 31.**

Clark, C.R. (1984). A close look at the standard Rebus system and Blissymbolics. *Journal of the Association for Persons with Severe Handicaps* 9: 37–48. **pp.18, 31.**

Clark, E.V. (1992). Conventionality and contrast: Pragmatic principles with lexical consequences. In: Lehrer, A. and Kittay, E.F. (Eds) *Frames, Fields and Contrasts*. Hove: Lawrence Erlbaum, pp. 171–188. **p.211.**

Clark, R. (1982). Theory and method in child-language research: Are we assuming too much? In Kuczaj, S., II (Ed.) *Language Development*, Volume 1: *Syntax and semantics*. Hillsdale, NJ: Erlbaum, pp. 1–36. **p.156.**

Clarke, S., Remington, B. and Light, P. (1986). An evaluation of the relationship between receptive speech skills and expressive signing. *Journal of Applied Behavior Analysis* 19: 231–239. **pp.158, 299, 313.**

Clarke, S., Remington, B. and Light, P. (1988). The role of referential speech in sign learning by mentally retarded children: A comparison of total communication and sign-alone training. *Journal of Applied Behavior Analysis* 21: 419–426. **p.313.**

Cline, T. and Baldwin, S. (1993). *Selective Mutism in Children*. London: Whurr. **p.100.**

Cohen, N.J., Davine, M. and Meloche-Kelly, M. (1989). Prevalence of unsuspected language disorders in a child psychiatric population. *Journal of the American Academy of Child and Adolescent Psychiatry* 28: 107–111. **p.65.**

Coleman, C.L., Cook, A.M. and Meyers, L.S. (1980). Assessing non-oral clients for assistive communication devices. *Journal of Speech and Hearing Research* 45: 515–526. **p.313.**

Collins, S. (1996). Referring expressions in conversations between aided and natural speakers. In: von Tetzchner, S. and Jensen, M.H. (Eds) *Augmentative and Alternative Communication: European perspectives*. London: Whurr, pp. 89–100. **pp.60, 277, 284, 291.**

Conway, N. (1986). My perceptions of communication aids. Presented at the 2nd Biennial Conference on Augmentative and Alternative Communication, Cardiff 1986. **pp.15, 23.**

Cook, A.M. and Coleman, C.L. (1987). Selecting augmentative communication systems by matching client skills and needs to system characteristics. *Seminars in Speech and Language* 8: 153–167. **p.313.**

Cregan, A. (1982). *Sigsymbol Dictionary*. Cambridge: LDA. **p.21.**

Cregan, A. (1993). Sigsymbol system in a multimodal approach to speech elicitation: Classroom project involving an adolescent with severe mental retardation.

Augmentative and Alternative Communication 9: 146–160. **pp.21, 313.**

Cregan, A. and Lloyd, L.L. (1984). *Sigsymbol Dictionary*, American edition. West Lafayette: Purdue University. **p.21.**

Cregan, A. and Lloyd, L.L. (1990). *Sigsymbol Dictionary*, American edition. Wauconda, IL: Don Johnston Developmental Equipment. **p.21.**

Crossley, R. (1994). *Facilitated Communication Training*. New York: Teachers College Press. **p.175.**

Crossley, R. and Remington-Gurney, J. (1992). Getting the words out: Facilitated communication training. *Topics in Language Disorders* 12: 2945. **pp.176, 177.**

Crystal, D. (1986). *Listen to Your Child*. Harmondsworth: Penguin. **p.251.**

Crystal, D. (1987). Towards a 'bucket' theory of language disability: taking account of interaction between linguistic levels. *Clinical Linguistics and Phonetics* 1: 7–22. **p.261.**

Culatta, B. and Blackstone, S. (1980). A program to teach non-oral communication symbols to multiply handicapped children. *Journal of Childhood Communication Disorders* 1: 29–55. **p.313.**

Cullen, K., Ollivier, H., Kubitschke, L., Clarkin, N., Darnige, A., Robinson, S. and Dolphin, C. (1995). Connecting the information superhighway: Access issues for elderly people and people with disabilities. In: Roe, P.R.W. (Ed.), *Telecommunications for All*. Luxembourg: Office for Official Publications of the European Communities, pp. 233–244. **p.282.**

Culp, D.M. (1982). Communication interactions – nonspeaking children using augmentative systems and their mothers. Unpublished manuscript. **pp.278, 286.**

Culp, D.M. (1989). Developmental apraxia and augmentative or alternative communication – a case example. *Augmentative and Alternative Communication* 5: 27–34. **pp.30, 313.**

Cumley, G.D. and Swanson, S. (1999). Augmentative and alternative communication options for children with developmental apraxia of speech: Three case studies. *Augmentative and Alternative Communication* 10: 161–168. **p.313.**

Dalhoff, F. (1986). *Forstår han hvad man sier?* Fredrikshavn: Dafolo Forlag. **p.221.**

Dattillo, J. and Camarata, S. (1991). Facilitating conversation through self-initiated augmentative communication treatment. *Journal of Applied Behavior Analysis* 24: 369–378. **p.313.**

Deacon, J. (1974). *Tongue Tied*. London: Spastics Society. **p.110.**

Deich, R.F. and Hodges, P.M. (1977). *Language without Speech*. London: Souvenir Press.

DeLoache, J. and Burns, N.M. (1994). Early understanding of the representational function of pictures. *Cognition* 52: 83–110. **pp.25, 29, 313.**

DeLoache, J., Miller, K.F. and Pierroutsakos, S.L. (1998). Reasoning and problem solving. In: Damon, W., Kuhn, D. and Siegler, R.S. (Eds) *Handbook of Child Psychology*, Volume 2. New York: John Wiley & Sons, pp. 801–850. **p.197.**

Dennis, R., Reichle, J., Wiliams, W. and Vogelsberg, R.T. (1982). Motoric factors influencing the selection of vocabulary for sign production programs. *Journal of the Association for Persons with Severe Handicaps* 7: 20–32. **p.33.**

Detheridge, T. and Detheridge, M. (1997). *Literacy Through Symbols*. London: David Fulton. **p.236.**

Dienes, Z. (1993). Implicit concept formation. In: Berry, D.C. and Dienes, Z. (Eds) *Implicit Learning. Theoretical and empirical issues*. Hove: Lawrence Erlbaum, pp. 37–61. **p.137.**

Dixon, H. (1996). Natalie and her ORAC: From babbling to custom scanning. *Communication Matters* 10(2): 13–16. **p.313.**

Dixon, L.S. (1981). A functional analysis of photo-object matching skills of severely retarded adolescents. *Journal of Applied Behavior Analysis* 14: 465–478. **pp.22, 197.**

Doherty, J.E. (1985). The effect of sign characteristics on sign acquisition and retention: An integrative review of the literature. *Augmentative and Alternative Communication* 1: 108–121. **p.201.**

Downing, J. (Ed.) (1973). *Comparative Reading*. New York: MacMillan. **p.10.**

Duker, P.C. and Michielsen, H.M. (1983). Cross-setting generalization of manual signs to verbal instructions with severely retarded children. *Applied Research in Mental Retardation* 4: 29–40. **p.314.**

Duker, P.C. and Moonen, X.M. (1985). A program to increase manual signs with severely/profoundly mentally retarded students in natural environments. *Applied Research in Mental Retardation* 6: 147–158. **p.314.**

Duker, P.C. and Moonen, X.M. (1986). The effect of two procedures on spontaneous signing with Down's syndrome children. *Journal of Mental Deficiency Research* 30: 335–364. **p.314.**

Duker, P.C. and Morsink, H. (1984). Acquisition and cross-setting generalization of manual signs with severely retarded individuals. *Journal of Applied Behavior Analysis* 17: 93–103. **p.314.**

Durand, M. (1993). Functional communication training using assistive devices: Effects on challenging behavior and affect. *Augmentative and Alternative Communication* 9: 168–176. **pp.89, 314.**

Elbro, C., Rasmussen, I. and Spelling, B. (1996). Teaching reading to disabled readers with language disorders: A controlled evaluation of synthetic speech feedback. *Scandinavian Journal of Psychology* 37: 140–155. **p.237.**

Elder, P.S. and Bergman, J.S. (1978). Visual symbol communication instruction with nonverbal, multiply-handicapped individuals. *Mental Retardation* 16: 107–112. **p.314.**

Elman, J.L., Bates, E.A., Johnson, M.H., Karmiloff-Smith, A., Parisi, D. and Plunkett, K. (1996). *Rethinking Innateness. A connectionist perspective on development*. London: MIT Press. **p.133.**

English, S.T. and Prutting, C.A. (1975). Teaching American Sign Language to a normally hearing infant with tracheostenosis. *Clinical Pediatrics* 14: 1141–1145. **pp.64, 314.**

Everson, J.M. and Goodwyn, R. (1987). A comparison of the use of adaptive microswitches by students with cerebral palsy. *American Journal of Occupational Therapy* 41: 739–744. **p.314.**

Facon, B., Bollengier, T. and Grubar, J-C. (1993). Overestimation of mentally retarded persons' IQ using the PPVT: a reanalysis and some implications for future research. *Journal of Intellectual Disability Research* 37: 373–379. **p.111.**

Faulk, J.P. (1988). Touch Talker: A case study. *Communication Outlook* 10: 8–11. **p.314.**

Fay, L. (1993). An account of the search of a woman who is verbally impaired for augmentative devices to end her silence. *Women and Therapy* 14: 105–115. **p.314.**

Feallock, B. (1958). Communication boards for the non-vocal individual. *American Journal of Occupational Therapy* 12: 60. **p.180.**

Fenn, G. and Rowe, J.A. (1975). An experiment in manual communication. *British Journal of Disorders of Communication* 10: 3–16. **p.314.**

Ferguson, C.A. (1978). Learning to pronounce: The earliest stages of phonological development in the child. In: Minifie, F.D. and Lloyd, L.L. (Eds) *Communicative and Cognitive Abilities – Early Behavioral Assessment*. Baltimore: University Park Press, pp. 273–297. **p.108.**

Ferguson, C.A. and Debose, C.E. (1977). Simplified registers, broken language, and pidginization. In: Valman, A. (Ed.) *Pidgin and Creole linguistics*. Bloomington, IN: Indiana University Press, pp. 99–125. **p.277.**

Ferrier, L. (1991). Clinical study of a dysarthric adult using a Touch Talker with Words Strategy. *Augmentative and Alternative Communication* 7: 266–274. **p.314.**

Fischer, U. (1994). Learning words from context and dictionaries: An experimental comparison. *Applied Psycholinguistics* 15: 551–574. **p.162.**

Fishman, I.R. (1987). *Electronic Communication Aids and Techniques: Selection and use*. San Diego, CA: College Hill. **pp.34 50.**

Flensborg, C. (1988). *Snak med mig*. København: Socialstyrelsen. **p.314.**

Foss, N.E. (1981). Tegnspråkopplæring av autister og psykisk utviklingshemmede (Teaching manual signs to people with autism and intellectual impairment). Thesis, University of Oslo. **p.314.**

Foxx, R.M., Kyle, M.S., Faw, G.D. and Bittle, R.G. (1988). Cues-pause-point training and simultaneous communication to teach the use of signed labeling repertoires. *American Journal of Mental Retardation* 93: 305–311. **pp.161, 314.**

Frafjord, F.D. and Brekke, K.M. (1997). *Bliss symbolkommunikasjon. Etablering av nettverkssamarbeid for fagpersoner i Rogaland*. Stavanger: Rehabiliteringstjenesten Østerlide. **p.16.**

Franklin, K., Mirenda, P. and Phillips, G. (1996). Comparison of five symbols assessment protocols with nondisabled preschoolers and learners with severe intellectual disabilities. *Augmentative and Alternative Communication* 12: 63–77. **p.167.**

Fried-Oken, M. and More, L. (1992). Initial vocabulary for nonspeaking preschool children based on developmental and environmental language samples. *Augmentative and Alternative Communication* 8: 1–16. **p.228.**

Fristoe, M. and Lloyd, L.L. (1980). Planning an initial expressive sign lexicon for persons with severe communication impairment. *Journal of Speech and Hearing Disorders* 45: 170–180. **pp.228, 229, 230, 231, 233.**

Frith, U. (1989). *Autism. Explaining the enigma*. Oxford: Blackwell. **p.180.**

Fry, D.B. (1966). The development of the phonological system in the normal and the deaf child. In: Smith, F. and Miller, G.A. (Eds) *The Genesis of Language*. London: MIT Press, pp. 187–206. **p.133.**

Fuller, D.R. (1997). Initial study into the effects of translucency and complexity on the learning of Blissymbols by children and adults with normal cognitive abilities. *Augmentative and Alternative Communication* 13: 14–29. **p.195.**

Fuller, D.R. and Lloyd, L.L. (1987). A study of physical and semantic characteristics of a graphic symbol system as predictors of perceived complexity. *Augmentative and Alternative Communication* 3: 26–35. **p.31.**

Fuller, P., Newcombe, F. and Ounsted, C. (1983). Late language development in a child unable to recognize or produce speech sounds. *Archives of Neurology* 40: 165–169. **pp.110, 314.**

Fulwiler, R.L. and Fouts, R.S. (1976). Acquisition of American sign language by a noncommunicating autistic child. *Journal of Autism and Childhood Schizophrenia* 6: 43–51. **pp.243, 314.**

Fundudis, T., Kolvin, I. and Garside, R. (Eds.) (1979). *Speech retarded and deaf children: Their psychological development*. London: Academic Press. **p70**.

Gandell, T. and Sutton, A. (1998). Comparisons of AAC interactions patterns in face-to-face and telecommunications conversations. *Augmentative and Alternative Communication*, 14, 3–10. **p.281**.

Gangkofer, M. and von Tetzchner, S. (1996). Cleaning-ladies and broken buses. A case study on the development of Blissymbol use. In: von Tetzchner, S. and Jensen, M.H. (Eds) *Augmentative and Alternative Communication: European perspectives*. London: Whurr, pp. 292–308. **pp.237, 314**.

Garber, N. and Veydt, N. (1990). Rett syndrome: A longitudinal developmental case report. *Journal of Communication Disorders* 23: 6175. **p.84**.

Garvey, C. (1977). The contingent query: A dependant act in conversation. In: Lewis, M. and Rosenblum, L.A. (Eds) *Interaction, Conversation and the Development of Language*. New York: Wiley, pp. 63–93. **p.293**.

Gee, K., Graham, N., Goetz, L., Oshima, G. and Yoshioka, K. (1991). Teaching students to request the continuation of routine activities by using time delay and decreasing physical assistance in the context of chain interruption. *Journal of the Association for Persons with Severe Handicaps* 16: 154–167. **p.314**.

Gibbon, F. and Grunwell, P. (1990). Specific developmental language learning disabilities. In: Grunwell, P. (Ed.), *Developmental speech disorders*. Edinburgh: Churchill Livingstone, pp. 135–161. **p.171**.

Glennen, S.L. and Calculator, S.N. (1985). Training functional communication board use: A pragmatic approach. *Augmentative and Alternative Communication* 1: 134–142. **pp.179, 278, 283, 314**.

Goldstein, H., Kaczmarek, L., Pennington, R. and Shafer, K. (1992). Peer-mediated intervention: Attending to, commenting on, and acknowledging the behavior of preschoolers with autism. *Journal of Applied Behavior Analysis* 25: 289–305. **p.307**.

Goodman, J. and Remington, B. (1993). Acquisition of expressive signing: Comparison of reinforcement strategies. *Augmentative and Alternative Communication* 9: 26–35. **p.314**.

Goodwin, C. and Duranti, A. (1992). Rethinking context: An introduction. In: Duranti, A. and Goodwin, C. (Eds) *Rethinking Context*. Cambridge: Cambridge University Press, pp. 1–42. **p.124**.

Goosens', C.A. (1983). The relative iconicity and learnability of verb referents represented in Blissymbolics, Rebus symbols, and manual signs: An investigation with moderately retarded individuals. Thesis, Purdue University. **p.192**.

Goosens', C.A. (1989). Aided communication intervention before assessment: A case study of a child with cerebral palsy. *Augmentative and Alternative Communication* 3: 14–26. **p.314**.

Goosens', C. and Crain, S.S. (1992). *Utilizing Switch Interfaces with Children who are Severely Physically Challenged*. Austin, TX: Pro-Ed. **p.50**.

Goosens', C., Crain, S.S. and Elder, P.S. (1992). *Engineering the Preschool Environment for Interactive, Symbolic Communication*. Birmingham, AL: Southeast Augmentative Communication Conference. **p.34**.

Goosens', C.A. and Kraat, A. (1985). Technology as a tool for conversation and language learning for the physically disabled. *Topics in Language Disorders* 6: 56–70. **p.314**.

Grandin, T. (1989). An autistic person's view of holding therapy. *Communication* 23: 75–78. **p.81**.

Granlund, M., Terneby, J. and Olsson, C. (1992). Creating communicative opportunities through a combined in-service training and supervision package. *European Journal of Special Needs Education* 7: 229–252. **p.308.**

Green, G. (1994). The quality of the evidence. In: Shane, H.C. (Ed.), *Facilitated Communication: The clinical and social phenomenon.* San Diego, CA: Singular Press, pp. 157–225. **p.177.**

Griffith, P.L. and Robinson, J.H. (1980). Influence of iconicity and phonological similarity on sign learning by mentally retarded children. *American Journal of Mental Deficiency* 85: 291–298. **p.193.**

Griffith, P.L. and Robinson, J.H. (1981). A comparative and normative study of the iconicity of signs rated by three groups. *American Annals of the Deaf* 126: 440–449 **p.193.**

Grove, N. (1990). Developing intelligible signs with learning-disabled students: A review of the literature and an assessment procedure. *British Journal of Disorders of Communication* 25: 265–294. **pp.30, 101, 188.**

Grove, N. (1998). *Literature for All.* London: David Fulton. **p.296.**

Grove, N. and Dockrell, J. (2000). Multi-sign combinations by children with intellectual impairments: An analysing of language skills. *Journal of Speech, Language and Hearing Research* 43: 309–323. **pp.143, 249.**

Grove, N., Dockrell, J. and Woll, B. (1996). The two-word stage in manual signs: Language development in signers with intellectual impairment. In: von Tetzchner, S. and Jensen, M.H. (Eds) *Augmentative and Alternative Communication: European perspectives.* London: Whurr, pp. 101–118. **pp.243, 244, 249, 300, 301.**

Grove, N. and Walker, M. (1990). The Makaton Vocabulary: Using manual signs and graphic symbols to develop interpersonal communication. *Augmentative and Alternative Communication* 6: 15–28. **p.229.**

Guillaume, P. (1971). *Imitation in Children.* Chicago: Chicago University Press. **p.171.**

Gustason, G., Pfetzing, D. and Zawolkow, E. (1980). *Signing Exact English*, 3rd edn. Los Alamitos, California: Modern Signs Press. **p.10.**

Guttentag, R.E., Ornstein, P.A. and Siemens, L. (1987). Children's spontaneous rehearsal: Transitions in strategy acquisition. *Cognitive Development* 2: 307–326. **p.261.**

Hagberg, B. (1995). Rett syndrome: Clinical peculiarities and biological mysteries. *Acta Pædiatrica* 84: 971–976. **p.82.**

Hagberg, B. (1997). Condensed points for diagnostic criteria and stages in Rett syndrome. *European Child and Adolescent Psychiatry* 6(suppl 1): 2–4. **pp.82, 83.**

Hagberg, B. and Hagberg, G. (1997). Rett syndrome: Epidemiology and geographical variability. *European Child and Adolescent Psychiatry* 6(suppl 1): 5–7. **p.83.**

Hagberg, B. and Skjeldal, O.H. (1994). Rett variant: A suggested model for inclusion criteria. *Pediatric Neurology* 11: 5–11. **p.83.**

Hagen, C., Porter, W. and Brink. J. (1973). Nonverbal communication: An alternate mode of communication for the child with severe cerebral palsy. *Journal of Speech and Hearing Disorders* 38: 448–455. **p.221.**

Halle, J.W., Alpert, C.L. and Anderson, S.R. (1984). Natural environment language assessment and intervention with severely impaired preschoolers. *Topics in Early Childhood Special Education* 4: 36–56. **p.215.**

Hamilton, B.L. and Snell, M.E. (1993). Using the milieu approach to increase spontaneous communication book use across environments by an adolescent with autism. *Augmentative and Alternative Communication* 9: 273–280. **pp.160, 314.**

Hansen, E.M. Jon lærer tegn. Thesis, Statens Spesiallærerhøgskole, 1986. **p.314.**

Hardy, J.C. (1983). *Cerebral Palsy*. Englewood Cliffs, NJ: Prentice-Hall. **p.67.**

Harris, D. (1982). Communicative interaction processes involving nonvocal physically handicapped children. *Topics in Language Disorders* 2: 21–37. **pp.179, 277, 280, 283, 286, 287, 314.**

Harris, L., Doyle, E.S. and Haaf, R. (1996). Language treatment approach for users of AAC: Experimental single-subject investigation. *Augmentative and Alternative Communication* 12: 230–243. **p.314.**

Harris, M. (1992). *Language Experience and Early Language Development. From input to uptake*. Hove: Lawrence Erlbaum. **pp.186, 240.**

Haskew, P. and Donnellan, A. (1992). *Emotional Maturity and Well Being: Psychological lessons of facilitated communication*. Madison, WI: DRI Press. **p.177.**

Hawkes, R. (1998). A visual communication-based intervention approach for challenging behaviour. Presented at the 8th Biennial Conference on Augmentative and Alternative Communication, Dublin, August 1998. **p.165.**

Healy, S. (1994). The use of a synthetic speech output communication aid by a youth with severe developmental disability. In: Linfoot, K. (Ed.) *Communication Strategies for People with Developmental Disabilities*. Baltimore, MA: Paul H. Brookes, pp. 156–176. **p.314.**

Heim, M.J.M. and Baker-Mills, A.E. (1996). Early development of symbolic communication and linguistic complexity through augmentative and alternative communication. In: von Tetzchner, S. and Jensen, M.H. (Eds) *Augmentative and Alternative Communication: European perspectives*. London: Whurr, pp. 232–248. **pp.181, 314.**

Heller, K.W., Allgood, M.H., Davis, B., Arnold, S.E., Castelle, M.D. and Taber, T.A. (1996). Promoting not task-related communication at vocational sites. *Augmentative and Alternative Communication* 12: 169–178. **pp.272, 314.**

Hermelin, B.A. and O'Connor, N. (1970). *Psychological Experiments with Autistic Children*. Oxford: Pergamon Press. **p.81.**

Higgins, J. and Mills, J. (1986). Communication training in real environments. In: Blackstone, S.W. (Ed.) *Augmentative Communication: An introduction*. Rockville: American Speech and Hearing Association, pp. 345–352. **p.280.**

Hill, S.D., Campagna, J., Long, D., Munch, J. and Naecker, S. (1968). An explorative study of the use of two response keyboards as a means of communication for the severely handicapped child. *Perceptual and Motor Skills* 26: 699–704. **p.314.**

Hind, M. (1989). Synrel: Programs to teach sequencing of Blissymbols. *Communication Outlook* 10: 6–9. **p.314.**

Hinderscheit, L.R. and Reichle, J. (1987). Teaching direct select color encoding to an adolescent with multiple handicaps. *Augmentative and Alternative Communication* 3: 137–142. **p.314.**

Hinerman, P.S., Jenson, W.R., Walker, G.R. and Petersen, P.B. (1982). Positive practice overcorrection combined with additional procedures to teach signed words to an autistic child. *Journal of Autism and Developmental Disorders* 12: 253–263. **p.314.**

Hjelmquist, E. and Sandberg, A.D. (1996). Sounds and silence: Interaction in aided language use. In: von Tetzchner, S. and Jensen, M.H. (Eds) *Augmentative and Alternative Communication: European perspectives*. London: Whurr, pp. 137–152. **p.291.**

Hobson, P.A. and Duncan, P. (1979). Sign learning and profoundly retarded people. *Mental Retardation* 17: 33–37. **p.314.**

Hodges, P.M. and Deich, R.F. (1978). Teaching an artificial language system to nonverbal retardates. *Behavior Modification* 2: 489–509. **p.28.**

Hodges, P.M. and Schwethelm, B. (1984). A comparison of the effectiveness of graphic symbol and manual sign training with profoundly retarded children. *Applied Psycholinguistics* 5: 223–253. **pp.28, 29.**

Hooper, J., Connell, T.M. and Flett, P.J. (1987). Blissymbols and manual signs: A multimodal approach to intervention in a case of multiple disability. *Augmentative and Alternative Communication* 3: 68–76. **p.314.**

Horn, E.M. and Jones, H.A. (1996). Comparison of two selection techniques used in augmentative and alternative communication. *Augmentative and Alternative Communication* 12: 23–31. **p.54.**

Horner, R.H. and Budd, C.M. (1985). Acquisition of manual sign use: Collateral reduction of maladaptive behavior, and factors limiting generalization. *Education and Training of the Mentally Retarded* 20: 39–47. **p.314.**

Howlin, P. (1997). *Autism: Preparing for adulthood*. London: Routledge. **p.77.**

Hsieh, M-C. and Luo, C-H. (1999). Morse code typing of an adolescent with cerebral palsy using computer technology: Case study. *Augmentative and Alternative Communication* 15: 216–221. **p.314.**

Hughes, J. (1974/75). Acquisition of a non-vocal 'language' by aphasic children. *Cognition* 3: 41–55. **pp.72, 314.**

Humphreys, G.W and Riddoch, M.J. (1987). *To see but not to see. A case study of visual agnosia*. London: Lawrence Erlbaum. **p.190.**

Hunt, P., Alwell, M. and Goetz, L. (1991). Establishing conversational exchanges with family and friends: Moving from training to meaningful communication. *Journal of Special Education* 25: 305–319. **pp.306, 314.**

Hurlbut, B.I., Iwata, B.A. and Green, J.D. (1982). Nonvocal language acquisition in adolescents with severe physical disabilities: Blissymbol vs. iconic stimulus formats. *Journal of Applied Behavior Analysis* 15: 241–258. **pp.31, 194, 195, 314.**

Iacono, T.A. and Duncom, J.E. (1995). Comparison of sign alone and in combination with an electronic communication device in early language intervention: Case study. *Augmentative and Alternative Communication* 11: 249–259. **p.314.**

Iacono, T.A., Mirenda, P. and Beukelman, D. (1993). Comparison of unimodal and multimodal AAC techniques for children with intellectual disabilities. *Augmentative and Alternative Communication* 9: 83–94. **p.314.**

Iacono, T.A. and Parsons, C.L. (1986). A comparison of techniques for teaching signs to intellectually disabled individuals using an alternating treatment design. *Australian Journal of Human Communication Disorders* 14: 23–34. **pp.171, 173, 315.**

Ingram, T.T.S. (1959). Specific disorders of speech in childhood. *Brain* 82: 450–467. **p.65.**

Ingram, T.T.S. (1975). Speech disorders in childhood. In: Lenneberg, E.H. and Lenneberg, E. (Eds) *Foundations of Language Development*. New York: Academic Press, pp. 195–261. **p.70.**

Johansson, I. (1987). Tecken – en genväg till tal (Signs – a short-cut to speech). *Down Syndrom: Språk ock tal*, No. 28. **pp.75, 157.**

Johnson, I. (1989). 'Hellish difficult to live in this world': The unexpected emergence of written communication in a group of severely mentally handicapped individuals.

Journal of Social Work Practice **1**: 13–23. **pp.175, 176.**

Johnson, R. (1981). *The Picture Communication Symbols*. Solana Beach, CA: Mayer-Johnson. **p.18.**

Johnson, R. (1985). *The Picture Communication Symbols – Book II*. Solana Beach, CA: Mayer-Johnson. **p.18.**

Johnson, R. (1992). *The Picture Communication Symbols – Book III*. Solana Beach, CA: Mayer-Johnson. **p.18.**

Jones, K. (1979). A Rebus system of non-fade visual language. *Child: Care, Health and Development* **5**: 1–7. **p.19.**

Jones, P.R. and Cregan, A. (1986). *Sign and Symbol Communication for Mentally Handicapped People*. London: Croom Helm. **p.21.**

Kahn, J.V. (1981). A comparison of sign and verbal language training with nonverbal retarded children. *Journal of Speech and Hearing Research* **24**: 113–119. **p.315.**

Kaiser, A.P., Ostrosky, M.M. and Alpert, C.I. (1993). Training teachers to use environmental and milieu teaching with nonvocal preschool children. *Journal of The Association for Persons with Severe Handicap* **18**: 188–199. **p.310.**

Karlan, G.R., Brenn-White, B., Lentz, A., Hodur, P., Egger, D. and Frankoff, D. (1982). Establishing generalized, productive verb-noun phrase usage in a manual language system with moderately handicapped children. *Journal of Speech and Hearing Disorders* **47**: 31–42. **p.315.**

Keogh, D., Whitman, T., Beeman, D., Halligan, K. and Starzynski, T. (1987). Teaching interactive signing in a dialogue situation to mentally retarded individuals. *Research in Developmental Disabilities* **8**: 39–53. **pp.271, 315.**

Kerr A.M. (1995). Early clinical signs in the Rett disorder. *Neuropediatrics* **25**: 67–71. **p.82.**

Kiernan, C. and Reid, B. (1987). *Pre-verbal Communication Schedule*. Windsor: NFER-Nelson. **p.94.**

Kiernan, C., Reid, B. and Jones, L. (1982). *Signs and Symbols*. London: Heinemann. **pp.19, 81, 229.**

Kirk, S.A., McCarthy, J.J. and Kirk, W.D. (1968). *The Illinois Test of Psycholinguistic Abilities*, revised edn. Urbana, IL: University of Illinois Press. **pp.93, 226.**

Kirman, B.H. (1985). Mental Retardation: Medical aspects. In: Rutter, M. and Hersov, L. (Eds) *Child and Adolescent Psychiatry*. Oxford: Blackwell, pp. 650–660. **p.74.**

Klewe, L., Starup, G., Cros, B., Andersen, J., Karpatschof, B. and Hansen, V.R. (1994). *Tro, håb og pædagogik* (Faith, hope and pedagogy). Herning: Systine. **p.177.**

Klima, E. and Bellugi, U. (1979). *The Signs of Language*. London: Harvard University Press. **pp.9, 101. 192, 193.**

Kobacker, N. and Todaro, M.P. (1992). Use of assistive devices by a preschooler with autism. Presented at the Fifth Biennial Conference of the International Society for Augmentative and Alternative Communication, Philadelphia, August, 1992. **p.56.**

Koerselman, E. (1996). Using Blissymbols to structure language. *Communication Matters* **10**(3): 13–14. **p.315.**

Koester, H.H. and Levine, S.P. (1996). Effect of word prediction features on user performance. *Augmentative and Alternative Communication* **12**: 155–168. **p.42.**

Kohl, F.L. (1981). Effects of motoric requirements on the acquisition of manual sign responses by severely handicapped students. *American Journal of Mental Deficiency* **85**: 396–403. **p.193.**

Koke, S. and Neilson, J. (1987). The effect of auditory feedback on the spelling of nonspeaking physically disabled individuals who use microcomputers. Unpublished manuscript, University of Toronto. p.237.

Kollar, Z. (1999). Growing up with Blissymbols. Paper at 2nd Regional Eastern and Central European Conference on Augmentative and Alternative Communication, Prague, Czech Republic, November 11–13th, 1999. p.11.

Kollinzas, G. (1984). The communication record: Sharing information to promote sign language generalization. *Journal of the Association for Persons with Severe Handicaps* 8: 49–55. pp.87, 117, 119, 315.

Konstantareas, M.M., Oxman, J. and Webster, C.D. (1977). Simultaneous communication with autistic and other severely dysfunctional nonverbal children. *Journal of Communication Disorders* 10: 267–282. p.315.

Konstantareas, M.M., Webster, C.D. and Oxman, J. (1979). Manual language acquisition and its influence on other areas of functioning in four autistic and autistic-like children. *Journal of Child Psychology and Psychiatry* 20: 337–350. pp.115, 315.

Koppenhaver, D. and Yoder, D. (1992). Literacy issues in persons with severe physical and speech impairments. In Gaylord-Ross, R. (Ed.) *Issues in Research and Special Education*, Volume 2. New York: Teacher's College Press, pp. 156–201. pp.16, 239.

Kose, G., Beilin, H. and O'Connor, J.M. (1983). Children's comprehension of actions depicted in photographs. *Developmental Psychology* 19: 636–643. pp.22, 197.

Kotkin, R.A., Simpson, S.B. and Desanto, D. (1978). The effect of sign language on the picture naming in two retarded girls possessing normal hearing. *Journal of Mental Deficiency Research* 22: 19–25. pp.157, 315.

Kouri, T. (1989). How manual sign acquisition relates to the development of spoken language: A case study. *Language, Speech, and Hearing Services in Schools* 20: 50–62. p.315.

Kozleski, E.B. (1991). Visual symbol acquisition by students with autism. *Exceptionality* 2: 173–194. p.315.

Kraat, A.W. (1985). *Communication Interaction Between Aided and Natural Speakers: A state of the art report.* Toronto: Canadian Rehabilitation Council for the Disabled. pp.57, 59, 60, 277, 291.

Kristen, U. (1997). Wie Kerstin lernt, über Bilder zu kommunizieren. *Unterstützte Kommunikation* 2–3: 18–25. p.315.

Kvale, A.M., Martinsen, H. and Schjølberg, S. (1992). Miljømessige betingelser for trivsel og læring hos autistiske barn og voksne. Oslo: Landsforeningen for Autister. p.79.

Lagergren, J. (1981). Children with motor handicaps. *Acta Paediatrica Scandinavia Supplementum* 289. p.67.

Lagerman, U. and Höök, O. (1982). Communication aids for patients with dys/anarthria. *Scandinavian Journal of Rehabilitational Medicine* 14: 155–158. p.315.

Lahey, M. and Bloom, L. (1977). Planning a lexicon: Which words to teach first. *Journal of Speech and Hearing Disorders* 42: 340–350. pp.199, 202, 229.

Lane, H. (1984). *When the Mind Hears.* London: Penguin. p.134.

Launonen, K. (1996). Enhancing communication skills of children with Down syndrome: Early use of manual signs. In: von Tetzchner, S. and Jensen, M.H. (Eds) *Augmentative and Alternative Communication: European perspectives.* London: Whurr, pp. 213–231. pp.64, 65, 75, 77, 134, 157, 298.

Launonen, K. (1998). *Eleistäsanoihin, viittomista kieleen.* Helsinki: Hehitysvammaliitto ry. pp.65, 75, 77, 134, 157, 298.

Layton, T.L. and Baker, P.S. (1981). Description of semantic–syntactic relations in an autistic child. *Journal of Autism and Developmental Disorders* 11: 385–399. **p.315.**

le Prevost, P. (1983). Using the Makaton vocabulary in early language learning with a Down's baby. *Mental Handicap* 11: 28–29. **pp.75, 157, 298, 315.**

Leber, I. (1994). *Nikki ist nicht Sprachlos!* Karlsruhe: von Loeper Literaturverlag. **p.315.**

Lees, J. and Urwin, S. (1997). *Children with Language Disorders*, 2nd edn. London: Whurr. **p.70.**

Lenneberg, E.H. (1967). *Biological Foundations of Language*. New York: Wiley. **p.133.**

Leonard, L.B. (1981). Facilitating linguistic skills in children with specific language impairment. *Applied Psycholinguistics* 2: 89–118. **p.157.**

Lesher, G.W., Moulton, B.J. and Higginbotham, D.J. (1998). Techniques for augmenting scanning communication. *Augmentative and Alternative Communication* 14: 81–101. **p.53.**

Light, J. (1985). *The Communicative Interaction Patterns of Young Nonspeaking Physically Disabled Children and Their Primary Caregivers*. Toronto: Blissymbolics Communication Institute. **pp.161, 162, 181, 241, 282, 283, 286, 288, 289, 290, 292.**

Light, J. (1988). Interaction involving individuals using augmentative and alternative communication systems: State of the art and future directions. *Augmentative and Alternative Communication* 4: 66–82. **p.60.**

Light, J., Binger, C., Agate, T.L. and Ramsay, K.N. (1999). Teaching partner-focused questions to individuals who use augmentative and alternative communication to enhance their communicative competence. *Journal of Speech, Language and Hearing Research* 42: 241–255. **pp.239, 315.**

Light, J., Binger, C. and Smith, A.K. (1994). Story reading interactions between preschoolers who use AAC and their mothers. *Augmentative and Alternative Communication* 10: 255–268. **p.239.**

Light, J., Dattilo, J., English, J., Gutierrez, L. and Hartz, J. (1992). Instructing facilitators to support the communication of people who use augmentative communication systems. *Journal of Speech and Hearing Research* 35: 865–875. **pp.307, 315.**

Light, J., Roberts, B., Dimarco, R. and Greiner, N. (1998). Augmentative and alternative communication to suport receptive and expressive communication for people with autism. *Journal of Communication Disorders* 31: 153–180. **p.315.**

Light, P., Remington, R.E. and Porter, D. (1982). Substitutes for speech? Nonvocal approaches to communication. In: Beveridge, M. (Ed.) *Children Thinking Through Language*. London: Arnold. **p.315.**

Lindberg, B. (1987). Retts syndrom – en kartlegging av psykologiske och pedagogiska erfarenheter i Sverige. Stockholm: Högskolan för lärarutbildning i Stockholm. **p.86.**

Lloyd, P., Camaioni, L. and Ercolani, P. (1995). Assessing referential communication skills in the primary school years: A comparative study. *British Journal of Developmental Psychology* 13: 13–29. **p.293.**

Lock, A. (1980). *The Guided Reinvention of Language*. London: Academic Press. **p.68.**

Locke, J.L. (1993). *The Child's Path to Spoken Language*. Cambridge: Harvard University Press. **p.133.**

Locke, J.L. (1994). Gradual emergence of developmental language disorders. *Journal of Speech and Hearing Research* 37: 608–616. **p.70.**

Locke, P.A. and Mirenda, P. (1988). A computer-supported approach for a child with severe communication, visual, and cognitive impairments: A case study. *Augmentative and Alternative Communication* 4: 15–22. **p.315.**

Lord, C. and Rutter, M. (1994). Autism and pervasive developmental disorders. In: Rutter, M., Taylor, E. and Hersov, L. (Eds) *Child and Adolescent Psychiatry*, 3rd edn. Oxford: Blackwell, pp. 569–593. **p.77.**

Lourenço, L., Faias, J., Afonso, R., Moreira, A. and Ferreira, J.M. (1996). Improving communication and language skills of children with developmental disorders: Family involvement in graphic language intervention. In: von Tetzchner, S. and Jensen, M.H. (Eds) *Augmentative and Alternative Communication: European perspectives*. London: Whurr, pp. 309–323. **p.302.**

Lovas, O.I., Koegel, R.L. and Schreibman, L. (1979). Stimulus overselectivity in autism: A review of research. *Psychological Bulletin* 86: 1236–1254. **p.190.**

Lucariello, J. (1987). Concept formation and its relation to word learning and use in the second year of life. *Journal of Child Language* 14: 309–332. **p.22.**

Luchsinger, R. and Arnold, G.E. (Eds) (1965). *Voice – Speech – Language*. Belmont: Wadsworth. **pp.65, 71.**

Luetke-Stahlman, B. (1985). Using single design to verify language learning in a hearing, aphasic boy. *Sign Language Studies* 46: 73–86. **p.315.**

Luftig, R.L. (1984). An analysis of initial sign lexicons as a function of eight learnability variables. *Journal of the Association for Persons with Severe Handicaps* 9: 193–200.

Luria, A.R. (1969). *The Mind of a Mnemonist*. London: Jonathan Cape. **pp.190, 193.**

Lyon, S.R. and Ross, L.E. (1984). Comparison scan training and the matching and scanning performance of severely and profoundly mentally retarded students. *Applied Research in Mental Retardation* 5: 439–449. **p.197.**

Lyons, J. (1977). *Semantics, Volume 1*. Cambridge, UK: Cambridge University Press. **p.4.**

McClenny, C.S., Roberts, J.E. and Layton, T.L. (1992). Unexpected events and their effect on children's language. *Child Language Teaching and Therapy* 8: 229–245. **p.160.**

McDonald, E.T. and Schultz, A.R. (1973). Communication boards for cerebral-palsied children. *Journal of Speech and Hearing Disorders* 38: 73–88. **p.180.**

McEwen, I.R. and Karlan, G.R. (1989). Assessment of effects of position on communication board access by individuals with cerebral palsy. *Augmentative and Alternative Communication* 5: 235–242. **p.315.**

McGregor, G., Young, J., Gerak, J., Thomas, B. and Vogelsbeerg, R.T. (1992). Increasing functional use of an assistive communication device by a student with severe disabilities. *Augmentative and Alternative Communication* 8: 243–250. **p.315.**

McIlvane, W.J., Bass, R.W., O'Brien, J.M., Gerovac B.J. and Stoddard, L.T. (1984). Spoken and signed naming of foods after receptive exclusion training in severe retardation. *Applied Research in Mental Retardation* 5: 1–27. **pp.211, 315.**

McKinnon, E., King, G., Cathers, T. and Scott, J. (1995). Electronic mail: Services from afar for individuals with physical disabilities. *Augmentative and Alternative Communication* 11: 236–243. **p.281.**

McLean, L.P. and McLean, J.E. (1973). A language training program for nonverbal autistic children. *Journal of Speech and Hearing Disorders* 39: 186–193. **p.315.**

McNaughton, D. and Light, J. (1989). Teaching facilitators to support the communication skills of an adult with severe cognitive disabilities: A case study. *Augmentative and Alternative Communication* 5: 35–41. **pp.22, 311, 315.**

McNaughton, D., Fallon, K., Tod, J., Weiner, F. and Neisworth, J. (1994). Effect of repeated listening experiences on the intelligibility of synthesized speech. *Augmentative and Alternative Communication* 10: 161–168. **p.44.**

McNaughton, S. (1998). Reading acquisition of adults with severe congenital speech and physical impairments: Theoretical infrastructure, empirical investigation, educational application. Thesis, University of Toronto. **pp.11, 236, 239.**

McNaughton, S. and Kates, B. (1974). Visual symbols: Communication system for the pre-reading physically handicapped child. Presented at the American Association on Mental Deficiency Annual Meeting, Toronto, 1974. **p.11.**

McNaughton, S. and Kates, B. (1980). The application of Blissymbolics. In: Schiefelbusch, R.L. (Ed.) *Nonspeech Language and Communication: Analysis and interventions*. Baltimore, Maryland: University Park Press, pp. 303–321. **p.12.**

McNaughton, S. and Lindsay, P. (1995). Approaching literacy with AAC graphics. *Augmentative and Alternative Communication* 11: 212–228. **p.236.**

McNaughton, S., Marshall, P., Millin, N., Baird, E. and Lindsay, P. (1996). The new highway for Bliss! Presented at the 7th Biennial Conference of the International Society for Augmentative and Alternative Communication, Vancouver, August 1996. **p.236.**

MacWhinney, B. (1982). Basic syntactic processes. In: Kuczaj, S. (Ed.), *Language Development*. Volume 1. *Syntax and semantics*. Hillsdale, NJ: Erlbaum, pp. 73–136. **p.264.**

Madge, N. and Fassam, M. (1982). *Ask the Children*. London: Batsford. **pp.69, 307.**

Magnusson, M. and Lundman, M. (1987). Datorkonferenser för talhandikappade (Computer conferences for speech-impaired people). Presented at Forskningskonferansen 'Människa – Miljö – Handikapp', Örebro 1987. **p.282.**

Maharaj, S.C. (1980). *Pictogram ideogram communication*. Regina, Canada: The George Reed Foundation for the Handicapped. **p.17.**

Marshall, N.R. and Hegrenes, J. (1972). The use of written language as a communication system for an autistic child. *Journal of Speech and Hearing Disorders* 37: 258–261. **p.315.**

Martinsen, H. (1980). Biologiske forutsetninger for kulturalisering (Biological prerequisites for culturalisation). *Tidsskrift for Norsk Psykologforening, Monografiserien* 6: 122–129. **p.68.**

Martinsen, H. and von Tetzchner, S. (1989). Imitation at the onset of speech. In: von Tetzchner, S., Siegel, L.S. and Smith, L. (Eds) *The Social and Cognitive Aspects of Normal and Atypical Language Development*. New York: Springer-Verlag, pp. 51–68. **p.252.**

Martinsen, H. and von Tetzchner, S. (1996). Situating augmentative and alternative communication intervention. In: von Tetzchner, S. and Jensen, M.H. (Eds) *Augmentative and Alternative Communication: European perspectives*. London: Whurr, pp. 37–48. **p.27, 136, 300.**

Masterson, J.J. (1997). Interrelationships in children's language production. *Topics in Language Disorders* 17(4): 11–22. **p.261.**

Masur, E. (1997). Maternal labelling of novel and familiar objects: Implications for children's development of lexical constraints. *Journal of Child Language* 24: 427–439. **p.168.**

Matas, J.A., Mathy-Laikko, P., Beukelman, D.R and Legresley, K. (1985). Identifying the nonspeaking population. *Augmentative and Alternative Communication* 1: 17–31. p.62.

Mathy-Laikko, P., Iacono, T., Ratcliff, A., Villarruel, F., Yoder, D. and Vanderheiden, G. (1989). Teaching a child with multiple disabilities to use a tactile augmentative communication device. *Augmentative and Alternative Communication* 5: 249–256. pp.26, 33, 190.

Meier, R.P. (1991). Language acquisition by deaf children. *American Scientist* 79: 60–70. p.240.

Mendes, E. and Rato, J. (1996). From system to communication: Staff training for attitude change. In: von Tetzchner, S. and Jensen, M.H. (Eds) *Augmentative and Alternative Communication: European perspectives*. London: Whurr, pp. 342–354. pp.309, 310.

Miller, M.S. (1987). Sign iconicity: Single-sign receptive vocabulary skills of nonsigning hearing preschoolers. *Journal of Communication Disorders* 20: 359–365. pp.192, 193.

Mills, J. and Higgins, J. (1984). An environmental approach to delivery of microcomputer-based and other communication systems. *Seminars in Speech and Language* 5: 35–45. pp.279, 315.

Mirenda, P. and Dattilo, J. (1987). Instructional techniques in alternative communication for students with severe intellectual handicap. *Augmentative and Alternative Communication* 3: 143–152. p.315.

Mirenda, P. and Santogrossi, J. (1985). A prompt-free strategy to teach pictoral communication system use. *Augmentative and Alternative Communication* 1: 143–150. p.315.

Møller, S. and von Tetzchner, S. (1996). Allowing for developmental potential: A case study of intervention change. In: von Tetzchner, S. and Jensen, M.H. (Eds) *Augmentative and Alternative Communication: European perspectives*. London: Whurr, pp. 249–269. pp.114, 165, 214, 273, 315.

Morley, M.E. (1972). *The Development and Disorders of Speech in Childhood*. Edinburgh: Churchill Livingstone. p.236.

Morgan, J.L and Demuth, K. (Eds) (1996). *Signal to Syntax: Bootstrapping from speech to grammar in early acquisition*. Mahwah, NJ: Lawrence Erlbaum. p.263.

Morningstar, D. (1981). Blissymbol communication: Comparison of interaction with naive vs. experienced listeners. Manuscript, University of Toronto. p.291.

Morris, S.E. (1981). Communication/interaction development at mealtimes for the multiple handicapped child: Implications for the use of augmentative communication systems. *Language, Speech, and Hearing Services in Schools* 12: 216–232. pp.68, 155, 290.

Murdock, J.Y. (1978). A non-oral expressive communication program for a nonverbal retardate. *Journal of Childhood Communication Disorders* 2: 18–25. p.315.

Murphy, J., Marková, I., Collins, S. and Moodie, E. (1996). AAC systems: Obstacles to effective use. *European Journal of Disorders of Communication* 31: 31–44. p.297.

Murphy, J., Marková, I., Moodie, E., Scott, J. and Boa, S. (1995). AAC systems used by people with cerebral palsy in Scotland: A demographic study. *Augmentative and Alternative Communication* 11: 26–36. p.15.

Murray-Branch, J, Udavari-Solner, A. and Bailey, B. (1991). Textured communication systems for individuals with severe intellectual and dual sensory impairments. *Language, Speech and Hearing Services in Schools* 22: 260–268. p.26.

Nadel, L. (Ed.) (1988). *The Psychobiology of Down Syndrome*. London: MIT Press. p.374.

Nelms, G. (1996). Tactile symbols: A case study. *Communication Matters* 10(3): 11–12. p.315.

Nelson, K. (Ed.) (1989). *Narratives from the Crib*. Cambridge, MA: Harvard University Press. p.237.

Nelson, K. (1996). *Language in Cognitive Development*. Cambridge: Cambridge University Press. pp.72, 157, 262, 269, 294.

Nelson, K.E., Camarata, S.M., Welsh, J., Butkovsky, L. and Camarata, M. (1996). Effects of imitative and conversational recasting treatment on the acquisition of grammar in children with specific language impairment and younger language-normal children. *Journal of Speech and Hearing Research* 39: 850–859. p.171.

Newell, A.F., Arnott, J.L., Booth, L., Beattie, W., Brophy, B. and Ricketts, I.W. (1992). Effect of the 'Pal' word prediction system on the quality and quantity of text generation. *Augmentative and Alternative Communication* 8: 304–311. p.42.

Newell, A.F., Booth, L. and Beattie, W. (1991). Predictive text entry with PAL and children with learning difficulties. *British Journal of Educational Technology* 22: 23–40. pp.43, 238.

Odom, A.C. and Upthegrove, M. (1997). Moving towards employment using AAC: Case study. *Augmentative and Alternative Communication* 13: 258–262. p.315.

O'Keefe, B.M. and Datillo, J. (1992). Teaching response-recode form to adults with mental retardation using AAC systems. *Augmentative and Alternative Communication* 8: 224–233. p.315.

Oliver, C.B. and Halle, J.W. (1982). Language training in the everyday environment. *Journal of the Association for Persons with Severe Handicaps* 8: 50–62. pp.160, 161, 315.

Olsson, B. and Rett, A. (1987). Autism and Rett syndrome: Behavioural investigations and differential diagnosis. *Developmental Medicine and Child Neurology* 29: 429–441. p.84.

Olsson, B. and Rett, A. (1990). A review of the Rett syndrome with a theory of autism. *Brain and Development* 12: 11–15. p.84.

Osguthorpe, R.T. and Chang, L.L. (1987). Computerized symbol processors for individuals with severe communication disabilities. *Journal of Special Education Technology* 8: 43–54. pp.39, 315.

Ottem, E., Sletmo, A. and Bollingmo, M. (1991). En analyse av WPPSI med relevans for barn med språk/talevansker. *Tidsskrift for Norsk Psykologforening* 28: 1079–1084. p.70.

Oxley, J.O. and von Tetzchner, S. (1999). Reflections on the development of alternative language forms. In: Loncke, F.T., Clibbens, J., Arvidson, H.H. and Lloyd, L.L. (Eds) *Augmentative and Alternative Communication: New directions in research and practice*. London: Whurr, pp. 62–74. p.197.

Paget, R. (1951). *The New Sign Language*. London: The Welcome Foundation. p.10.

Paget, R., Gorman, P. and Paget, P. (1976). *The Paget Gorman Sign System*, 6th edn. London: Association for Experiment in Deaf Education. p.10.

Park, K. (2000). The object of communication. Unpublished manuscript. p.296.

Parkinson, E., Royal, L. and Darvil, G. (1995). Does augmentative communication improve communication and reduce frustration? *Communication Matters* 9(2): 17–21. p.315.

Pecyna, P.M. (1988). Rebus symbol communication training with a severely handicapped preschool child: A case study. *Language, Speech, and Hearing Services in Schools* 19: 128–143. **p.315.**

Peirce, C.S. (1931). *Collected Papers*. Cambridge, MA: Harvard University Press. **p.4.**

Percy, A.K. (1997). Neurobiology and neurochemistry of Rett syndrome. *European Child and Adolescent Psychiatry* 6(suppl 1): 80–82. **p.84.**

Peters, A.M. (1983). *The Units of Language Acquisition*. Cambridge: Cambridge University Press. **p.260.**

Peters, A.M. (1986). Early syntax. In: Fletcher, P. and Garman, M. (Eds) *Language Acquisition*, 2nd edn. Cambridge: Cambridge University Press, pp. 307–325. **p.240.**

Peters, A.M. (1995). Strategies in the acquisition of syntax. In: Fletcher, P. and MacWhinney, B. (Eds) *The Handbook of Child Language*. Oxford: Basil Blackwell, pp. 462–482. **p.260.**

Peters, L.J. (1973). Sign language stimulus vocabulary learning of a brain-injured child. *Sign Language Research* 3: 116–118. **p.315.**

Peterson, S.L., Bondy, A.S., Vincent, Y. and Finnegan, C.S. (1995). Effects of altering communicative input for students with autism and no speech: Two case studies. *Augmentative and Alternative Communication* 11: 93–100. **pp.65, 316.**

Petretic, P.A. and Tweeney, R.D. (1977). Does comprehension precede the production? The development of children's responses to telegraphic sentences of varying grammatical adequacy. *Journal of Child Language* 4: 201–209. **p.300.**

Phillips, W., Gómez, J.C., Baron-Cohen, S. Laá, V. and Rivière, A. (1995). Treating people as objects, agents, or 'subjects': How young children with and without autism make requests. *Journal of Child Psychology and Psychiatry* 36: 1383–1398. **p.108.**

Piaget, J. and Inhelder, B. (1969). *The psychology of the child*. London: Routledge & Kegan Paul. **p.167.**

Pinker, S. (1984). *Language Learnability and Language Development*. Cambridge, MA: Harvard University Press. **p.263.**

Pinker, S. (1990). Language acquisition. In: Osherson, D.N. and Lasnik, H. (Eds) *Language*. Cambridge, MA: MIT Press, pp. 199–241. **p.291.**

Premack, D. (1971). Language in a chimpanzee? *Science* 172: 808–822. **p.24.**

Prinz, P.M. and Prinz, E.A. (1979). Acquisition of ASL and spoken English in a hearing child of a deaf mother and hearing father: Phase I – Early lexical development. *Papers and Reports on Child Language Development* 17: 139–146. **p.134.**

Prinz, P.M. and Prinz, E.A. (1981). Acquisition of ASL and spoken English in a hearing child of a deaf mother and hearing father: Phase II – Early combinatorial patterns. *Sign Language Studies* 30: 78–88. **p.134.**

Prior, M. and Ozonoff, S. (1998). Psychological factors on autism. In: Volkmar, F.R. (Ed.), *Autism and Pervasive Developmental Disorders*. Cambridge: Cambridge University Press, pp. 64–108. **p.80.**

Quist, R.W. and Lloyd, L.L. (1997a). Principles and use of technology. In: Lloyd, L.L., Fuller, D.R. and Arvidson, H.H. (Eds) *Augmentative and Alternative Communication. A handbook of principles and practices*. Boston: Allyn & Bacon, pp. 107–126. **p.34.**

Quist, R.W. and Lloyd, L.L. (1997b). High technology. In: Lloyd, L.L., Fuller, D.R. and Arvidson, H.H. (Eds) *Augmentative and Alternative Communication. A handbook of principles and practices*. Boston: Allyn & Bacon, pp. 137–168. **p.34.**

Raghavendra, P. and Allen, G.D. (1993). Comprehension of synthetic speech with three text-to-speech systems using a sentence verification paradigm. *Augmentative and Alternative Communication* 9: 126–133. **p.44**.

Raghavendra, P. and Fristoe, M. (1990). 'A spinach with a $\underline{V}$ on it': What 3-year-olds see in standard and enhanced Blissymbols. *Journal of Speech and Hearing Disorders* 55: 149–159. **p.14**.

Raghavendra, P. and Fristoe, M. (1995). 'No shoes; they walked away?': Effects of enhancement on learning and using Blissymbols by normal 3-year-old children. *Journal of Speech and Hearing Research* 38: 174–188. **p.14**.

Ramer, A. (1976). Syntactic styles in emerging language. *Journal of Child Language* 3: 49–62. **p.240**.

Rankin, J.L., Harwood, K. and Mirenda, P. (1994). Influence of graphic symbol use on reading comprehension. *Augmentative and Alternative Communication* 10: 269–281. **p.237**.

Ratcliff, A. (1994). Comparison of relative demands implicated in direct selection and scanning: Considerations from normal children. *Augmentative and Alternative Communication* 10: 67–74. **p.54**.

Ratusnik, C.M. and Ratusnik, D.L. (1974). A comprehensive communication approach for a ten-year-old nonverbal autistic child. *American Journal of Orthopsychiatry* 44: 396–403. **p.316**.

Reichle, J., Barrett, C., Tetlie, R.R. and McQuarter, R.J. (1987). The effect of prior intervention to establish generalized requesting on the acquisition of object labels. *Augmentative and Alternative Communication* 3: 3–11. **p.316**.

Reichle, J. and Brown, L. (1986). Teaching the use of a multipage direct selection communication board to an adult with autism. *Journal of the Association for Persons with Severe Handicaps* 11: 68–73. **p.316**.

Reichle, J. and Karlan, G. (1985). The selection of an augmentative communication system in communication intervention: A critique of decision rules. *Journal of the Association for Persons with Severe Handicaps* 10: 146–156. **p.167**.

Reichle, J., Rogers, N. and Barrett, C. (1984). Establishing pragmatic discriminations among the communicative functions of requesting, rejecting, and commenting in an adolescent. *Journal of the Association for Persons with Severe Handicaps* 9: 31–36. **p.316**.

Reichle, J. and Ward, M. (1985). Teaching discriminative use of an encoding electronic communication device and Signing Exact English to a moderately handicapped child. *Language, Speech, and Hearing Services in Schools* 16: 58–63. **p.30**.

Reichle, J. and Yoder, D.E. (1985). Communication use in severely handicapped learners. *Language, Speech, and Hearing Services in Schools* 16: 146–157. **p.316**.

Reid, D.H. and Hurlbut, R. (1977). Teaching nonvocal communication skills to multi-handicapped retarded adults. *Journal of Applied Behavior Analysis* 10: 591–603. **p.316**.

Remington, B. and Clarke, S. (1983). Acquisition of expressive signing by autistic children: An evaluation of the relative effects of simultaneous communication and sign-alone training. *Journal of Applied Behavior Analysis* 16: 3154–3328. **p.316**.

Remington, B. and Clarke, S. (1993a). Simultaneous communication and speech comprehension. Part l: Comparison of two methods of teaching expressive signing and speech comprehension skills. *Augmentative and Alternative Communication* 9: 36–48. **p.316**.

Remington, B. and Clarke, S. (1993b). Simultaneous communication and speech comprehension. Part II: Comparison of two methods of overcoming selective attention during expressive signing training. *Augmentative and Alternative Communication* 9: 49–60. p.316.

Reynell, J. (1985). *Reynell Developmental Language Scales – Revised.* Windsor: NFER-Nelson. p.92.

Reynolds, M.E., Bond, Z.S. and Fucci, D. (1996). Synthetic speech intelligibility: Comparison of native and non-native speakers of English. *Augmentative and Alternative Communication* 12: 32–36. p.44.

Rimland, B. (1971). The differentiation of childhood psychosis: An analysis of checklists for 2,218 psychotic children. *Journal of Autism and Childhood Schizophrenia* 1: 161–174. p.94.

Robinson, L.A. and Owens, R.E. (1995). Functional augmentative communication and positive behaviour change. *Augmentative and Alternative Communication* 11: 207–211 p.316.

Roe, P.R.W. (Ed.) (1995). *Telecommunications for All.* Luxembourg: Office for Official Publications of the European Communities. p.45.

Romaine, S. (1988). *Pidgin and Creole Languages.* London: Longman. p.291.

Romski, M.A. and Ruder, K.F. (1984). Effect of speech and speech and sign instruction on oral language learning and generalization of action + object combinations by Down's syndrome children. *Journal of Speech and Hearing Research* 49: 293–302. p.316.

Romski, M.A. and Sevcik, R.A. (1989). An analysis of visual-graphic symbol meanings for two nonspeaking adults with severe mental retardation. *Augmentative and Alternative Communication* 5: 109–114. p.316.

Romski, M.A. and Sevcik, R.A. (1993). Language comprehension: Considerations for augmentative and alternative communication. *Augmentative and Alternative Communication* 9: 281–285. p.65.

Romski, M.A. and Sevcik, R.A. (1996). *Breaking the Speech Barrier.* Baltimore: Paul H. Brookes. pp.21, 34, 56, 64, 66, 134, 244, 299, 300, 301, 307.

Romski, M.A., Sevcik, R.A. and Pate, J.L. (1988). Establishment of symbolic communication in persons with severe retardation. *Journal of Speech and Hearing Disorders* 53: 94–107. pp.134, 316.

Romski, M.A., White, R.A., Millen, C.E. and Rumbaugh, D.M. (1984). Effects of computer-keyboard teaching on the symbolic communication of severely retarded persons: Five case studies. *The Psychological Record* 34: 39–54. pp.31, 316.

Rosenberg, S. and Abbeduto, L. (1993). *Language and Communication in Mental Retardation.* Hillsdale, NJ: Lawrence Erlbaum. p.241.

Rosenblum, S.M., Arick, J.R., Krug, D.A. Stubbs, E.G., Young, N.B. and Pelson, R.O. (1980). Auditory brainstem evoked responses in autistic children. *Journal of Autism and Childhood Disorders* 10: 215–225. p.104.

Rostad, A.M. (1989). Erfaringer med tegnopplæring av psykisk utviklingshemmede småbarn. Levanger: Unpublished manuscript. pp.75–76.

Rotholz, D.A., Berkowitz, S.F. and Burberry, J. (1989). Functionality of two modes of communication in the community by students with developmental disabilities: A comparison of signing and communication books. *Journal of the Association for Persons with Severe Handicaps* 14: 227–233. pp.29, 316.

Rowe, J.A. and Rapp, D.L. (1980). Tantrums: Remediation through communication. *Child: Care, Health, and Development* 6: 197–208. p.316.

Rowland, C. and Schweigert, P. (1989). Tangible symbols: Symbolic communication for individuals with multisensory impairments. *Augmentative and Alternative Communication* 5: 226–234. **p.24.**

Rutter, M. (1985). Infantile autism and other pervasive developmental disorders. In: Rutter, M. and Hersov, L. (Eds) *Child and Adolescent Psychiatry*. Oxford: Blackwell, pp. 545–566. **p.133.**

Rutter, M., Mawhood, L. and Howlin, P. (1992). Language delay and social development. In: Fletcher, P. and Hall, D. (Eds) *Specific Speech and Language Disorders in Children*. London: Whurr , pp. 63–78. **p.72.**

Ryan, J. (1974). Early language development: Towards a communication analysis. In: Richards, M.P.M. (Ed.) *The Integration of a Child into a Social World*. London: Cambridge University Press, pp. 185–213. **p.68.**

Ryan, J. (1977). The silence of stupidity. In: Morton, J. and Marshall, (J.C. Eds) *Psycholinguistic Series*, Volume 1. *Developmental and pathological*. London: Elek Science, pp. 99–124. **pp.68, 75, 147.**

Salvin, A., Routh, D.K., Foster, R.E. Jr. and Lovejoy, K.M. (1977). Acquisition of modified American Sign Language by a mute autistic child. *Journal of Autism and Childhood Schizophrenia* 7: 359–371. **p.316.**

Sandberg, A.D. (1996). Literacy abilities in nonvocal children with cerebral palsy. Thesis, Gothenburg University. **pp.236, 239.**

Sandberg, A.D. and Hjelmquist, E. (1992). Blissanvändare i förskola, skola och efter avslutad skolgång. Inventering an antall och skattning av grad av Blissanvänding. *Rapport från Psykologiska Institutionen*, No. 6. **pp.12, 15.**

Sarriá, E., Gómez, J.C. and Tamarit, J. (1996). Joint attention and alternative language intervention in autism: Implications of theory for practice. In: von Tetzchner, S. and Jensen, M.H. (Eds) *Augmentative and Alternative Communication: European perspectives*. London: Whurr, pp. 49–64. **pp.79, 168.**

Schaeffer, B., Kollinzas, G., Musil, A. and McDowell, P. (1977). Spontaneous verbal language for autistic children through signed speech. *Sign Language Studies* 17: 387–328. **p.316.**

Schaeffer, B., Musil, A. and Kollinzas, G. (1980). *Total Communication*. Champaign, IL: Research press. **p.81.**

Schaeffer, B., Raphael, A. and Kollinzas, G. (1994). *Signed Speech for Nonverbal Students*. Seattle, Washington: Educational Achievement Systems. **p.170.**

Schaffer, H.R. (1989). Language development in context. In: von Tetzchner, S., Siegel, L.S. and Smith, L. (Eds) *The Social and Cognitive Aspects of Normal and Atypical Language Development*. New York: Springer-Verlag, pp. 1–22. **p.123.**

Schank, R.C. and Abelson, R.P. (1977). *Scripts, Plans, Goals, and Understanding*. Hillsdale, NJ: Lawrence Erlbaum. **p.269.**

Schepis, M.M., Reid, D.H. and Behrman, M.M. (1996). Acquisition and functional use of voice output communication by persons with profound multiple disabilities. *Behavior Modification* 20: 451–469. **pp.56, 316.**

Schepis, M.M., Reid, D.H., Behrman, M.M. and Sutton, K.A. (1998). Increasing communicative interactions of young children with autism using a voice output communication aid and naturalistic teaching. *Journal of Applied Behavior Analysis* 31: 561–578. **p.316.**

Schepis, M.M., Reid, D.H., Fitzgerald, J.R., Faw, G.D., Pol, A. van der and Welty, P.A. (1982). A program for increasing manual signing by autistic and profoundly retarded youth within the daily environment. *Journal of Behavior Analysis* **15**: 363–379. **p.316.**

Scherz, J.W. and Beer, M.M. (1995). Factors affecting the intelligibility of synthesized speech. *Augmentative and Alternative Communication* **11**: 74–78. **p.44.**

Schjølberg, S. (1984). Forståelighet av talen til barn med språkvansker. Thesis, University of Oslo. **pp.71, 274.**

Schlosser, R.W. (1997a). Nomenclature of category levels in graphic symbols, Part I: Is a flower a flower a flower? *Augmentative and Alternative Communication* **13**: 4–13. **pp.12, 31.**

Schlosser, R.W. (1997b). Nomenclature of category levels in graphic symbols, Part II: The role of similarity in categorization. *Augmentative and Alternative Communication* **13**: 14–29. **pp.12, 31.**

Schlosser, R.W., Blischak, D.M., Belfiore, P.J., Bartley, C. and Barnett, N. (1998). Effects of synthetic speech output and orthographic feedback on spelling in a student with autism: A preliminary study. *Journal of Autism and Developmental Disorders* **28**: 309–319. **pp.237, 316.**

Schlosser, R.W. and Lloyd, L.L. (1997). Effects of paired-associate learning versus symbol explanations on Blissymbol comprehension and production. *Augmentative and Alternative Communication* **13**: 226–238. **p.14.**

Schopler, E., Reichler, R.J., DeVellis, R.F. and Daly, K. (1980). Toward objective classification of childhood autism: Childhood Autism Rating Scale (CARS). *Journal of Autism and Developmental Disorders* **10**: 91–103. **p.94.**

Scollon, R. (1976). *Conversations with a One Year Old*. Honolulu: University of Hawaii Press. **p.251.**

Sellin, A. (1992). Bericht über die Arbeit mit Birger nach der Methode ‛Facilitated Communication’ vom 2. August 1990 bis November 1990. *Autismus* **33**: 2–4. **p.176.**

Shane, H.C. and Bashir, A.S. (1981). Election criteria for the adoption of an augmentative communication system: Preliminary considerations. *Journal of Speech and Hearing Disorders* **45**: 408–414. **p.167.**

Shane, H.C. and Cohen, C.G. (1981). A discussion of communicative strategies and patterns by nonspeaking persons. *Language, Speech, and Hearing Services in Schools* **12**: 205–210. **pp.224, 277, 282.**

Shane, H.C., Lipschultz, R.W. and Shane, C.L. (1982). Facilitating the communicative interaction of nonspeaking persons in a residential setting. *Topics in Language Disorders* **2**: 73–84. **p.288.**

Sharpe, P.A. (1992). Comparative effects of bilateral hand splints and an elbow orthosis on stereotypic hand movements and toy play in two children with Rett syndrome. *American Journal of Occupational Therapy* **46**: 134–140. **p.85.**

Sheehy, E., Moore, K. and Tsamtsouris, A. (1993). Augmentative communication for the non-speaking child. *Journal of Clinical Pediatric Dentistry* **17**: 261–264. **p.221.**

Shepherd, T.C. and Haaf, R.G. (1995). Comparison of two training methods in the learning and generalization of Blissymbolics. studies. *Augmentative and Alternative Communication* **11**: 154–164. **p.14.**

Shere, B. and Kastenbaum, R. (1966). Mother–child interaction in cerebral palsy: Environmental and psychosocial obstacles to cognitive development. *Genetic Psychology Monographs* **73**: 255–335. **p.67.**

Shipley, E., Gleitman, L.R. and Smith, C. (1969). A study in the acquisition of language: Free responses to commands. *Language* **45**: 322–342. **p.300.**

Sigafoos, J., Laurie, S. and Pennell, D. (1996). Teaching children with Rett syndrome to request preferred objects using aided communication: Two preliminary studies. *Augmentative and Alternative Communication* 12: 88–96. **pp.86, 316.**

Sigafoos, J. and Roberts-Pennell, D. (1999). Wrong-item format: A promising intervention for teaching socially appropriate forms of rejecting to children with developmental disabilities? *Augmentative and Alternative Communication* 15: 135–140. **p.316.**

Silverman, H., Kates, B. and McNaughton, S. (1978). The formative evaluation of the Ontario Crippled Children's Centre symbol communication program. In: Silverman, H., McNaughton, S. and Kates, B. (Eds) *Handbook of Blissymbolics*. Toronto: Ontario Crippled Children's Centre. **p.60.**

Siple, P. and Fischer, S. (Eds) (1991). *Theoretical Issues in Sign Language Research*, Volume 2: *Psychology*. Chicago: University of Chicago Press. **p.9.**

Sisson, L.A. and Barrett, R.P. (1984). An alternating treatment comparison of oral and total communication training with minimally verbal children. *Journal of Applied Behavior Analysis* 17: 559–566. **p.316.**

Skinner, B.F. (1957). *Verbal Behavior*. New York: Appleton-Century-Crofts. **p.167.**

Skjeldal, O.H., von Tetzchner, S., Asplund, F., Herder, G.A. and Lofterød, B. (1997). Rett syndrome: geographic variation in prevalence in Norway. *Brain and Development* 19: 258–261. **p.83.**

Skjelfjord, V.J. (1976). *Fonemlæring i skolen* (Phoneme learning in school). Oslo: Universitetsforlaget. **p.20.**

Smeets, P.M. and Striefel, S. (1976). Acquisition of sign reading by transfer of stimulus control in a retarded deaf girl. *Journal of Mental Deficiency Research* 20: 197–205. **p.316.**

Smith, A.K., Thurston, S., Light, J., Parnes, P. and O'Keele, B. (1989). The form and use of written communication produced by physically disabled individuals using microcomputers. *Augmentative and Alternative Communication* 5: 115–124. **pp.15, 236, 238.**

Smith, L. and von Tetzchner, S. (1986). Communicative, sensorimotor, and language skills of young children with Down syndrome. *American Journal of Mental Deficiency* 91: 57–66. **p.75.**

Smith, M.M. (1991). Assessment of interaction patterns and AAC use: A case study. *Journal of Clinical Speech and Language Studies* 1: 76–102. **pp.288, 316.**

Smith, M.M. (1992). Reading abilities of nonspeaking student: Two case studies. *Augmentative and Alternative Communication*, 8, 57–66. **p.316.**

Smith, M.M. (1994). Speech by another name: The role of communication aids in interaction. *European Journal of Disorders of Communication*, 29, 25–240. **p.316.**

Smith, M.M. (1996). The medium or the message: A study of speaking children using communication boards. In: von Tetzchner, S. and Jensen, M.H. (Eds) *Augmentative and Alternative Communication: European perspectives*. London: Whurr, pp. 119–136. **pp.22, 243, 262, 301.**

Smith, M.M. and Grove, N. (1999). The bimodal situation of children learning language using manual and graphic signs. In: Loncke, F.T., Clibbens, J., Arvidson, H.H. and Lloyd, L.L. (Eds) *Augmentative and Alternative Communication: New directions in research and practice*. London: Whurr, pp. 8–30. **pp.242, 262.**

Smith-Lewis, M. (1994). Discontinuity in the development of aided augmentative and alternative communication systems. *Augmentative and Alternative Communication* 10: 14–26. **p.52**

Smith-Lewis, M. and Ford, A. (1987). A user's perspective on augmentative communication. *Augmentative and Alternative Communication* 3: 12–17. **p.316.**

Snow, C.E. and Ferguson, C.A. (Eds) (1977). *Talking to Children.* Cambridge: Cambridge University Press. **p.262.**

Sommer, K.S., Whitman, T.L. and Keogh, D.A. (1988). Teaching severely retarded persons to sign interactively through the use of a behavioral script. *Research in Developmental Disabilities* 9: 291–304. **pp.270, 272, 316.**

Soro, E., Basil, C. and von Tetzchner, S. (1992). *Teaching Initial Communication and Language Skills to AAC Users.* Part 1: *Children and adolescents with impairment of language comprehension and expression.* Video presented at Fifth Biennial Conference on Augmentative and Alternative Communication, Philadelphia, August 1992. **p.280.**

Soto, G., Belfiore, P.J., Schlosser, R.W. and Haynes, C. (1993). Teaching specific requests: A comparative analysis on skill acquisition and preference using two augmentative and alternative communication aids. *Education and Training in Mental Retardation* 28: 169–178. **p.316.**

Sparrow, S.S., Balla, D.A. and Cicchetti, D.V. (1984). *Vineland Adaptive Behavior Scales.* Circle Pines: American Guidance Service. **p.94.**

Spiegel, B.B., Benjamin, B.J. and Spiegel, S.A. (1993). One method to increase spontaneous use of an assistive communication: case study. *Augmentative and Alternative Communication* 9: 111–118. **p.316.**

Stephenson, J. and Linfoot, K. (1996). Pictures as communication symbols for students with severe disability. *Augmentative and Alternative Communication* 12: 244–255. **pp.24, 167.**

Stokes, T.F., Baer, D.M. and Jackson, R.L. (1974). Programming the generalization of a greeting response in four retarded children. *Journal of Applied Behavior Analysis* 7: 599–610. **p.129.**

Stone, W.L., Ousley, O.Y., Yoder, P.J., Hogan, K.L. and Hepburn, S.L. (1997). Nonverbal communication in two- and three-year-old children with autism. *Journal of Autism and Developmental Disorders* 27: 677–696. **p.79.**

Sutton, A.C. (1982). Augmentative communication systems: The interaction process. Presented at the Annual Convention of the American Speech-Language-Hearing Association, Toronto, 1982. **pp.280, 282, 285, 286.**

Sutton, A. (1999). Linking language learning experience and grammatical acquisition. In: F.T. Loncke, J. Clibbens, H.H. Arvidson and L.L. Lloyd (Eds) *Augmentative and Alternative Communication: New directions in research and practice.* London: Whurr, pp. 49–61. **p.242.**

Sutton, A. and Morford, J.P. (1998). Constituent order in picture pointing sequences produced by speaking children using AAC. *Applied Psycholinguistics,* 19, 525–536. **p.243.**

Sweeney, L.A. (1999). Moving forward with families: Perspectives on augmentative and alternative communication research and practice. In: F.T. Loncke, J. Clibbens, H.H. Arvidson and L.L. Lloyd (Eds) *Augmentative and Alternative Communication: New directions in research and practice.* London: Whurr, pp. 231–254. **pp.306, 308.**

Sweidel, G.B. (1989). Stop, look and listen! When vocal and nonvocal adults communicate. *Disability, Handicap and Society* 4: 165–175. **p.282.**

Taylor, H.G. and Alden, J. (1997). Age-related differences in outcomes following childhood brain insults: An introduction and overview. *Journal of the International Neuropsychological Society* 3: 555–567. **p.133.**

Tomasello, M. (1992). *First Verbs: A case study of early grammatical development*. Cambridge: Cambridge University Press. **p.247.**

Tomasello, M. (1995). Joint attention as social cognition. In: Moore, C. and Dunham, P. (Eds) *Joint Attention*. Hillsdale, NJ: Erlbaum, pp. 103–133. **p.123.**

Topper, S.T. (1975). Gesture language for a non-verbal severely retarded male. *Mental Retardation* 13: 30–31. **p.316.**

Trasher, K. and Bray, N. (1984). Effects of iconicity, taction, and training technique on the initial acquisition of manual signing by the mentally retarded. Presented at the 17th Annual Gatinburg Conference on Research in Mental Retardation, Gatinburg, 1984. **p.192.**

Trefler, E. and Crislip, D. (1985). No aid, an Etran, a Minspeak: A comparison of efficiency and effectiveness during structured use. *Augmentative and Alternative Communication* 1: 151–155. **p.316.**

Trevarthen, C. (1986). Notes on the psychology and developmental neurobiology of Rett syndrome. *Journal of Mental Deficiency Research* 31: 106–108. **p.85.**

Trevathan, E. and Moser, H.W. (1988). Diagnostic criteria for Rett syndrome. *Annals of Neurology* 23: 425–428. **p.83.**

Trevinarus, J. and Tannock, R. (1987). A scanning computer access system for children with severe physical disabilities. *The American Journal of Occupational Therapy* 41: 733–738. **p.316.**

Tronconi, A. (1989). Blissymbolics-based telecommunications. *Communication Outlook* 11: 8–11. **p.281.**

Udwin O. and Yule, W. (1990). Augmentative communication systems taught to cerebral palsy children – a longitudinal study. 1. The acquisition of signs and symbols and syntactic aspects of their use over time. *British Journal of Disorders of Communication* 25: 295–309. **p.241.**

Udwin, O. and Yule, W. (1991). Augmentative communication systems taught to cerebral-palsied children – A longitudinal study. 3. Teaching practices and exposure to sign and symbol use in schools and homes. *British Journal of Disorders of Communication* 26: 149–162. **p.244.**

Undheim, J.O. (1978). *Håndbok til Wechsler Intelligence Scale for Children – Revised*. Oslo: Norsk Psykologforening. **p.94.**

Van Acker, R. (1991). Rett syndrome: A review of current knowledge. *Journal of Autism and Developmental Disorders* 21: 381–406. **p.85.**

van Oosterom, J. and Devereux, K. (1985). *Learning with Rebus Glossary*. Back Hill: Earo, The Resource Centre. **p.19.**

Vance, M. and Wells, B. (1994). The wrong end of the stick: Language-impaired children's understanding of non-literal language. *Child Language Teaching and Therapy* 10: 23–46. **p.228.**

Vanderheiden, D.B., Brown, W.P., MacKenzie, P., Reinen, S. and Scheibel, C. (1975). Symbol communication for the mentally handicapped. *Mental Retardation* 13: 34–37. **pp.146, 167, 316.**

Vanderheiden, D.B. and Lloyd, L.L. (1986). Communication systems and their components. IN: Blackstone, S.W. (Ed.) *Augmentative Communication: An introduction*. Rockville, MD: American Speech and Hearing Association, pp. 49–161. **p.316.**

Vaughn, B. and Horner, R.H. (1995). Effects of concrete versus verbal choice systems on problem behavior. *Augmentative and Alternative Communication* 11: 89–92. **p.316.**

Venkatagiri, H.S. (1993). Efficiency of lexical prediction as a communication acceleration technique. *Augmentative and Alternative Communication* 9: 161–167. **p.42.**

Venkatagiri, H.S. (1994). Effect of sentence length and exposure on the intelligibility of synthesized speech. *Augmentative and Alternative Communication* 10: 96–104. **p.44.**

Venkatagiri, H.S. and Ramebadran, T.V. (1995). Digital speech synthesis: A tutorial. *Augmentative and Alternative Communication* 11: 14–25. **p.43.**

Villiers, J.G.D. and McNaughton, J.M. (1974). Teaching a symbol language to autistic children. *Journal of Consulting and Clinical Psychology* 42: 111–117. **p.316.**

von Tetzchner, S. (1984a). Facilitation of early speech development in a dysphasic child by use of signed Norwegian. *Scandinavian Journal of Psychology* 25: 265–275. **pp.64, 72, 316.**

von Tetzchner, S. (1984b). Tegnspråksopplæring med psykotiske/autistiske barn: Teori, metode og en kasusbeskrivelse. *Tidsskrift for Norsk Psykologforening* 21: 3–15. **pp.81, 317.**

von Tetzchner, S. (1985). Words and chips – pragmatics and pidginization of computer-aided communication. *Child Language Teaching and Therapy* 1: 295–305. **p.253.**

von Tetzchner, S. (1987). *Testprogrammer for barn med bevegelseshemning.* Oslo: Sentralinstituttet for Cerebral Parese. **p.111.**

von Tetzchner, S. (Ed.) (1991). *Issues in Telecommunication and Disability.* Luxembourg: Office for Official Publications of the European Communities. **pp.45, 281.**

von Tetzchner, S. (1996a). Facilitated, automatic and false communication: Current issues in the use of facilitating techniques. *European Journal of Special Needs Education* 11: 151–166. **pp.176, 177.**

von Tetzchner, S. (1996b). The contexts of early aided language acquisition. Presented at the 7th Biennial Conference of the International Society for Augmentative and Alternative Communication, Vancouver, August 1996. **pp.219, 250, 253, 304.**

von Tetzchner, S. (1997a). The use of graphic language intervention among young children in Norway. *European Journal of Disorders of Communication* 32: 217–234. **pp.14, 15, 16, 217, 236, 305.**

von Tetzchner, S. (1997b). Communication skills of females with Rett syndrome. *European Child and Adolescent Psychiatry* 6(suppl 1): 33–37. **pp.85–86, 158.**

von Tetzchner, S. (1997c). Historical issues in intervention research: Hidden knowledge and facilitating techniques in Denmark. *European Journal of Disorders of Communication* 32: 1–18. **p.174.**

von Tetzchner, S., Dille, K., Jørgensen, K.K., Ormhaug, B.M., Oxholm, B. and Warme, R. (1998). From single signs to relational meanings. Presented at the 8th Biennial Conference of the International Society for Augmentative and Alternative Communication, Dublin, August 1998. **pp.24, 29, 254, 260, 262, 264.**

von Tetzchner, S., Jacobsen, K.H., Smith, L., Skjeldal, O.H., Heiberg, A. and Fagan, J.F. (1996b). Vision, cognition and developmental characteristics of girls and women with Rett syndrome. *Developmental Medicine and Child Neurology* 38: 212–225. **p.84.**

von Tetzchner, S. and Jensen, K. (1999). Communicating with people who have severe communication impairment: Ethical considerations. *International Journal of Disability, Development and Education* 46: 453–462. **pp.61, 285.**

von Tetzchner, S. and Jensen, M.H. (1996). Introduction. In: von Tetzchner, S. and Jensen, M.H. (Eds) *Augmentative and Alternative Communication: European perspectives*. London: Whurr, pp. 1–18. **pp.5, 10, 15, 81.**

von Tetzchner, S. and Martinsen, H. (1980). A psycholinguistic study of the language of the blind: I. Verbalism. *International Journal of Psycholinguistics* 19: 49–61. **p.198.**

von Tetzchner, S. and Martinsen, H. (1996). Words and strategies: Communicating with young children who use aided language. In: von Tetzchner, S. and Jensen, M.H. (Eds) *Augmentative and Alternative Communication: European perspectives*. London: Whurr, pp. 65–88. **pp.38, 48, 59, 61, 241, 252, 278, 283, 286, 290, 294, 301.**

von Tetzchner, S. and Øien, I. (1989). *Rett syndrom: Forløp og tiltak*. Video. Oslo: Norsk forening for Rett syndrom. **p.86.**

von Tetzchner, S., Rogne, S.O. and Lilleeng, M.K. (1997). Literacy intervention for a deaf child with severe reading disorders. *Journal of Literacy Research* 29: 25–46. **pp.43, 236, 238.**

Vygotsky, L. (1962). *Thought and Language*. Cambridge, MA: MIT Press. **p.96.**

Wagner, K.R. (1985). How much do children say in a day? *Journal of Child Language* 12: 475–487. **p.60.**

Walker, M. (1976). *Language Programmes for Use with the Revised Makaton Vocabulary*. Surrey: M. Walker. **pp.228, 229.**

Walker, M. and Ekeland, J. (1985). *The Revised Makaton Vocabulary*, Norsk versjon (foreløpig utgave). Klæbu: Vernepleierhøgskolen i Sør-Trøndelag. **pp.229, 230, 231, 232.**

Walker, M., Parson, P., Cousins, S., Carpenter, B. and Park, K. (1985). *Symbols for Makaton*. Back Hill: Earo, The Resource Centre. **p.19.**

Warren, D.H. (1994). *Blindness and Children*. Cambridge: Cambridge University Press. **p.198.**

Warren, S.F. and Kaiser, A.P. (1986). Incidental teaching: A critical review. *Journal of Speech and Hearing Disorders* 51: 291–299. **p.160.**

Watson, M.M. and Leahy, J. (1995). Multimodal therapy for a child with developmental apraxia for speech: A case study. *Child Language Teaching and Therapy* 11: 264–272. **p.317.**

Watters, R.G. Wheeler, L.J. and Watters, W.E. (1981). The relative efficiency of two orders for training autistic children in the expressive and receptive use of manual signs. *Journal of Communication Disorders* 14: 273–285. **p.157.**

Webster, C.D., McPherson, L., Evans, M.A. and Kuchar, E. (1973). Communication with an autistic boy by gesture. *Journal of Autism and Childhood Schizophrenia* 3: 337–346. **p.317.**

Weir, R.H. (1966). Some questions on the child's learning of phonology. In: Smith, F. and Miller, G.A. (Eds) *The Genesis of Language*. London: MIT Press, pp. 153–168. **p.237.**

Weis, D.A. (1967). Cluttering. *Folia Phoniatrica* 19: 233–263. **p.71.**

Wells, M.E. (1981). The effect of total communication training versus traditional speech training on word articulation in severely mentally retarded individuals. *Applied Research in Mental Retardation* 2: 323–333. **pp.134, 317.**

Wexler, K., Blau, A., Leslie, S. and Dore, J. (1983). Conversational interaction of nonspeaking cerebral palsied individuals and their speaking partners, with and without augmentative communication aids. Manuscript, West Haverstraw, Helen Hayes Hospital. **pp.286, 288.**

Whedall, K. and Jeffree, D. (1974). Criticisms regarding the use of PPVT in subnormality research. *British Journal of Disorders of Communication* 9: 140–143. **p.111.**

Wherry, J.N. and Edwards, R.P. (1983). A comparison of verbal, sign, and simultaneous systems for the acquisition of receptive language by an autistic boy. *Journal of Communication Disorders* 16: 201–216. **p.317.**

Wilken-Timm, K. (1997). *Kommunikationshilfen zur Persönlichkeitsentwicklung.* Karlsruhe: von Loeper Literaturverlag. **p.317.**

Wilkinson, K.M., Romski, M.A. and Sevcik, R.A. (1994). Emergence of visual-graphic symbol combinations by youth with moderate or severe mental retardation. *Journal of Speech and Hearing Research* 37: 883–895. **pp.243, 246.**

Wills, K.E. (1981). Manual communication for nonspeaking hearing children. *Journal of Pediatric Psychology* 6: 15–27. **p.205.**

Woll, B. and Barnett, S. (1998). Toward a sociolinguistic perspective on augmentative and alternative communication. *Augmentative and Alternative Communication* 14: 200–211. **pp.291, 302.**

Woll, B., Kyle, J.G. and Deuchar, M. (1981). *Perspectives on British Sign Language and Deafness.* London: Croom Helm. **p.9.**

Woodcock, R.W., Clark, C.R. and Davies, C.O. (1969). *Peabody Rebus Reading Program.* Circle Pines: American Guidance Service. **p.18.**

Woodyatt, G.C. and Ozanne, A.E. (1992). Communication abilities in a case of Rett syndrome. *Journal of Intellectual Disability Research* 36: 83–92. **p.84.**

Woodyatt, G.C. and Ozanne, A.E. (1993). A longitudinal study of communication behaviours in children with Rett syndrome. *Journal of Intellectual Disability Research* 37: 419–435. **p.84.**

World Health Organization (1993). The ICD-10 classification of mental and behavioural disorders: Diagnostic criteria for research. Geneva: World Health Organization. **pp.73, 77–79.**

Yoder, D.E. and Kraat, A. (1983). Intervention issues in nonspeech communication. In: Miller, J., Yoder, D.E. and Schiefelbusch, R.L. (Eds) *Contemporary Issues in Language Intervention.* Rockville, MD: American Speech and Hearing Association, pp. 27–51. **pp.288, 290, 292.**

York, J., Nietupski, J. and Hamre-Nietupski, S. (1985). A decision-making process for using microswitches. *Journal of the Association for Persons with Severe Handicaps* 10: 214–223. **p.50.**

Yorkston, K.M., Honsinger, M.J., Dowden, P.A. and Marriner, N. (1989). Vocabulary selection: A case report. *Augmentative and Alternative Communication* 5: 101–109. **pp.233, 235, 317.**

Subject index

abbreviation 21, 41–2, 44
aided
    communication 8, 26, 28-29, 53,
      57–61, 85, 101, 262, 280, 291
    language 47
    play 38
    speaker 5, 59, 61, 242, 253, 278,
      280, 282–283, 285–6, 289–90,
      292–3, 301
    alternative language group 62, 64–6,
      70, 74, 81, 88, 100, 107–8, 116,
      122, 128, 131, 146, 151, 178,
      180, 185, 205, 207, 236, 260,
      267–73, 275, 279, 295, 298, 300
      (*see also* expressive language
      group and supportive language
      group)
American Sign Language 9, 10, 26,
    191–3.
analogy 12, 14, 226–8, 238–9, 249–50,
    284, 310
anarthria 63, 67
articulation 9, 43, 57, 63–4, 70–2, 75,
    101, 106, 108, 172, 187–188, 228,
    236–7, 240, 261, 263, 274–5, 288,
    293, 309
artificial speech 5, 8, 27, 34, 40, 43–5,
    52–3, 55–7, 86, 134, 190, 221,
    228, 234, 237–8, 281, 288, 292
    digitised 5, 43–4, 53, 57, 86, 152,
      221
    synthetic 8, 27, 43–5, 52–3, 55, 57,
      221, 234, 237–8, 281, 288, 292

assessment 4, 16, 21, 52, 85, 90–121,
    126, 130–2, 265, 308
assistive technology
    aid 2, 8, 27, 37, 54–5, 82, 221, 225,
      228, 277, 306
    environmetal control 38, 174
    switch 35, 38–39, 50–1, 53–5, 85,
      101, 104, 111, 140, 174, 190, 289
    technical device 56, 101
at risk 16, 82, 134, 298
attention 1, 27, 34, 41, 47, 57–8, 61,
    79, 83, 85, 87, 89, 99–100, 107–8,
    115, 125–8, 137, 148, 167, 179,
    187, 215, 221, 237, 242, 246,
    252–3, 261, 264, 267, 288, 295,
    301
    joint 79, 122–4, 168
    visual 7, 46–7
attitude 69, 126, 177, 291, 305, 311
auditory
    agnosia 65
    disorder 104
    perception 104
    scanning 221
    screening 176
autism 1, 29, 34, 38, 77–82, 84, 100,
    105, 137, 141, 148–50, 154,
    165–8, 170, 209, 241, 254, 258,
    295, 307, 313–7
automaticy 35–7, 45, 55, 57, 126, 128,
    174, 176

babbling 53, 237
behavioural disorders 3, 77, 87, 89, 94,

96–97, 107–8, 114, 148, 165, 172,
180, 206, 209
bilingualism 134
second language learning 137
Blissymbols (*see* graphic sign systems)
bootstrapping 247, 249, 257, 261, 263
British Sign Language 9, 21, 26

cerebral palsy 38, 48, 54, 63, 66–7,
233, 279–80, 285, 292
chaining 32, 149–150, 167, 170–1,
257–8, 276
challenging behaviour (*see* behavioural
disorders)
check list 94–5
chinese writing 11
co-construction 252, 294
coding 43, 47, 243
cognition 22, 42, 52, 54, 57, 74, 84–5,
111, 135, 155, 160, 174, 228,
240–2, 258, 260–1
communication
aid 2–5, 8, 10, 14, 24, 28–30, 34–61,
66–7, 69, 85–6, 96, 101, 107, 116,
123, 134, 152, 154, 167, 174,
190, 217–9, 221–2, 224–8, 234,
242, 252–3, 259, 277, 279–83,
285–9, 291, 294–5, 301, 307,
309–10
board 11, 14, 23, 30, 32, 38, 46, 56,
59, 105, 174, 178–9, 189–90,
218–20, 223–6, 239, 255, 273,
279, 284, 286, 290, 301, 304, 309
book 254–5, 279–80, 294
breakdown 37, 60, 291–3
competence 66, 74, 99, 124
disorder 1, 2, 4, 10, 27, 31, 45, 66,
77, 82, 87, 90, 108, 118, 124, 140,
174–5, 178, 188, 198–200, 202,
205, 211, 213, 229, 266, 269,
297, 300
function 1, 37, 138, 155 (*see also*
pragmatic)
idiosyncratic 108
intentional 136, 168
nonverbal 113
partner 27, 37–8, 57, 60–1, 64, 101,
123, 137, 140, 148, 161, 179,

189, 215, 228, 244, 250, 263–4,
276–7, 282–93, 297, 299, 307,
310
record 117–8
style 40, 69, 277, 287, 307
task 114
total 85, 136, 134, 264, 310
competence 16, 66, 99, 176, 223, 249,
282, 287, 308
complement 61, 156, 287
complexity 12, 14, 30, 63, 71, 109, 136,
188, 198–204, 237, 240, 243, 253,
256–7, 271, 286, 300, 304
comprehension
of language 2, 31, 56, 63, 69, 81, 91,
107, 110–2, 122, 136–7, 163, 171,
205, 243, 266, 298
of sign 27, 30, 63, 110, 124, 137–40,
144–6, 156, 156, 199, 208–9, 241,
263–4, 273, 309
of spoken language 14, 43, 61, 64,
66, 68–70, 109, 124, 137–8, 152,
217–8, 241–2, 250, 260–2, 264–5,
273–4, 277, 285, 293–4, 297,
299–301, 311
of pictures 22, 197
problem 44, 91, 300
training 64–5, 140–6, 155, 157–8,
210–11, 229, 257
concept keyboard 38, 49–50, 55, 190,
237
context 5, 48, 79, 124, 127, 144, 160,
168, 202, 240, 248, 250, 264–5,
278
decontextualisation 124
frame 124, 164
recontextualisation 124
shared 79, 123, 158, 253
conversation 14–6, 37, 43, 45, 69, 71,
95, 115, 124, 179, 184, 207,
218–20, 222, 225–6, 252–4, 258
page 254–7, 261–2
partner 5, 8, 14, 27, 41, 46, 48, 57,
59–61, 72, 138–40, 150, 174, 187,
189, 198, 215–6, 219, 223–4, 226,
228, 251, 254, 267–8, 274, 276–9,
282–7, 290, 292–3, 297, 299, 301
skills 208, 23, 266–96

stratgies 177, 278–93, 310 (*see also* dialogue)
creative 11, 15
cue 56, 68, 100–1, 111–3, 123, 125, 130, 132–3, 158, 188, 190, 198, 201–2, 218, 226, 237, 269, 274–5, 279

day clock 97–9
deaf 1–2, 4, 9–10, 30, 63, 65, 74, 80, 104, 134, 192–3, 214, 240, 299, 309
deaf-blind 1, 189
dependency 2, 3, 14, 22, 84, 87–8, 113, 122, 129–30, 170, 223, 233, 266, 277, 281, 285, 307
   learned 88–9, 100–1, 164, 205, 277
dependent
   communication 8, 36
   mode 38, 174
developmental
   delay 75, 79
   disorder 1, 5, 16, 62, 70–73, 75, 87, 107, 199, 208, 273–4
   dysphasia 64, 191
   group 63–64
   path 66, 77
diagnosis 65, 70, 73, 77, 81–3, 94, 100, 104–5, 192
dialogue 40, 60–1, 176, 242, 252, 260, 267–72, 275, 284, 294–5, 302, 306
Down's syndrome 63, 65, 74–7, 118, 134, 157, 276, 297
drawing 14, 17–8, 22–3, 27, 31–2, 58, 91–2, 118, 146, 153, 165, 194–5, 198, 214, 216, 248, 273
dyspraxia 30, 71–2, 84–6, 158

echolalia 79
epilepsy 82
expressive language group 63–4, 70, 74, 86, 88, 100, 11, 116, 122–3, 131, 146, 151, 161, 168, 179, 184, 199, 205, 207, 217–228, 241–2, 265–6, 275–293, 307, 311 (*see also* alternative language group and supportive language group)

explicit 108–9, 113, 122, 124, 136–8, 226, 229, 237, 248, 257, 264–5
eye
   blinking 8
   contact 45, 80, 113, 167
   gaze 48, 100, 123, 167–9
   pointing 35, 47–8, 50, 54, 58, 85, 105, 113, 168–9, 181, 189, 219
   switches 50–1

facial expression 6, 37, 41, 181, 289, 299
facilitating techniques 174–177
family 5, 42, 46, 90, 97, 10, 105–6, 111, 121, 175, 179, 181, 213, 282, 297–8, 302–6, 311
fill-in 256–7, 263

generalization 88, 114–5, 127–30, 171, 272
gesture 6, 8, 59, 77, 101, 108–10, 113, 123, 172, 181, 308
   deictic 123
gloss 5, 11, 17–21, 118, 191–2, 195, 216–7, 238–9, 262, 309
grammar 9, 10, 247 (*see also* 'morphology' and 'syntax')
graphic sign 2, 4–8, 10–22, 24, 26–7, 29–38, 41, 43, 45–50, 52–56, 58–60, 63–4, 67, 72, 81–2, 85, 109, 113–4, 118, 124, 127, 133–8, 140–1, 144–6, 149–52, 159–60, 162, 165, 167–9, 171–2, 174, 179, 181, 183, 186, 188–91, 194–8, 205–6, 214, 216–9, 221–4, 226, 228–9, 236–44, 250–1, 253–7, 259–64, 268, 273–5, 281–7, 289, 292–3, 295, 298–302, 304–10.
graphic sign system
   Blissymbols 8, 10–18, 27, 31–2, 38, 57, 60, 63, 146, 163, 195–6, 220, 226, 233, 236–9, 281–4, 286, 288, 292, 304, 310, 313–7
   lexigram 20–1, 31–2, 134, 195
   PIC 4–5, 8, 14, 16–8, 22, 27, 29, 31–3, 38, 58, 63, 142, 152, 154, 159, 190, 195–7, 220, 227, 254, 294, 304–5, 313–7

PCS 8, 14, 18, 22, 27, 32–3, 38, 63,
    195–7, 273, 304–5, 313–7
Rebus 8, 18–20, 27, 31, 38, 195–6,
    226–7, 238, 279, 313–7
Sigsymbols 21, 313–7
guessing 37–8, 58, 60–1, 127, 176–7,
    191–3, 278–9, 282–3, 285, 290,
    309–10

habilitation 3, 16, 91, 95, 121,
    plan 91, 95, 121
hand-guidance 151–2, 171–3, 176
hearing 1–2, 7, 62, 67, 81, 104, 134,
    193
    aid 34, 133
    impairment 27, 62, 74, 91, 104, 133,
        233 (see also deaf)
hierarchy 31
high-technology system 34, 37–46, 69
horizontal structure 250–3, 295

iconicity 4, 21–2, 25, 191–8
    transluency 191–5, 198
    transparency 191–5, 198
Illinois Test of Psycholinguistic Abilities
    93, 111, 226
imitation 80, 101, 160, 167, 171–3
implicit 108–9, 122, 124, 136–9, 232,
    247–8, 253, 284
independence 3, 96, 131, 170, 185,
    266, 278, 282
instruction (see teaching)
intellectual impairment (see learning
    disability)
intelligence 28, 63, 70, 73–4 91–5
    quotient (IQ) 28, 73–4, 92
    test 70, 73–4, 91–4
intention 85, 89, 108, 114, 12, 136,
    143, 162, 247–8
interaction 2–3, 46, 57, 68, 71–3, 75,
    80, 95, 114, 124, 181, 184, 209,
    242, 256, 266–8, 271–2, 277, 280,
    287, 295, 298–9, 303, 306–8,
    310–11

key-word signing 300

learning
    disability 1, 12, 14–5, 17, 19, 22–4,
        27, 30–1, 36, 38, 45–6, 53, 56,
        63–6, 73–7, 84, 87, 92, 95, 101,
        104, 110, 117, 129, 133–4, 136,
        239–40, 142–3, 145, 147–8,
        159–61, 169–71, 175, 190, 192–5,
        197, 206, 208–9, 211, 213–4, 217,
        249–50, 256, 267–8, 270, 272–3,
        295–6, 300, 302, 304, 307–8
    explicit 136–8
    implicit 136–8
    patten 137
    situation 63, 87, 128, 137, 160
    spontaneous 126
    strategy 137
lexigram (see graphic sign system)
literacy 236, 239 (see also reading and
    writing)
logographic 10, 18
low–technology aid 137

Makaton 19, 229, 230
manual sign 1–2, 4–10, 21, 26–30,
    32–3, 38, 45, 51, 63–4, 66–7, 72,
    75, 77, 79, 81–2, 85, 101, 105,
    109, 113–4, 117–8, 123–4, 127,
    133–8, 140–2, 144–6, 148–52,
    157–60, 163–8, 170–2, 181–3,
    186–90, 192–5, 205–6, 208–9,
    211, 214–7, 221, 226, 229, 240,
    243, 249, 253, 256, 262, 268,
    270, 273–5, 280, 287, 294–5,
    297–302, 304, 306–9
manual sign language
    American 9, 10, 26, 191–3.
    British 9, 21, 26
    Norwegian 9
manual sign system
    Paget Gorman Sign System 10
    Signed English 21
    Signed Norwegian 7, 10
    Signing Exact English 7, 10
memory 27, 44, 154, 193, 261
metaphor 14, 113, 137, 228
Minspeak 43, 225, 227
morphology 111
Morse 7–8

motor impairment 1–3, 16, 34, 38, 46,
54, 63, 67, 70, 74, 100–1, 104–5,
155, 161, 163, 168, 171, 218–20,
228, 239, 242, 266, 276–7, 281,
288–9, 299
multi-sign utterance 24, 47, 240–265,
306

naming 14, 22–3, 145, 162–3, 209,
214–5, 231, 265, 267
narrative 294–6
negation 256
Norwegian Sign Language 9
notation 5–6
noun 25, 226

orthography 16, 18, 24, 41, 60, 63,
236–9, 281 (see also reading and
writing)
overinterpretation 68, 85, 112, 136,
146, 298
structured 85, 136, 146

Paget Gorman Sign System (see manual
sign system)
paraphrase 226, 292
parent   2, 15–7, 23, 38, 59, 63,
67–70, 75, 80, 88, 93, 95–7,
105–6, 109, 111–3, 121, 134,
147, 160, 162, 179, 222, 228,
239, 245, 252–3, 268, 274,
278–9, 287, 298, 302–6
participation 3, 16, 31, 45, 69, 71, 73,
75, 89, 97, 105, 113–4, 121–3,
126–7, 131, 144, 163, 178, 207,
218–9, 268, 271, 273–4, 276, 278,
280–3, 302–3, 306, 310
model 126–7
passivity
learned 3, 88–9, 161, 205
problem 146, 164, 277
Peabody Rebus Reading Program 18
perspective
language 263–4
metapersective 137
shared 263
photograph 22–4, 29, 32, 58, 85, 154,
214, 253–5, 268, 273, 294, 313–7

Pictogram Ideogram Communication
(PIC) (see graphic sign system)
pictographic 14, 18, 20–1, 33, 194–5,
305
Picture Communication Symbols (PCS)
(see graphic sign system)
Picture Exchange Communication
System 47, 134
pidgin language 291
pivot 245–7, 258
pragmatic 43, 109, 114, 240, 262, 295
prediction 41–4, 238
Premack's word bricks 8, 24–9, 31, 33,
190, 195, 198, 313–7
proper names 23, 213–4

question
clarification 292–3
open 301
probing 14
rhetorical 279
yes/no 232, 274, 283, 285–6, 301,
305
twenty 69

reading
disorder 12, 16, 57, 71, 236–8
instruction 16, 71, 123, 236–9
skills 19–20, 57, 236, 238
receptive language (see comprehension)
relevance 79, 123–5, 158, 202, 253
relief service 97, 105–6, 308
request 209, 263, 280, 285–6, 291,
293–4
responsibility 5, 91, 97, 117–21, 132,
281, 301, 304, 306, 308, 311
communicative 276–9
Rett's syndrome, 71, 82–7, 105, 132,
136, 158
Reynell Developmental Language
Scales 92, 111, 262, 264
routine 22, 80, 87, 97, 124, 130–1, 141,
143–4, 149–50, 164–5, 186, 201,
209, 268–73, 278, 283, 295, 299,
303

scaffold 64

scanning 33–7, 39–40, 50, 53–56, 58,
    126, 128, 174, 197, 211, 219,
    221, 223, 237, 261
    auditory 221
    automatic 35–7, 45, 55, 126, 128,
       174, 211, 237, 261
    dependent 36–7, 56, 58, 174, 219,
       221
    directed 35–6, 55
    independent 36–7, 56, 174
screening 136
script 268–73, 275
self-help skills 91, 94, 96–7, 100, 229,
    232
semantic
    agent 213, 232, 240, 253–6
    category 116
    patient 255, 265
    relation 240, 243
    role 213, 232, 240, 253–6, 265, 295
sentences 5, 6, 9, 12, 14, 17, 24–6, 36,
       37, 41, 43–4, 46, 53, 60, 70–1, 81,
       86, 111–4, 176. 183, 203, 207,
       213, 232, 240–2, 244–8, 250–3,
       255–65, 271, 280, 282–4, 290–1,
       294–5, 301–2, 310.
    ready–made 5, 8, 259–60, 288
shared
    attention 123
    context 79, 123, 158, 253
    experience 64
    focus 2, 45, 123, 250, 252–3, 263
    perspective 263
    topic 252
sigsymbols (see graphic sign systems)
staff training 297–8, 307–11
structure
    frame 131, 141, 144, 150, 164
    situational 131–2, 163–4, 231, 267,
       269 (see also cues)
structured waiting 160–2
supportive language group 62–6, 70,
       72, 100, 108, 117, 122, 128, 138,
       146, 151, 169, 178, 185, 202,
       207–17, 236, 260, 267, 273–6
       (see also alternative language
       group and expressive language
       group)

switch (see assistive technology)
symbol 4, 24, 33, 48, 123, 142 (see also
    sign)
syntax 9–10, 12, 26, 71, 79, 111, 240,
    242–3, 246–7, 253, 260–2, 264
    (see also grammar)

tactile signs 1, 8, 26
tangible signs 4–5, 7–8, 24–9, 33, 105,
    109, 113–4, 118, 127, 133, 135–8,
    140, 144–6, 149–52, 159–60, 165,
    171–2, 181, 183, 186, 190, 198,
    214, 216, 229, 240, 299, 302,
    306–8
teaching
    domain-oriented 207–9, 225
    experimental 95–6
    explicit 136–8, 199
    implicit 136–8, 237
    incidental 158–61
    material 10
    milieu 125
    situation 29, 88, 97, 114–6, 122–34,
       140, 145, 159–65, 186, 199, 202,
       207, 209, 215–6, 219, 233–4, 244,
       270, 297, 304, 309
    staff 297–8, 307–11
    strategy 14, 28–9, 125, 130, 135–77,
       207, 229, 238, 272, 305
telecommunication 45–6, 281–2
topic-comment 252–3, 257, 264–5,
    275–6, 282–3, 290–1, 295
total communication 85, 136, 134, 264,
    310
    structured 85, 136, 134,
turn
    conversational 60–1, 161, 215, 267,
       269, 276, 283, 287–90, 307, 310

unaided 8, 26, 28
uptake 122

verb island constructs 247–8
vertical structure 250–3, 255, 295
videotelephone 45
vision 12, 104, 190
    impairment 190
vocable 108–9

vocabulary 16, 22, 24, 29–30, 32, 36,
    40–1, 44, 52–3, 56, 70, 72, 77, 79,
    81, 110–1, 114, 123, 178–240,
    243–50, 254, 257, 262, 270, 273,
    286, 306

writing
    automatic 177

Chinese 11
disorder 1, 7, 42, 71, 236–7
ideograpgic 10
logographic 10, 18
orthographic 4, 236–9
skills 38, 236, 239
(*see also* reading)

9 781861 561879

Printed in the United States
by Baker & Taylor Publisher Services

Printed in the United States
by Baker & Taylor Publisher Services